Praise for *Madness Contested*

Madness Contested is a thought-provoking, informed manifesto for rethinking what we call madness and how best to treat such psychiatric distress. As the writers of this book convincingly argue, science, philosophy, and the lived experience of those who have known such states all tell of how our current 'medical model' of madness fails us, and of the benefit that could come from a reconceptualization of what it means to be 'mad'.

Robert Whitaker, journalist and author of *Mad in America* and *Anatomy of an Epidemic*

This impressive volume not only comprehensively critiques the simplistic, pessimistic medical model that dominates the mental health world, but provides an array of exciting exceptions and alternatives. A must-read for all interested in creating more effective, humane, evidence-based approaches to madness.

Professor John Read, Psychology Department, University of Auckland, co-editor of *Models of Madness* and editor of the journal *Psychosis: Psychological, Social and Integrative Approaches*

This inspiring collection of essays is a welcome addition to the growing literature on critical and alternative approaches to psychiatry. The authors, some well-known and some speaking out for the first time, cover topics ranging from the experience of taking neuroleptics to new ways of understanding paranoia.... The book is particularly strong on service user perspectives and projects. In fact, there is something for everyone here ... it is unfailingly lively, challenging and thought-provoking.

Lucy Johnstone, clinical psychologist and author of *Users and Abusers of Psychiatry*

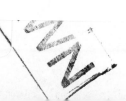

Madness Contested

Power and Practice

edited by

Steven Coles, Sarah Keenan & Bob Diamond

PCCS Books
Ross-on-Wye

Dedication

From the past to the present.

From our parents, partners and to our children:
Abigail, Anna, Cesca, Dylan, Isaac, Laura, Sam.

A thank you to all those we have learnt from.

This collection first published 2013

PCCS BOOKS
2 Cropper Row
Alton Road
Ross-on-Wye
Herefordshire
HR9 5LA
UK
Tel +44 (0)1989 763900
contact@pccs-books.co.uk
www.pccs-books.co.uk

Madness Contested: Power and practice

British Library Cataloguing in Publication Data.
A catalogue record for this book is available from the British Library.

ISBN 978 1 906254 43 8

Cover image 'Environment' by Susan Hammami
Cover designed in the UK by Old Dog Graphics
Printed in the UK by Ashford Colour Press, Gosport, Hants

Contents

Introduction

Steven Coles, Sarah Keenan & Bob Diamond

This book brings together the ideas and actions of authors who are searching for changes in the way we currently understand and respond to madness.[1] Many of these concepts and approaches were first shared at two national conferences in Nottingham in 2008 and 2010. Together they represent a questioning of dominant theories and frameworks, and a commitment to introduce changes and development, both inside and outside of mental health services. In this collection, madness is contested out of necessity. There is a stranglehold around open discussion in mental health services, which is maintained by a variety of interest groups including psychiatry, government, the pharmaceutical industry, and to a lesser extent, psychology. Dominant concepts not only shape practice within mental health services, but influence how the wider public understands and responds to fear, misery and madness.

Contesting the dominant understanding and approaches to madness requires reflection on the question: what constitutes the conventional paradigm? Whilst the dominant framework is not entirely homogenous, the current paradigm centres on the technical scientific expert, who utilises the tools of biological treatments and cognitive therapies. It is predicated on an individualistic conceptualisation of madness, where people are diagnosed with disorders of assumed biological origin or as having psychological deficits or distortions. The emphasis on technical expertise and use of an individualist framework not only obscures people's social-material world in our understanding of people's experiences, behaviour and distress, it also marginalises the lived experience and knowledge of those deemed mad. Mental health services offer a paternalistic form of care to people viewed as suffering from an illness and in need of treatment.

---

1 We have utilised the word 'madness' as we wish to detach ourselves from the restriction of medicalised conceptualisations of experience and behaviour, so to allow space to explore alternative ideas.

Whilst not denying that, in the main, the intention of staff working within mental health services is to offer a benign form of care, a key function of services is social control. Although some form of social control is perhaps at times a necessity, currently such state coercion lacks the usual legal and public scrutiny afforded to the rest of the population when civil liberties are curtailed. The paternalism and coercion of services restrict the voices and decision making of those deemed mad, and limit their abilities to resist and negotiate often misguided and potentially harmful treatments.

The chapters in this book challenge the dominant paradigm's conceptualisation and approaches to madness. The current hierarchy and hegemony have received sustained criticisms from the fields of academia, social care, survivor groups, practitioners and often from within psychiatry. This collection has its roots in bringing together people who share our concerns, questions, and discontent about dominant ideas and practices, as well as our hopes and strivings for something better. This reflects our belief that we wield greater power and resistance if we stand together. Acting collectively was the energy behind the two aforementioned national conferences, Psychosis in Context I and II, which considered the relationship between power and the much-used psychiatric term 'psychosis'. The first conference had the aim of moving away from the individualistic models of madness, and instead to contextualise people's experiences, to create equity and openness in sharing ideas between professionals, academics and survivors, and to consider how we might put these ideas into practice. The second conference shared this ethos, but started to analyse the reasons for the status quo persisting, the barriers to putting ideas into practice and ways to overcome them. The book is written by many who presented at the conference and additional authors who share our concerns.

We are committed to seeking and supporting much-needed development and change in the way we currently understand and respond to madness. However, we wish to present the ideas collected here with a degree of modesty, openness and critical reflection; we do not believe there is a definitive way forward, though there are many worthwhile paths to pursue. Part of the resistance to development of the current system is that its ideas and practices are presented as definitive, factual and beyond question. There is always need for thoughtful and reflective development and evolution, and systems and ideas need to be open to such change, including those which present themselves as alternatives. The process of moving away from established and conventional knowledge bases inevitably involves experiencing less familiarity and more uncertainty. We hope this collection provides some signposts in searching for new pathways that will lead to a more enlightened understanding of madness. The collection is broken into two separate but overlapping sections, which look at the domination and liberation of our conceptualisation of, and actions taken towards, madness.

Questioning the domination of madness

We believe the dominant ideology in mental health services has restricted our collective and individual conceptualisation, discourse and action regarding madness. The domination of madness is not just the direct control by professional and social hierarchies of those deemed mad; the dominant paradigm shapes our very notions of what madness is, who the mad are and how to respond to those in distress. The chapters in this section analyse and question the multiple functions, processes and forms of power involved in the realm of madness, including the interests at play in maintaining dominant theories, practices and social hierarchies. The constructive criticism residing in these chapters opens up space for a diversity of perspectives and exploration of new pathways to conceptualise and approach madness. Indeed many of the chapters modestly signpost possible pathways forward. A key theme in this section is the need to look outward in understanding people's experiences, and to theorise madness in relation to wider society.

Mary Boyle's chapter, 'The Persistence of Medicalisation', discusses that one of the reasons biomedical models dominate madness is due to processes that attempt to invalidate, assimilate and neutralise alternative conceptualisations. The chapter highlights that the construction and presentation of alternative understandings of madness are often not as robust as they could be. Due to alternative models often ignoring issues of embodiment, social responsibility and blame, they are more easily co-opted and neutralised into the dominant narrative. Boyle makes suggestions as to how alternatives need to be presented so that they can resist co-option.

As noted in Boyle's chapter, reductionist biological understandings of madness are dominant within services and alternative models often neglect biology, limiting their ability to challenge the dominant framework. However, the chapter by John Cromby and Dave Harper offers a model of paranoia that incorporates biology in a non-reductionist manner. Their chapter looks at how feelings (feedback from our bodies) are shaped by our social and material circumstances, and complex blends of feelings (such as anger, shame and fear) drive experiences which are labelled as paranoia. It notes how such feelings are often shaped by experiences of disempowerment and marginalisation, which are obscured by reductionist biological models.

In 'Meaning, Madness and Marginalisation', Steven Coles also discusses how biomedical models purport the content of madness to be meaningless within a person's biographical and social context, and highlights how decontextualising madness maintains a societal and professional hierarchy. The chapter argues that the process of psychiatric diagnosis is a key practice in concealing, reaffirming and initiating relationships of domination and submission. It looks at how professionals could start to practise more progressively by critiquing and speaking up against the dominant hierarchy and by being more open, questioning and modest in our practice.

Alastair Morgan and Anne Felton's chapter considers the rhetoric and discourse behind the utilisation of power in mental health services. Their chapter considers how notions of recovery abound in mental health services, the aspiration of such an approach being of services evolving to encourage service users' development, hopes, strengths and agency; values which are much needed in paternalistic and deficit-orientated mental health services. However, the chapter highlights the contradiction between the rise of the concept of recovery and an increase in coercion within mental health services (in particular in terms of community treatment orders). The chapter highlights several discourses that justify such coercion, a key one being that of risk. The authors note how the notion of recovery is co-opted to justify increasing coercion: 'You will recover, and we have ways of making you recover'.

David Pilgrim and Floris Tomasini advocate that we need to look at madness from a socio-ethical perspective, including the social control function of mental health services. Their chapter argues that post-enlightenment society has emphasised rationality and reason, which, by definition, people deemed mad are seen to lack. It also notes that many people in society act in unreasonable ways, but are not subject to the same coercion as those deemed mad; therefore society is acting discriminatorily towards such people. The chapter highlights that there are many nuances around being unreasonable, such as a distinction between being a nuisance and a danger, however, professionals and society ignore such nuances when it comes to madness. The chapter notes that society and professionals have been myopic to the ethical challenges of reasonableness. It argues that these issues can no longer be confined to mental health professionals, but need to be openly discussed and debated by all in society.

There are a number of competing interest groups within the field of mental health; Joan Busfield's chapter discusses how the economic interests of the pharmaceutical industry have shaped our understanding and response to madness and misery. The power of the pharmaceutical industry has encouraged mental health services and madness to be dominated by biological understandings and treatments, therefore marginalising social perspectives. By allying with the shared interests of biological psychiatry, the pharmaceutical industry has expanded the range of what is deemed mental illness, so to increase its potential market for psychiatric drugs.

Steven Coles, Bob Diamond and Sarah Keenan discuss how professional interests shape our conceptualisation and approach to madness. The chapter discusses how psychiatry dominates madness with individualistic understandings of distress and claims to expertise, and how professional interests within mainstream clinical psychology have led to the discipline perpetuating this understanding, as well as making its own claims to therapeutic expertise. The chapter highlights how both professions obscure social models of causation. It concludes in thinking about how clinical psychology could challenge dominant models, highlight the social material nature of distress and create space for alternative voices and perspectives.

The Midlands Psychology Group presents a 'Manifesto for a Social Materialist Psychology of Distress', highlighting how the dominant assumptions and philosophical underpinnings of mainstream psychology are individual and idealist. Conventional psychology emphasises the individual as the main unit of analysis and minimises the importance of the social. They note how psychology subordinates the material world to ephemeral and immaterial cognitions, in turn maintaining social hierarchies. As an alternative, the group's twelve-point manifesto grounds psychology in the social material world, an approach that highlights and questions the use and misuse of power.

Philip Thomas argues that the technological paradigm gripping mental health provision and research leaves little space for human experience and subjectivity. This technological paradigm in the main is being driven by the financial interests of the pharmaceutical industry and professional anxieties. A limited form of science has been applied to madness and one that excludes other forms of knowledge and philosophical understandings. In particular, such reductionism excludes a search for meaning and connection with madness, and increases isolation and marginalisation. His chapter expounds philosophical existentialism and the practice of Soteria as a much-needed antidote.

Exploring the liberation of madness

The chapters in this section explore new pathways away from conventional discourse, theorising and actions of the mental health services. They represent an attempt to liberate our conceptualisation and approach to madness from the restriction of the dominant paradigm discussed in the previous section. Attempts at embedding new ideas and practice face many barriers because of limited resources and the lack of broader political apparatus to make whole system change. However, such attempts at progress do act as beacons of what is possible, challenge the status quo and offer hope for evolution. The chapters are diverse in range; however, they often share values of openness, reflection, striving for equality and a commitment to democratic decision making. They also highlight the potential power of bringing together and connecting with like-minded individuals with shared interests. Freeing ourselves from established conventions of ideas, actions and professional customs can leave people feeling anxious and uncertain in how to make sense of madness, and how to help and offer support. It is hoped that the following chapters offer points of reference in exploring roads previously untaken.

The chapter 'Recovery, Discovery and Revolution', by Eleanor Longden, Dirk Corstens and Jacqui Dillon, highlights how the Hearing Voices Network was born out of and in reaction to the oppression and stranglehold of the biomedical paradigm of hearing voices. It parallels Intervoice and the Hearing Voices movements with other social movements, where communal protest, solidarity and action work to challenge the status quo. The chapter also discusses how the movement maintains itself, the continuing challenges, and describes its model of making sense of voices and supporting people with such experiences.

Peter Beresford highlights that we need to liberate and develop the experiential knowledge of people who experience madness. His chapter argues that this experiential knowledge is a unique contribution to the field of mental health, one often ignored and marginalised; this is a theme common to a number of chapters in this section. Beresford notes the current contributions of lived experience in attempting to shape madness and responses to madness, such as research, survivor histories and peer support. Looking to the future, Beresford suggests the need for a network of survivor-led organisations that will make it possible to form alliances and equal relationships with other services, rather than relationships based upon assimilation and co-option.

Continuing from the themes of the previous chapter, Jan Wallcraft looks at attempts to combat the marginalisation of survivor knowledge and research, and to give it credibility and legitimacy. The chapter links efforts to progress service user-led research to service users' struggle to gain civil liberties and social standing in wider society. The chapter shows how the questioning of the epistemology of mainstream research, service users gaining research skills, setting research agendas and publishing research can all be seen as part of the process of emancipating those deemed mad.

In 'The Patient's Dilemma', Joanna Moncrieff, David Cohen and John Mason also highlight the importance of service user knowledge and experience regarding the effects of psychiatric drugs. They argue that our conceptualisation of psychiatric drugs needs to be freed from a disease-centred model of psychiatric medication, and replaced with a drug-centred model. The latter would necessitate paying more attention to the subjective experience of taking psychiatric drugs, and necessitate greater participation of service users in decision making. They argue for a more a more open, honest and democratic approach to psychiatric drug use.

Rufus May introduces a collection of voices of people who speak out against the discrimination and marginalisation of those with mental health problems. The chapter notes that madness hold truths about the relational and social difficulties we all face, and so such madness and distress needs to be heard. The chapter argues for building 'emancipatory communities' to combat attempts to separate madness from our collective consciousness. It argues that we need to create space for a diversity of voices to speak and be listened to, so that people can share their commonalities and celebrate their differences.

Guy Holmes highlights how many of the proximal stressors (such as housing, relationships and money) and distal influences (culture, big business, government policy) in people's lives are often concealed. Instead society places emphasis on the individual's responsibility to find inner resources in order to achieve change. The chapter describes how 'Psychology in the Real World' groups have encouraged people to free up their thinking about the causes of distress, so to consider a range of social and material influences. Holmes encourages us to acknowledge when we see social injustice and rather than feeling overwhelmed by the enormity of trying to challenge entire systems, to 'think small' in making a difference. In doing so, the chapter outlines some practical steps that collectives can make to counter the stigma that is attached to the experiences of mental distress.

The Nottingham Mind Medication Group and the Leicester Living with Psychiatric Medication Group were partially inspired to form by one of the aforementioned Psychology in the Real World groups. Across two chapters, members have written about their experiences of taking psychiatric medication and feeling trapped within the psychiatric system. Each group is an attempt to open up a space beyond the constraints of mental health services, where people have greater freedom to ask questions, debate and express a range of opinions about medication and alternatives. The chapters emphasise the importance of access to information about medication, and also of acting together to challenge the dominant medicalised understandings of madness which necessitate the use of psychiatric drugs. They illustrate these points through descriptions of their projects, groups and developments, and conclude with their hopes that other groups might develop and form a wider network.

Becky Shaw discusses the importance of peers joining together to lend each other social, emotional and practical support, and to share experiences, ideas and knowledge. Peer support groups can facilitate a redefinition of participants, from the role of passive and disordered patient to a person who has knowledge to share and who supports others. The chapter also notes that as a collective such groups have more power and influence to try to challenge some of the dominant narratives and power structures by taking on roles such as peer advocates, linking with other groups, and sharing resources and knowledge.

The final three chapters reflect on attempts to evolve services from positions inside and outside of the dominant service structures. Theo Stickley, from his perspective as Lecturer in Nursing, accounts how he came to question the practice of user involvement. Whilst retaining many of the values and philosophy of user involvement, he argues that such involvement is often assimilated and co-opted into the dominant hierarchy. The chapter advocates for emancipation through collaboration, where service users establish a power position outside the traditional hierarchy, and whose services are commissioned as consultants. In terms of teaching nurses, this would mean service users devising and running whole modules, rather than be brought in for one-off lectures.

In 'Rebuilding the House of Mental Health Services with Home Truths', Bob Diamond critically reflects on the current structures and foundations of mental health services. He looks at how services could be reshaped and rebuilt utilising values and ideas from critical and community psychology, such as modesty, liberation, innovation and critical reflection. The chapter argues that services need to free themselves from expert-driven approaches, a reductionist science and paternalism, and instead base themselves more on ideas such as the importance of connecting with others, helping people make sense of their lives, and looking outwards to changes in social and material circumstances. Redesigned services would also include more honesty and shared decision making around psychiatric drugs, and more open debate and scrutiny of the controlling function of services, including its conflict of interest between care and control.

Several chapters have advocated for an emancipatory approach, where service users and survivors form organisations and services outside of the traditional hierarchy. The Leeds Survivor Led Crisis Service (LSLCS) is an example of this in action. Fiona Venner and Michelle Noad detail how LSLCS eschews common facets of mainstream services, such as diagnosis, oppressive control and an obsession with risk. Instead they offer a service based on: listening; treating people with warmth, kindness and respect; not judging or categorising people; peer support; and a calm environment. They highlight how the organisation maintains its autonomy and philosophy, whilst also maintaining relationships with mainstream services.

Critical reflection

By going beyond the current restricted thinking about madness and acknowledging that distress, fear and madness are never far from any of us, we start to see that madness signifies a message: the social structures and the hierarchies we all live under are not fit for purpose and are damaging for many. Currently we are living in a time of economic crisis, where those with least are likely to get less, leading to ever-increasing levels of fear, misery and madness. The current government refers to rebuilding the economy; however they appear to have very little idea as to the function of the economy, except perhaps to maintain the self-interest of the rich. We have lost the idea that an economy should serve the good of society, and that the economy is not an end in itself.[2] Questions such as, 'what constitutes a healthy society and how should we strive towards it?' no longer exist in the public domain and have been supplanted by shallow meaningless concepts such as 'The Big Society' and the pursuit of happiness. What form of society do we wish to live within? What sort of society will nurture, rather than harm individuals? The neoliberal policies and values of the past 30 years have placed a burden of responsibility on isolated individuals and taken us further away from building a society which works for the public good, as well as nurturing individual development. We need to fundamentally grapple with restructuring society and envisioning a better world if we are to significantly advance the future of those suffering from the sharpest end of what society has to offer. As this collection highlights, such a burdensome goal should not stop us as individuals, small groups, networks and communities striving and searching for something better; however, it does caution us against looking for solutions in internal cognitive distortions and neurochemical imbalances. There is much we can do to improve how we conceptualise and respond to madness, including many of the ideas shared here. Liberation of madness will only occur once we free ourselves to imagine a different form of society and find the collective political will to enact change.

---

2 See Galbraith, J. K. (1992). *The Culture of Contentment*. London: Sinclair-Stevenson Ltd.; Tawney, R. H. (1920). *The Acquisitive Society*. New York: Harcourt, Brace and Howe.

Part One

Questioning the Domination of Madness

Chapter 1

The Persistence of Medicalisation: Is the presentation of alternatives part of the problem?

Mary Boyle

As many of the chapters of this book point out, the most common way of presenting those behaviours and experiences called psychosis[1] – for example, hearing voices or expressing highly unusual beliefs – is as if they were the same kind of phenomena as physical problems such as diabetes or rheumatoid arthritis. It is this claimed similarity between certain behaviours and psychological experiences and bodily problems, the application of the theoretical terms and practices of medicine to people's behaviour, thoughts and feelings, which is often referred to as the 'medical model'. This model is, of course, applied not only to psychosis but to many other forms of emotional distress and problematic behaviour. If versions of the model include social or interpersonal factors, these will always be seen as secondary to the more fundamental biological factors. The model operates and is disseminated through medical language (e.g., symptoms, disorders, treatment), through practice (e.g., diagnosis, hospitalisation, administration of drugs) and through a research agenda which privileges genetic, biological and pharmaceutical research.

Members of the public and professionals are often surprised to be told that there is no direct evidence for this model of problematic behaviour and experience. Despite this lack of evidence and many detailed critiques, medicalised accounts of psychosis and other forms of emotional distress persist. Explanations of this persistence have highlighted factors such as entrenched professional and corporate interests; a highly sophisticated public relations industry supportive of medicalisation and largely funded by pharmaceutical companies; systematic misrepresentation of research

---

1 The term 'psychosis' has become more popular in the face of increasing criticism of 'schizophrenia'. Although I am using the term here as neutrally and descriptively as possible, it is notable that clinical and research use of 'psychosis' often replicates the problems of the concept of schizophrenia and that the relationship of the two concepts is complex and problematic (Boyle, 2006).

data; media credulity in the face of claims about brain research; a cultural milieu supportive of biological and individualistic accounts of human behaviour; habits of thought and cognitive biases which lead us to question medical explanations far less than we should; a training system which makes it difficult for professionals even to imagine, far less implement, a different way of thinking; and the capacity of medical accounts of distress to deflect attention from the harm done to the (relatively) powerless by the (relatively) powerful (Ross & Pam, 1995; Johnstone, 2000; Boyle, 2002a, 2011; Pilgrim, 2007; Moncrieff, 2008; Whitaker, 2010).

Important though these factors are, I will focus here on an explanation for the persistence of medicalised accounts of psychosis which has been given rather less attention. That is the possibility that what are intended as alternatives to medical accounts may sometimes be presented in ways which actually contribute to the persistence of a medical model. Before I discuss this in detail, I'll suggest a possible framework for thinking about this issue.

It has often been pointed out that when any group is faced with new ideas which threaten its dominance it can respond in one of several ways. It can, first, ignore the ideas but this will be difficult if the ideas are persistent or taken up by other powerful groups. Second, the dominant group can accept the new ideas and change its own stance, a paradigm shift in scientific terms. Kuhn (1970) has argued that such shifts are crucial to scientific progress, as happened, for example, when Einsteinian physics replaced Newtonian physics. Kuhn has also noted, however, that matters are very different when we leave the world of the natural sciences for a world where social, economic, political and psychological factors may play a major role in judgements about the worth of alternative theories. While Kuhn's sharp separation of the natural sciences from other disciplines may be rather idealistic, it is certainly true that in the case of psychosis, and regardless of the evidence for non-medicalised accounts, there is little sign of a paradigm shift in their direction.

If ignoring or fully accepting new and potentially threatening ideas is not feasible, there are at least two further possibilities. The dominant group can misrepresent, attack, ridicule or otherwise try to invalidate the ideas – make them seem unreasonable or unnecessary – or it can question the abilities, motives or knowledge of those who propagate them. Finally, new ideas can be assimilated into the dominant way of thinking. This can sometimes be done constructively but where there is much at stake, as there certainly is in the case of theories of psychosis, financially, professionally and socially, what is more likely is that potentially threatening ideas will be assimilated in a way which neutralises them, takes away their most critical elements, leaving the 'old' worldview intact. This strategy may have the further advantage of presenting the dominant group in a positive light, open to new thinking, while at the same time ensuring that nothing fundamentally changes.

I would argue that it is the last two of these – invalidation and assimilation/neutralisation – which characterise mainstream responses to alternative ideas about psychosis and other forms of emotional problems. In fact, these processes are so widespread as to suggest that, far from being ignored, challenges to medicalisation have been enormously influential but often in ways that show themselves in increasing efforts to neutralise the challenge and ensure that traditional ideas remain more or less intact.

In this chapter, I'll discuss how some aspects of the presentation of alternatives might actually make these processes of invalidation, assimilation and neutralisation easier than they could be. I'll also suggest some additional steps we might take to make non-medicalised theories of psychosis more robust. Let me emphasise that this is not an exercise in criticism or blame; we inhabit a professional, social and political culture which is immensely supportive of simplistic, individualised and medicalised approaches to distress and most especially to psychosis. Even if alternatives manage to avoid being ignored or ridiculed, it is very difficult indeed for them to avoid being more subtly invalidated or at least to some extent assimilated and neutralised. However, by keeping these processes to the forefront of our thinking it may be possible to block at least some attempts to implement them. With this in mind I'll first address the problem of alternatives being invalidated before discussing assimilation and neutralisation.

Preventing invalidation

It is not unusual for attempts at invalidation to involve subtly or not so subtly denigrating those who put forward non-medical accounts of psychosis often via suggestions that they are out of touch with the latest research or even with the reality of psychosis. For example, when asked in a recent interview what he thought of suggestions that 'schizophrenia' was on a continuum with 'normal' behaviour and experience, Chris Frith, a professor at the Wellcome Trust Centre for Neuroimaging, replied, 'If I was feeling aggressive I would say I suspect these people have never actually worked with anyone with schizophrenia!' (*The Psychologist*, October, 2010, p. 816). It is not easy to avoid these personalised attempts at invalidation but there are aspects of the presentation of non-medical approaches which can make it easier for others to invalidate them and which could be changed. I'll discuss two of these: lack of attention to biology and embodiment, and to questions of blame and responsibility.

Invalidation and the missing body

Alternatives to medical accounts have placed great emphasis on the importance of people's life experiences and social context in the development of psychosis and other forms of mental distress. This has been necessary not only because of the strength of evidence supporting these arguments but as a counter to far less evidence-based biological accounts. One consequence of this, however, has been a relative neglect of the fact that mental distress of all kinds is an embodied experience. This was well illustrated by participants in a recent study:

> What a lot of people don't know about depression is that it's as though somebody's borrowed your brain ... a little thing like vacuuming is a big chore.

> Because you don't only have these depression and anxiety, it also causes physical pain all over the body. I used to have bad earaches ... headaches, sleeplessness, no appetite, you know there's so much involved in it, this mental health.
> (Leeming, Boyle & Macdonald, 2009, p. 15)

Similarly, personal accounts of psychosis emphasise sleep disturbances and unusual states of consciousness or arousal, while seemingly bizarre beliefs about the body, which may be derived from actual bodily experiences, are not uncommon. And it may seem that we cannot 'really' explain hearing voices without involving the brain. Any account of psychosis or other emotional problems which does not include the body in one way or another is therefore likely to seem at best incomplete or at worst simply wrong and to risk invalidation. But there are considerable challenges to incorporating bodies and biology into non-medicalised accounts of emotional distress. Modern Western culture is highly reductionist in the sense that explanations of emotion or behaviour involving brain or biology are routinely presented and accepted as more fundamental, more 'real', and are accorded higher status, than accounts involving social context, psychological processes or life experiences. Some people have tried to redress the balance by pointing out that the physical and mental interact but this modest claim has already been exploited through its conflation with the entirely different claim that emotional and behavioural problems are the same sort of phenomena as bodily disease, that they require the same kind of theoretical and therapeutic approach. *The Diagnostic and Statistical Manual of Mental Disorders* (*DSM*) makes this conflation – and its purpose in justifying the medicalisation of distress – quite explicit:

> … the term *mental disorder* unfortunately implies a distinction between 'mental' disorders and 'physical' disorders that is a reductionist anachronism of mind/body dualism. A compelling literature documents that there is much 'physical' in 'mental' disorders and much 'mental' in 'physical' disorders. (APA, 1994, p. xxi)

It is a considerable conceptual leap from this to the conclusion on which the *DSM* is based – that emotional distress and behavioural problems should be theorised and responded to in the same way as bodily disorders. Unfortunately, it is not difficult to find more everyday examples of this kind of thinking. The following is from a magazine in which readers put questions to a doctor. One reader asks:

> How true is it that your mental state – depression or anxiety for example – can make a difference to you physically? If true in what ways do they do so? Or is the connection simply fanciful?

And the doctor's rather aggressive reply to this perfectly reasonable question is:

> Are you suggesting that so-called mental problems have no physical basis and that they are different from other illnesses? Well, they aren't. Altered mood is just as physical, biochemical and electrical an entity as so-called physical or bodily disorders. (*Guardian Weekend*, 27 February 2010)

These arguments, like those of the *DSM*, are of course absurd. The mere fact that the physical and mental interact can no more justify the wholesale application of a medical framework to certain kinds of behaviour and emotion than it could justify the wholesale application of a psychological framework to cancerous tumours or infected tissue. But even if the *DSM*'s and the magazine doctor's claims lack logic or evidence, they have a powerful cultural allure which creates formidable obstacles for any attempt to integrate the body into accounts of mental distress. As we will see, models which may seem to offer a way of doing this, such as the biopsychosocial or vulnerability-stress models, have done nothing to counter the privileging of biology, while their psychosocial or stress aspects have been effortlessly assimilated leaving the medical framework intact (Boyle, 2002a; Read, 2005).

What is needed instead are more sophisticated models which take account of the inseparable, reciprocal relationships amongst the social, psychological and biological; models which, unlike most versions of the biopsychosocial or vulnerability-stress models, actually conceptualise the nature of these relationships rather than listing factors in a framework which always accords biology the most privileged and fundamental status. As Cromby (2006) notes, mainstream psychology has done little to promote such models and indeed has structured itself and its relationship to other disciplines in such a way as to make their development unlikely. Some progress, however, has been made. Cromby (2004) has proposed a 'socio-neural' perspective on feelings of depression which attempts to link social inequality, psychological experience and embodied processes (see also Cromby, Harper & Reavey, 2013, Chapter 4). Discussing people with a diagnosis of schizophrenia, Harrop, Trower and Mitchell (1996) subvert the usual practice of asserting any claimed biological difference between those diagnosed as schizophrenic and so-called normal comparison groups as evidence of a biological cause of 'schizophrenia'. Instead, they argue that to the extent that such differences are reliable, they may be a consequence of social and psychological experiences such as specific traumas or occupying subordinate social roles. They also note that psychotic experiences themselves, for example, those involving high levels of fear, are likely to produce biological changes. Like Cromby, they emphasise reciprocal relationships amongst the social, psychological and biological. Given the strong relationship between mental distress, including psychosis, and social disadvantage, it is interesting that all of these authors draw attention to possible biological and psychological consequences of the powerlessness and subordination which social disadvantage entails.

It is not necessary to wait for fully formed truly interactionist models; we can challenge the reductionism inherent in the medicalisation of psychosis, suggest alternative interpretations of biological data and provide examples of reciprocal relationships amongst the social, psychological and biological so as to open discussion and debate. For example, much has been made of structural brain abnormalities found in a minority of those with a diagnosis of schizophrenia, including claims that they are evidence of 'schizophrenia' being a neurodevelopmental disorder. But these abnormalities are found in other groups and are linked to the use of minor and major tranquillisers. They may also be linked to a mother's social disadvantage or drug and alcohol misuse during pregnancy, to childhood abuse and neglect or to later drug and alcohol misuse. In turn, these brain abnormalities may set the scene for problems in school, relationships and work, creating or adding to the kinds of highly stressful environments linked to psychotic experiences. Similarly, drug misuse is often suggested as a 'trigger' of psychosis, and indicative of its biological nature, when it may be more a way of trying to cope with the kinds of adverse environments associated with psychosis. What is important here is to demonstrate another way of thinking about the possible relationships between biology, the body and psychosis and to emphasise repeatedly how different this is from a medical model.

There is also an emerging literature (see Moncrieff, Cohen and Mason in this collection) which complements this approach and which could provide added protection from invalidation for non-medicalised accounts of psychosis. Moncrieff and Cohen (2005) and Moncrieff (2008) have strongly criticised disease-centred models of psychotropic drug action, i.e., the assumption that these drugs 'work' by acting on a disease process – as reflected in the renaming of major tranquillisers as 'antipsychotics' and some sedatives and stimulants as 'antidepressants'. Part of the importance of these critiques is that disease-centred models of drug action and the linguistic impression they create of specific diseases being targeted by specific biological agents have played a vital role in supporting medicalised accounts of mental distress in the absence of any reliable evidence of their validity. Moncrieff and Cohen argue instead for a drug-centred approach which assumes that psychotropic drugs create abnormal brain states with a wide range of behavioural and psychological outcomes, some of which may be seen as positive, although what counts as positive may be very different for the person taking the drugs, professionals and relatives (see also Whitaker, 2010). The importance of a drug-centred approach is that it can accommodate both positive and negative effects of psychotropic drugs without any assumption of disease, illness or the need for diagnosis; it is therefore entirely compatible with non-medical accounts of psychosis.

Invalidation via blame and responsibility

Medicalisation of problematic behaviour and emotions locates their primary causes in faulty genes or biology rather than in social structures, power relations or life experience. One of the most important functions of this approach is that of seeming to remove blame or responsibility for behaviour that may attract very negative judgements. It is difficult to overstate the significance of this function and how far it is exploited in encouraging acceptance of the idea of behaviour and emotion as illness.

The process of involving blame and responsibility in mental distress and seeming to remove it through medicalisation operates partly within a culture which places a high value on the ideas of free will and personal responsibility. It also operates more explicitly through the frequent use of a 'mad or bad' dichotomy whose more modern version might better be described as 'brain or blame'. What this implies is that, in the face of behavioural or emotional problems, and most especially of psychosis, we have only two choices: either someone's brain is faulty or the person themselves or those close to them, especially relatives, must be to blame. This way of thinking operates as an extremely powerful means of invalidating alternatives to medicalisation because it depicts them as somehow judgemental and inhumane.

The brain-or-blame dichotomy operates most obviously at the level of families of those diagnosed as schizophrenic and has been very influential in shaping mainstream research and clinical practice in this area; accusations of 'family blaming' are also routinely used as a way of preventing open discussion of research which challenges medicalised approaches. Similarly, biological and genetic researchers often claim that their research 'exonerates families' or 'relieves them of feelings of guilt'; apart from the many critiques of biological and genetic data, such claims imply that the purpose of research is to enable moral judgements and that those who disagree with a medical approach are eager to attribute blame (see Johnstone, 2000 and Boyle, 2002a for more detailed discussion).

Censoring of social and psychological accounts of psychosis via the brain-or-blame dichotomy can also happen more privately at the level of individuals. This was very apparent in the Leeming et al. (2009) study mentioned earlier, in which participants seemed very aware that events and people in their lives were in some ways implicated in their distress but were equally aware that saying this could imply blaming others and a reluctance to take personal responsibility. For example, one participant who had been given a diagnosis of bipolar disorder said:

> I'd got the issue of abuse to deal with ... I thought well maybe that caused it ... I certainly wasn't forced to work to a resolution and a forgiveness but I did get there in the end, but ... of course I was blaming the person that perpetuated [sic] the abuse um for my mental health problems as well. I mean I understand now that it can actually be a trigger but it's actually a trigger for something that's already there. (Leeming et al., 2009, p. 14)

Through her contact with mental health services, and by drawing on the vulnerability-stress model, this woman has reformulated the sexual abuse she suffered as a child so that it is no longer – as she had thought – the possible primary factor in her later difficulties, but a 'triggering' event which led to the expression of pre-existing and presumably biological tendencies to psychosis. I'll return in the next section to the importance of the idea of vulnerability-stress in maintaining medicalised approaches to psychosis; for the moment what is notable is the woman's assumption that positing a direct relationship between what is done to you as a child and how you feel and behave as an adult must involve attributing blame ('of course I was blaming the person ...') and her acceptance ('I mean I understand now ...') of her susceptibility to 'mental illness' as a valid way of seeming to avoid blaming others. In our culture, the implication either that you are trying to blame others for your problems or that you have not been a 'good parent' seem to be especially dreaded (Coulter & Rapley, 2011). The strength of desire to avoid the latter judgement can perhaps be gauged by a psychiatrist's comment to the media, following one of many unsubstantiated claims to have shown that 'schizophrenia is a brain disease': 'Those who take comfort from the evidence that schizophrenia has a biological basis should be further reassured ... [T]he study should relieve any feelings of guilt. Families cannot be blamed ...' (Jablensky, *The Times*, 3 March 1986). Apart from the implication that the brain-or-blame dichotomy is the only framework for interpreting this kind of research, what is actually being claimed here is that it is preferable for your child to have an incurable brain disease than for your behaviour as a parent to be linked to their psychosis. It is these fears that some supporters of medicalisation so skilfully exploit in their pretence that the only alternative to biology-as-primary-cause is to attribute blame.

In spite of the importance of the brain-or-blame dichotomy in maintaining the credibility of medical approaches to psychosis, alternative approaches do not often engage directly with this issue, although there are exceptions, for example, Johnstone, 1999; Read, Seymour & Mosher, 2004; Coulter & Rapley, 2011. But unless this engagement is strengthened and becomes routine, it is difficult to see how non-medical approaches can protect themselves from invalidation. We can challenge the brain-or-blame dichotomy and expose these strategies of invalidation as often and as publicly as possible, persistently assert the right to discuss research evidence on family interaction and psychosis, including that showing likely causal links between childhood abuse and neglect and adult psychosis (Read, van Os, Marken & Ross, 2005) and insist that those who challenge the research do so with appropriate arguments and not through accusations of 'blaming families'. That, however, may not be enough unless we can also make very clear that carrying out research which examines the links between social and family structures, life experiences and psychosis is not necessarily the same as finding fault or blaming people or, indeed, of denying personal agency. While we may wish with Coulter and Rapley to make exceptions in instances of 'unequivocal and deliberate abuse', we can still discuss the involvement of parents and others in the development of psychosis in a way which recognises that 'being in some way responsible' for an outcome does not necessarily imply the intent to cause it (2011, p. 172). But it will not be easy. The brain-or-blame dichotomy, in one guise or another, is not only central to medical accounts of distress; it is culturally embedded and has long informed criminal justice systems (Reznek, 1997). Its frequent use in presenting medical theories of psychosis to the media and public and its impact on research and practice also highlight the wider issue of the ways in which knowledge is socially produced (Foucault, 1972) in contrast to the value-free scientific objectivity so often asserted for statements about the biological basis of 'abnormal' behaviour.

Preventing assimilation and neutralisation

Although persistent attempts are made to invalidate alternatives to medicalised accounts of psychosis, I'd argue that it is largely the more subtle means of assimilation and neutralisation which have been used to reduce the threat from alternatives. And if there is one practice more than any other which fosters the assimilation of alternative ideas back into the medical model, and the neutralisation of any threat they present to it, it is the continued reliance on medical language. Supposed alternatives to medicalisation are routinely couched in a language which seems to accept it, a language of diagnostic categories, and of symptoms, disorders, illness, treatment and even that ubiquitous term mental health. Of course, some of those who focus on psychological factors, but use medical language, clearly intend to offer not an alternative to medicalisation but a complementary approach where cognitive or, less often, social factors are simply added to a basic medical understanding. Some versions of these are explicitly medical, for example, Frith (1992); others are more subtly so, for example, a good deal of the literature on cognitive approaches to psychosis or on cognitive behavioural therapy (CBT) remains highly individualistic and within what we might call a metaphorical medical model, where some form of cognitive disorder or deficit is substituted for biological disorder or inserted between biology and behaviour (Boyle, 2002a). But the use of medical language is still widespread even amongst those who clearly intend to offer a more fundamental challenge to the medical model. There are at least three closely related reasons for this. First, supporters of medicalisation have put a great deal of effort into presenting medical language not as a particular way of *thinking* about emotional distress or problematic behaviour but as a way of *describing* them. The devisers of the *DSM* have strongly asserted this descriptive claim as a way of fielding criticism of diagnosis and diagnostic categories and as a way of obscuring their problematic theoretical assumptions. A second reason for the continued use of medical language is the difficulty of finding an alternative language which seems satisfactorily to convey what we want to say; third, there is the risk that if we move too far from what Smart (2002) has called the epistemological space of those we are trying to influence, then we will not be listened to, far less understood.

In the face of these difficulties, the continued use of medical language even by those who want to challenge medical assumptions is perhaps not surprising. But why is it such a problem? A major reason is that using medical language can make any disagreement with the medical model seem relatively superficial, just a matter of emphasis: you study single symptoms of schizophrenia, I'll study schizophrenia as a whole; you study psychological aspects of bipolar disorder, I'll study biological aspects of bipolar disorder; you provide psychological treatments for mental disorders, I'll provide drug treatments for mental disorders, and so on.

This use of language can make it trivially easy to assimilate alternatives, to make it look as if they are simply part of the same larger medicalised picture, as if we are all talking about the same thing – the causes and treatment of mental illness and mental disorders – just emphasising different aspects. Even placing a strong emphasis on psychological and social factors in mental distress is no barrier to assimilation because the medical model has developed a range of very effective ways of assimilating and neutralising these kinds of challenge and of ensuring that medicalised approaches will always take precedence. One of the most important functions of these assimilation tactics is to ensure that social and psychological factors do not appear to be primary causes of mental distress and therefore primary targets for intervention (Boyle, 2002b, 2011). For example, the fact that social class is very strongly related to psychosis and other forms of distress (Bentall, 2003; Tew, 2005) is assimilated via the claim that people with serious mental illness slide down the social scale. This makes lower social class look as if it is only a consequence of 'mental illness' rather than also, as the evidence suggests, a cause. Similarly, mainstream literature often pays more attention to 'trauma' as a consequence rather than a cause of psychosis. Psychological therapy is assimilated by calling it an 'adjunct', that is subordinate, to drug interventions; the evidence that family interactions influence psychosis is assimilated by claiming that this influence operates only after the 'illness' shows itself (i.e., families may contribute to 'relapse'), and not before (Johnstone, 1993; Boyle, 2002a). Perhaps most pervasively, the vast amount of evidence on the links between life experiences and mental distress, including psychosis, is assimilated and neutralised via the idea of vulnerability-stress. In this framework, negative life experiences are reduced to triggers of an assumed pre-existing genetic, biological or, in more modern parlance, neural vulnerability to 'mental illness'. Even the emotion-laden and personally meaningful content of psychotic experiences – always a problem for the medical model and usually ignored – can be accommodated. Fowler

(2000), for example, talks of the 'neural basis of psychotic disorder' and suggests that the form and content of 'psychotic symptoms' can be understood as deriving from both 'biological predisposition and personal adaptation (appraisal, meaning and emotion)' (pp. 108–109). So, even when the content of voices or beliefs is acknowledged as important, it remains secondary ('personal adaptation') to a supposed biological predisposition to illness.

These methods of assimilation owe much of their success to the widely held belief that although social and psychological processes may influence the development of psychosis and other forms of mental distress, the *end point* of these processes is still an 'illness', to be understood in much the same way as we understand the possible physical end points of, say, living in poor housing or working under pressure. This analogy was recently made explicit by the Vice-Chair of the *DSM-5* task force, in response to some UK psychologists' criticism of the *DSM*: '… [the group] wants to exclude the possibility of mental disorders being independently present in the person – the way that cancer or heart disease may be affected by social and psychological realities but nevertheless exist within individuals as discrete states' (*The Psychologist*, August 2011, p. 566). If we want to avoid assimilation of alternatives to medicalisation, it is therefore not enough for them to emphasise social and psychological processes; they must also offer an explicit and fundamental reconceptualisation of the 'end point', that is the behaviours and psychological experiences currently conceptualised as illness. I would argue that it is this reconceptualisation which is difficult if not impossible so long as medical language is used.

The problem of medical language and potential ways of reconceptualising the 'end point' can be clarified by focusing on the two key assumptions which the medical model makes about emotional and behavioural problems and which it passes off as taken-for-granted facts. The first assumption, already mentioned, is that certain psychological, emotional and behavioural difficulties are the same kind of phenomena as physical problems and can be understood in the same terms. The second assumption, which follows from the first, is that, while the form and content of these difficulties may be influenced by social context, the difficulties can still be organised and recognised as mental disorders with an existence independent of context or culture in the same way as, for example, cancer or diabetes. Included in this assumption is the idea that these mental disorders are distinguishable from 'normal' behaviour and experience by their lack of cultural sanction, that they are not justifiable reactions to adversity; in other words they are not socially or psychologically intelligible in terms of someone's life experience (Jacobs, 2009; Jacobs & Cohen, 2010). The first assumption of identity between physical and psychological problems is, of course, built into medical language. This language also to some extent conveys the second assumption of lack of intelligibility – after all, why would we need to see someone's beliefs as symptoms of a brain disorder if they might be expected from their life experience? Medical language, however, may not provide strong enough protection for the idea of unintelligibility because people's accounts of what has happened in their lives and the effect it has had on them constantly threaten to make mental distress and behavioural problems intelligible and expose the assumption as invalid. The assimilation tactics I described earlier function to neutralise this threat by 'reducing' these life experiences either to *consequences* rather than causes or to *triggers* of biological predispositions which act as the primary cause. It is the fact that medical language implies one or both of the two assumptions about mental distress, together with the availability of these assimilation tactics, which make it almost impossible to use medical language to convey what may be intended as alternatives to medicalisation (e.g., a 'single symptom' approach or psychological models of bipolar disorder) without potential confusion and almost certain assimilation back into the medical model.

What can be done about this? It seems reasonable to suggest that if we are to develop alternatives which are difficult to assimilate and neutralise then they should be presented in ways which clearly do not accept the assumption of equivalence between emotional/behavioural and physical problems or the assumption of unintelligibility. The most explicit way of doing this would be to abandon medical language completely. As I discussed earlier, however, this may be difficult but a first step would be to describe behaviour and experiences as neutrally as possible; some progress has already been made with the terms 'hearing voices', 'unusual beliefs' or 'extreme mood states'. But if medical language is difficult to avoid, then it should always be used in a way which makes clear that it involves a particular way of *thinking about* problematic behaviour and experience and not a way of *describing* them – 'what some people think of as symptoms of bipolar disorder' rather than 'symptoms of bipolar disorder'. In this way, people can be encouraged to see medical language as an optional way of thinking rather than a description of reality. Of course, some medical language has been taken from ordinary speech – for example, anxiety, depression, hyperactivity – and medicalised partly by adding 'disorder'. This converts what would have been a culturally shaped expression of feeling or behaviour into a universal mental disorder with an independent existence within the person. Some of this language can be reclaimed, for example, 'she felt very depressed' rather than 'she has depression'.

Important though it is to avoid medical language or to make clear that it is a way of thinking, it is if anything even more important to convey explicitly and persistently the intelligibility and meaningfulness of 'abnormal' behaviour and experience if we want to protect non-medical accounts of psychosis and other forms of distress from assimilation. This is because it is the intelligibility of any behaviour or psychological experience which renders, if not redundant then very problematic, the idea that they are merely surface manifestations – symptomatic – of an underlying brain disorder. It is important to emphasise that biology and embodiment are not separate from intelligibility but, as in some of the ways I mentioned earlier, contribute to it; this is quite different from the way in which the medical model uses biology to nullify intelligibility.

The understandability of any form of distress can be conveyed for a particular individual through formulation or – an idea popular in the 'schizophrenia' literature – normalisation. But these are often private transactions which offer little challenge to medicalised accounts in the public realm and, in any case, neither formulation nor normalisation offers any guarantee that the account will not in one way or another be based on the medical model (Boyle, 2002a; Johnstone, 2006; and see Fowler, 2000, above). It is therefore vitally important that understandability and meaning are emphasised whenever and wherever psychosis and other forms of distress are talked or written about, as well as the fact that these phenomena can be understood in the same terms as so-called normal behaviour and experience. This can be done in several ways. The first is by setting psychotic behaviour and experience in the context of 'normal' responses to 'abnormal' events. This would include descriptions of the scale of adversity many people experience, its cumulative impact and meaning. It is otherwise very easy to assume that frequently used words like 'stress', 'trauma' or 'life events' refer to relatively ordinary adversity or single events, leaving the way open for explanations based on genetic or biological predisposition, whose credibility depends on the assumption that the 'stress' is not sufficient to account for psychosis.

A second way of conveying understandability is by highlighting links between psychotic experiences such as hearing voices or holding highly unusual beliefs and 'normal' experiences widely distributed in the general population. Third, more attention needs to be paid to the fact that psychotic behaviour and experiences, like any other, may fulfil important functions in people's lives. Fourth, strong links should be made between the content of psychotic experiences, for example, what voices say and what people believe, and particular life experiences.

Finally, we need a stronger focus on why only some people who hear voices or hold highly unusual beliefs experience distress or come to the attention of psychiatric services. It is often simply assumed that it is because they are self-evidently mentally ill or their experiences pathological, rather than because, say, the content of their experiences is more negative, those around them are less tolerant of their experiences, or they lack the personal, social or material resources to manage the experiences or incorporate them into their lives. Taken together, it is these aspects of psychosis which represent the reconceptualisation of the 'end point' I discussed earlier, a reconceptualisation which rejects the notion that psychosis is culturally not understandable, and which has intelligibility and meaning at its centre. There is a great deal of research and personal narratives to support these ways of talking and thinking about psychosis, but it is remarkable how little of this filters through to the media or mainstream research and practice, and how often psychotic experiences and other forms of distress are talked about, implicitly and explicitly, as if they were only tangentially if at all connected to events and situations in people's lives (Roberts, 1991; Johnstone, 2000; Boyle, 2002a; Bentall, 2003; Read, Mosher & Bentall, 2004; Read, van Os, Marken & Ross, 2005; Schreier et al., 2009; British Psychological Society, 2010; Harper, 2011; Romme & Escher, 2011).

Although it is not directly concerned with reconceptualising psychosis or with assimilation or invalidation, it is worth mentioning one further way in which non-medical approaches to psychosis can be made more credible and robust and that is by persistently challenging the assumed explanatory power of psychiatric diagnoses. It is striking how frequently diagnoses are talked about as if they answered the question 'why' about mental distress, for example, 'I was relieved to get a diagnosis ... there's a reason for my difficulties' (Leeming et al., 2009, p. 15). The myth that psychiatric diagnoses explain distress comes from the assumed similarity between medical and psychiatric diagnoses, when in fact the two are quite different and not only in that one is based on bodily phenomena and the other on behaviour and psychological experience (Boyle, 1999, 2007). While some medical diagnoses (e.g., dermatitis) are little more than technical language re-descriptions, a great many more bring with them information about bodily events or processes which help account for a patient's complaints or symptoms. For example, a diagnosis of diabetes tells a patient that their bodily experience, perhaps tiredness or thirst, is caused by abnormal pancreatic function and blood sugar levels, in the sense that these are antecedents of the patient's complaints and linked to them by strong theoretical networks. Yet with very few exceptions, for example, where an assumed cause is included in the diagnostic label, as in 'substance-induced disorders', psychiatric diagnoses offer nothing by way of explanation. Instead, any attempt to invoke a diagnosis as an explanation leads to tautology: 'Why does this person hear voices?' 'Because they have schizophrenia.' 'How do you know they have schizophrenia?' 'Because they hear voices.' This circular explanation arises from psychiatry's failure to show reliable links between the behaviours and experiences on which its diagnoses are based and any biological antecedents.

Of course, it is not simply a matter of 'educating' people about the explanatory bankruptcy of psychiatric diagnoses. While they may lack any scientific support, diagnoses serve important personal and social functions for those who receive them, such as suggesting that professionals are familiar with this kind of problem and that there might be a remedy; they provide access to services, appear to lessen personal responsibility and may help to manage a potentially damaged identity in interaction with others (Leeming et al., 2009). Some of these functions, however, depend on the assumed explanatory power of diagnostic labels and as long as these appear to explain distress then alternative, non-medical accounts may seem at best supplementary and at worst completely unnecessary. By contrast, the more we point out the explanatory emptiness of diagnoses, the more we encourage people to ask for and expect different kinds of explanation.

Conclusions

The medical model of psychosis works by persistently shifting our attention from people's lives to their brains; many psychological models do exactly the same either by simply inserting 'cognitive disorder' between brain and behaviour or by focusing on 'deficits of the mind'. It is because there is so much evidence that attention should be focused on people's life experience and that psychotic experiences do not fit a medical framework, that the medical model, in order to persist, has had to develop so many ways of shifting our attention back to brain and biology. I am not arguing that taking up all the suggestions I've made here would easily or quickly result in non-medical accounts of psychosis becoming mainstream – there are still those external obstacles I mentioned in the introduction and which are discussed elsewhere in this book. It is easy, however, to underestimate the sheer adaptability of the medical model and its power to shift our attention, to invalidate, assimilate and neutralise challenges through the devices I've discussed. I would argue that we should acknowledge how far it has already done this and in what ways the presentation of alternatives has made these processes easier than they might otherwise have been. At the least, the suggestions made here could make it more likely that non-medical accounts will be listened to and understood and more difficult for them to be ignored or rejected.

References

American Psychiatric Association. (1994). *The Diagnostic and Statistical Manual of Mental Disorders* (4th ed.). Washington, DC: APA.

Bentall, R. P. (2003). *Madness Explained: Psychosis and human nature*. London: Allen Lane.

Boyle, M. (1999). Diagnosis. In C. Newnes, G. Holmes & C. Dunn (Eds.), *This is Madness: A critical look at psychiatry and the future of mental health services* (pp. 75–90). Ross-on-Wye: PCCS Books.

Boyle, M. (2002a). *Schizophrenia: A scientific delusion?* (2nd ed.). London: Routledge.

Boyle, M. (2002b). It's all done with smoke and mirrors. Or, how to create the illusion of a schizophrenic brain disorder. *Clinical Psychology, 12*, 9–16.

Boyle, M. (2006). *From Schizophrenia to Psychosis: Paradigm shift or more of the same?* Paper presented at the Annual Conference of the British Psychological Society Division of Clinical Psychology, London, December 2006.

Boyle, M. (2007). The problem with diagnosis. *The Psychologist, 20*, 290–292.

Boyle, M. (2011). Making the world go away, and how psychology and psychiatry benefit. In M. Rapley, J. Moncrieff & J. Dillon (Eds.), *De-medicalizing Misery: Psychiatry, psychology and the human condition*. Basingstoke: Palgrave Macmillan.

British Psychological Society. (2010). *Understanding Bipolar Disorder: Why some people experience extreme mood states and what can help*. Leicester: British Psychological Society.

Coulter, C., & Rapley, M. (2011). 'I'm just, you know, Joe Bloggs': The management of parental responsibility for first-episode psychosis. In M. Rapley, J. Moncrieff & J. Dillon (Eds.), *De-medicalizing Misery: Psychiatry, psychology and the human condition*. Basingstoke: Palgrave Macmillan.

Cromby, J. (2004). Depression and social inequality: A 'socio-neural' perspective. *Clinical Psychology, 38*, 15–17.

Cromby, J. (2006). Fundamental questions for psychology. *Clinical Psychology Forum, 162*, 9–12.

Cromby, J., Harper, D., & Reavey, P. (2013). *Psychology, Mental Health and Distress*. Basingstoke: Palgrave Macmillan.

Foucault, M. (1972). *The Archaeology of Knowledge*. London: Tavistock.

Fowler, D. (2000). Psychological formulation of early episodes of psychosis: A cognitive model. In M. Birchwood, D. Fowler & C. Jackson (Eds.), *Early Intervention in Psychosis: A guide to concepts, evidence and interventions*. Chichester: Wiley.

Frith, C. D. (1992). *The Cognitive Neuropsychology of Schizophrenia*. Hillsdale, NJ: Erlbaum.

Harrop, C. E., Trower, P., & Mitchell, I. J. (1996). Does biology go around the symptoms? A Copernican shift in schizophrenia paradigms. *Clinical Psychology Review, 16*, 641–654.

Harper, D. (2011). The social context of paranoia. In M. Rapley, J. Moncrieff & J. Dillon (Eds.), *De-medicalizing Misery: Psychiatry, psychology and the human condition*. Basingstoke: Palgrave Macmillan.

Jacobs, D. H. (2009). Is a correct psychiatric diagnosis possible? Major depressive disorder as a case in point. *The Journal of Ethical Human Psychology and Psychiatry, 11*, 83–96.

Jacobs, D. H., & Cohen, D. (2010). Does 'psychological dysfunction' mean anything? A critical essay on pathology versus agency. *The Journal of Humanistic Psychology, 50*, 312–334.

Johnstone, L. (1993). Family management in 'schizophrenia': Its assumptions and contradictions. *Journal of Mental Health, 14*, 255–261.

Johnstone, L. (1999). Do families cause 'schizophrenia'? Revisiting a taboo subject. *Changes, 17*, 77–90.

Johnstone, L. (2000). *Users and Abusers of Psychiatry*. London: Routledge.

Johnstone, L. (2006). Controversies and debates in formulation. In L. Johnstone & R. Dallos (Eds.), *Formulation: Making sense of people's problems*. Hove: Brunner-Routledge.

Kuhn, T. S. (1970). *The Structure of Scientific Revolutions* (2nd ed.). Chicago: University of Chicago Press.

Leeming, D., Boyle, M., & Macdonald, J. (2009). Accounting for psychological problems: How user-friendly are psychosocial formulations? *Clinical Psychology Forum, 200*, 12–17.

Moncrieff, J. (2008). *The Myth of the Chemical Cure: A critique of psychiatric drug treatment*. Basingstoke: Palgrave Macmillan.

Moncrieff, J., & Cohen, D. (2005). Rethinking models of psychotropic drug action. *Psychotherapy and Psychosomatics, 74,* 145–153.

Pilgrim, D. (2007). The survival of psychiatric diagnosis. *Social Science & Medicine, 65,* 536–547.

Read, J. (2005). The bio-bio-bio model of madness. *The Psychologist, 18,* 596–597.

Read J., Seymour, F., & Mosher, L. R. (2004). Unhappy families. In J. Read, L. R. Mosher & R. P. Bentall (Eds.), *Models of Madness: Psychological, social and biological approaches to schizophrenia.* Hove: Brunner-Routledge.

Read, J., Mosher, L. R., & Bentall, R. P. (Eds.). (2004). *Models of Madness: Psychological, social and biological approaches to schizophrenia.* Hove: Brunner-Routledge.

Read, J., van Os, J., Marken, A., & Ross, C. A. (2005). Childhood trauma and schizophrenia: A literature review with theoretical and clinical implications. *Acta Psychiatrica Scandinavica, 112,* 330–350.

Reznek, L. (1997). *Evil or Ill? Justifying the insanity defence.* London: Routledge.

Roberts, G. (1991). Delusional belief systems and meaning in life: A preferred reality? *British Journal of Psychiatry, 159*(Suppl. 14), s19–28.

Romme, M., & Escher, S. (Eds.). (2011). *Psychosis as a Personal Crisis: An experience-based approach.* Hove: Brunner-Routledge.

Ross, C. A., & Pam, A. (1995). *Pseudoscience in Biological Psychiatry: Blaming the body.* New York: Wiley.

Schreier, A., Wolke, D., Thomas, K., Horwood, J., Hollis, C., Gunnell, D., et al. (2009). Prospective study of peer victimization in childhood and psychotic symptoms in a nonclinical population at age 12 years. *Archives of General Psychiatry, 66,* 527–536.

Smart, C. (2002). *Feminism and the Power of the Law.* London: Routledge.

Tew, J. (Ed.). (2005). *Social Perspectives in Mental Health: Developing social models to understand and work with mental distress.* London: Jessica Kingsley.

Whitaker, R. (2010). *Anatomy of an Epidemic: Magic bullets, psychiatric drugs, and the astonishing rise of mental illness in America.* New York: Crown.

Chapter 2

Paranoia: Contested and contextualised

John Cromby & Dave Harper

In this chapter we discuss how paranoia might best be conceptualised and responded to. By paranoia we mean experiences of perceiving and relating to others that are characterised by suspicion, mistrust or hostility. Whilst such experiences are common in the general population, amongst people who receive clinical interventions they often include complex, self-insulating belief systems, distorted perceptions and marked distress. In psychiatry these experiences are usually associated with diagnoses of schizophrenia, delusional disorder and paranoid personality disorder. The problems with the reliability and validity of these diagnostic categories are well known (Bentall, 2004; Boyle, 2002; Pilgrim, 2001). One alternative approach is to focus on specific problematic experiences and behaviours (Boyle, 2002) or 'complaints' (Bentall, 2004) rather than heterogeneous diagnostic categories. Doing so addresses the problem of heterogeneity – but how might we then conceptualise these experiences? Drawing on a discussion of Bleuler's notion of schizophrenia, we present an approach to paranoia that considers both its social context and its embodied character. We then investigate the notion of 'distress'. Given the well-established finding that many people have experiences similar in content to those of mental health service users but without any accompanying distress, we discuss the importance of context in the generation of distress – in particular how it may arise because of a lack of 'fit' in the way they negotiate their beliefs and unusual experiences with their social world. Finally, we discuss how one might offer help or support differently in relation to paranoia.

Conceptualising paranoia

Clinicians might usefully reflect upon what paranoia is, because how they conceptualise it will influence the interventions they offer. In recent writings we have proposed that paranoia can be understood as constituted most crucially from complex mixtures of feelings (Cromby & Harper, 2009). By feelings we mean embodied states that can be subjectively experienced: emotions fall into this category, as do states like pain and fatigue, alongside more subtle states such as 'feeling certain'. These states constantly reflect our social and material situation and are the basis of all of our more formal thought processes (Langer, 1967).

Here, we introduce this approach, contrasting it with one of the foundational accounts of schizophrenia: Eugene Bleuler's work, which also gave a prominent role to feelings. We are cautious not to over-extend this comparison, partly because interpretations even across such relatively short periods of historical time are fraught, and partly because there is evidence that the population studied by Bleuler (and Kraepelin, the other architect of schizophrenia) was fundamentally different from today's. Substantial numbers of these early patients probably suffered from undiagnosed encephalitis lethargica, the symptoms of which (e.g., cyanosis, disorders of balance and gait, tremors) were also recorded as symptoms of schizophrenia but which (excluding the Parkinsonian effects of medication) are rarely seen today (Boyle, 2002). We also recognise that in examining Bleuler's concept we might appear to give it further legitimacy by reifying schizophrenia. However, many concepts in psychiatry are of this nature – reified categories that have become separated from the experiences they were originally designed to understand. Moreover, Bleuler's work is still cited by psychiatric textbooks to legitimate the schizophrenia diagnosis (e.g., Burton, 2006) and continues to inform research (Andreasen, 2000; Kraus & Keefe, 2007; Park & Thakkar, 2010). So it is both timely and appropriate to revisit Bleuler; having done so, we describe some differences between his account and ours, then identify some clinical implications of our discussion.

The disease of schizophrenia

The invention of schizophrenia is a seminal moment in the history of psychiatry, and the basics of the story are well known. In 1896 Emil Kraepelin claimed to have identified a subset of patients who shared similarities in the onset, course and outcome of their difficulties. He argued that these patients were reliably distinguishable from others (for example, those he described as having manic-depressive disorders) and concluded that all had the same disease, dementia praecox. Subsequently, Bleuler gave this disease its modern name: schizophrenia. The new name reflected two major differences from Kraepelin's conception. First, Bleuler's observation that – unlike in dementia – outcomes were not always negative, and deterioration was not inevitable and irreversible. Second, his view that the core symptom of this disease was a 'loosening of associations' between the various elements of thought, a 'weakening' of mental energy.

For Bleuler, this loosening or weakening causes a shattering of the psyche – a 'split mind'. The usual processes that link thinking, feeling, memory, identity and perception, enabling them to work together seamlessly, are pathologically impaired: consequently, these functions get dissociated or disconnected from each other. Bleuler describes how the product of this splitting is an excess of feeling that then gets associated in a relatively fixed way with a particular idea – an 'idea complex' – but that 'behind this systematic splitting into definite idea complexes, we have found a previous primary loosening of the associational structure which can lead to an irregular fragmentation of such solidly established elements as concrete ideas' (Bleuler, 1911/1950, p. 362). Schizophrenia, then, impairs the usual power of rational thought to inhibit, control and regulate affect: 'What is pathological in the organic psychoses, so far as the feelings are concerned, is that they dominate the thoughts more strongly than in healthy individuals. Their inhibitory and helping influence on associations is rendered stronger by the faultiness of intellectual function' (Bleuler, 1912, p. 34).

Historically, at least, this is the sense in which schizophrenia is portrayed primarily as a cognitive disorder, a disease of thought. A weakening of cognitive processes, caused by an organic impairment, is seen as the fundamental cause of schizophrenia. The subsequent imbalance of thinking and feeling (for Bleuler, disorders of affect, autism and ambivalence), along with delusions and hallucinations, are merely derivative or secondary symptoms. As Andreasen (2000, p. 107) puts it, 'For both Kraepelin and Bleuler, the most important defining feature was an impairment in the ability to think in a clear, fluent and logical way.' To summarise, then: Bleuler proposed that in schizophrenia, an organic deficit impairs the ability to think. This causes an excess of feeling, which allows idea complexes to form; these idea complexes are the basis of the delusions and hallucinations often associated with the diagnosis.

This very brief account of Bleuler's concept of schizophrenia allows us to make comparisons and contrasts with recent work of our own (Cromby & Harper, 2009). We have argued that experiences of paranoia for which a person might receive professional help are produced when complex mixtures of feelings produce very high states of arousal. When a person is highly aroused in this way, perceptions – which are usually simply tinged by feelings – can become powerfully influenced by them. Proximally, these states of heightened arousal may happen as a consequence of feeling traps (Scheff, 2003): arrangements of social, relational and material circumstances which cause mixtures of feelings to persist. This can cause the feelings involved to sustain, intensify and generalise, making it harder for the person to interpret or understand them, or to recognise their origins or causes, and so – in turn – producing additional feelings of anxiety, confusion or excitement that further complicate the person's experience.

Scheff proposes that, because of its specific qualities, shame will often be a component of feeling traps. He also discusses evidence suggesting that experiences of shame are frequently 'disavowed' – that is, people simply avoid recognising them. Shame itself is shameful, and the feelings associated with it are highly toxic; as a consequence, people frequently avoid all reference to their own experiences of shame and try to act as though they did not happen. Whilst for any specific individual very many different feelings might be involved, shame is frequently discussed in relation to paranoia, and our reading of the literature suggests that shame, fear and anger might all typically be important.

In paranoia, then, fear might cause shame (in men, for example, because of normative gender expectations); this in turn could lead to anger, especially if the shame is disavowed (Lewis, 1971); and this anger could be frightening, so magnifying the initial state of fear. Importantly, though, this is a schematic summary: at every moment, the precise way such feeling dynamics are enacted will continuously be influenced by fluctuating social and material circumstances. Feelings also influence – and are reciprocally influenced by – the narratives we tell others and ourselves, the 'inner speech' we experience, and the discursive constructions of world and self that, in everyday life, we constantly construct, update and revise. In paranoia these narratives are often conspiratorial and may refer to security services, aliens, secret organisations, surveillance and military technologies, or obscure or extreme religious or political groups.

Paranoia is likely to be characterised both by complex, shifting mixtures of feeling and by obstacles to their interpretation: where people believe they are not allowed to have or express certain feelings; where having or being seen to have certain feelings is dangerous; where it is adaptive not to feel, or at least appear not to feel; where feelings are difficult to identify or acknowledge because they run counter to the expectations or strictures of powerful others, and so on. In such circumstances, personal narratives may become somewhat complex and convoluted, occasionally lacking in overt logical coherence whilst retaining a deeper metaphorical or affective structure. Some of the typical features of the narratives of people experiencing distressing forms of paranoia – rapid speech, and an obsessive concentration on particular themes – are often associated with the presence of disavowed feelings (Scheff, 2003), suggesting that these may be particularly important. Moreover, the well-documented associations between paranoia, poor attachment, victimisation, powerlessness and marginalisation mean that paranoid narratives may often be managing some degree of exclusion or disenfranchisement: consequently, they may frequently serve a compensatory function that would (if accurate) endow the speaker with arcane knowledge or privileged insight (Bentall, 2004; Cromby & Harper 2009).

Beyond notions of disease

So there are similarities between our account and Bleuler's, since both are concerned with the relations between thinking and feeling, but there are also differences. Most fundamentally, Bleuler is explaining a putative disease, schizophrenia, whereas our aim is to understand an experience; consequently, our account is not confined to a single diagnostic category and recognises that paranoia is associated with numerous diagnoses (and with no diagnosis at all). Also, by comparison to our notion of feeling, Bleuler's conceptualisation of affect is on balance narrower, more sharply distinguished from cognition, and more interchangeable with emotion. But there are also other differences, and we will now explore three that are especially significant.

First, our account does not presuppose an organic impairment which gives rise to a cognitive deficit. Since Bleuler proposed this, more than a hundred years of generously funded research, using ever more sophisticated technologies, has failed to find consistent evidence for any such pathology. As eminent biological psychiatrist Kenneth Kendler (2005, pp. 434–435) puts it:

> We have hunted for big, simple, neuropathological explanations for psychiatric disorders and have not found them. We have hunted

for big, simple, neurochemical explanations for psychiatric disorders and have not found them. We have hunted for big, simple genetic explanations for psychiatric disorders, and have not found them.

Importantly, though, whilst our account does not presume an organic deficit, nor does it *ignore* the body, as social science and cognitive psychology so often do: instead, we emphasise embodied feelings as the medium through which paranoia is primarily constituted.

Second, Bleuler's account posits an imbalance between thinking and feeling, arising as a consequence of weakened cognitive function. However, not only is the organic impairment purported to cause this initial weakening still elusive, we also question whether there can actually be an 'imbalance' of this kind. There is a contemporary movement within the humanities and social sciences known as the 'affective turn' (e.g., Athanasiou, Hantzaroula & Yannakopoulos, 2008; Clough & Halley, 2007). Whilst the diversity of this work is such that even the basic terms, affect, emotion and feeling, are disputed, scholars associated with this movement agree that affective phenomena are hugely significant in human life; cannot sensibly be reduced to language, discourse or representation; and, conversely, cannot simply be treated as separable biological causes. From the perspective of the affective turn, *no* cognition is free of affect. Every thought is simultaneously both a movement of feeling and an associated fragment of inner speech that, to borrow Vygotsky's terminology, 'completes' it, making it fully sensible and available for reflection upon by ourselves, and (if we speak it aloud) by others (Cromby, 2007; Johnson, 2007; Vygotsky, 1962).

Frequently, the experiences associated with psychiatric diagnoses get related to neural structures and processes. Notwithstanding the well-documented dangers of individualism, reductionism and reification of diagnostic categories associated with such inferences (Bennett & Hacker, 2003), neuroscience itself provides evidence suggesting that thinking and feeling are not actually separable. Panksepp's (1998) studies of the mammalian brain identify a set of evolutionary older affect structures that he calls 'basic operating system circuits' that, once engaged, set the imperative and tone of cognitive processing. Similarly, Damasio (1999) proposes that feelings – feedback from the body – are the raw stuff of consciousness itself, which he suggests is generated in pulses that consist of the *difference* between the body in one somatic state and then, momentarily later, in another. Both of these neuroscientists (and others, e.g., LeDoux, 1999) provide arguments and evidence indicating that thinking and feeling are always thoroughly intertwined. On the basis of this evidence, *all* thinking – whether or not it is associated with mental health difficulties – is already *felt thinking*.

All of this evidence suggests that, rather than being capable of getting stuck in a state of imbalance, feeling and thinking are in a continuous, dialectical relation, each with the other. Additionally, both are constantly open to external influence, so experiences of paranoia ebb and flow according to circumstance and situation. Even during intensely distressing episodes (so-called florid paranoia), when sustained, complex mixtures of feeling have temporarily generated highly aroused states, it does not seem that thinking somehow stops: on the contrary, individuals continue to generate narratives by which to understand their experience. These narratives may become rapid (so-called 'pressure of speech') as the person strives to keep toxic feelings out of awareness (cf. Scheff, 2003). They may become disjointed as the person struggles to make sense of their multiple, fluctuating feelings and the fragments of meaning they are able to attach to them (so-called 'thought disorder'). Likewise, their logic – reflecting the complex, mobile, partially unspeakable mix of feelings within it – may defy some everyday conventions whilst entirely according with others, and indeed whilst reflecting in important ways the events, people and circumstances with which the person is currently preoccupied. But even during these intensely distressing episodes, feeling does not simply prevent or overwhelm thinking. In fact, it seems equally plausible to suggest that these are experiences where people are thinking *too much*: one way of understanding paranoia is to see it as a determined search for meanings and significances where none may actually exist.

A third difference between Bleuler's account and ours is that we do not see the origin of paranoia as a cognitive deficit within the individual. Instead, we propose that toxic social and material circumstances combine to produce feeling traps which position individuals in ways that engender self-amplifying mixtures of shame, fear, anger and other feelings, mixtures that – if they persist – can induce extreme levels of arousal. Arguably, Bleuler's view that paranoia (at least in association with diagnoses of schizophrenia) is caused by individual cognitive deficits is mirrored by recent innovations in clinical psychology which emphasise the role of cognitive processes (e.g., attentional biases and jumping to conclusions) in producing experiences such as voice-hearing and delusional beliefs (Bentall, Corcoran, Howard, Blackwood & Kinderman, 2001; Bentall, Kinderman & Kaney, 1994). This work is a valuable advance upon Bleuler's because it emphasises experiences that can be identified relatively reliably, rather than being dependent upon unreliable diagnostic categories, and also because it is associated with psychological rather than pharmaceutical interventions. Nevertheless, it is conceptually similar in that it posits a cognitive disorder as the root cause of these problems.

By contrast, we propose that the cause of intensely distressing episodes of paranoia is not an individual disorder or deficit, whether cognitive or organic, but a set of circumstances in the world itself. By virtue of their immersion in environments, individuals acquire habits of feeling, alongside habits of making sense both of their feelings and of the circumstances which generated them. If acquired in toxic circumstances, or alternately if acquired in benign environments but subsequently transferred to toxic ones, these habits may themselves become unhelpful. But even where this occurs, the origin of these habits is the social and material circumstances that gave rise to them, not some intrinsic cognitive flaw. As Jacqui Dillon, chair of the UK Hearing Voices Network puts it 'instead of asking people – what is wrong with you? We ask people – what has happened to you?' (2011, p. 155).

So it is not necessarily that these habits of thinking and feeling are themselves unhelpful, so much as their 'goodness of fit' with the situations within which they are now enacted is not optimal. Strikingly, however, this issue of fit is rarely discussed, even though the context of experience is hugely influential on whether distress is associated with it.

Context, 'fit' and paranoia

One of the problems facing clinicians is that the vast majority of people they see because of paranoia are either in distress themselves or causing distress to others. Consequently, they might fall prey to the clinician's fallacy: the assumption that unusual experiences are necessarily associated with distress. A number of studies challenge this assumption, notably those using the PDI (Peters et al., Delusions Inventory), a self-report questionnaire which asks questions about beliefs drawn from schedules of psychiatric symptoms but uses everyday rather than psychiatric language. Items include questions like 'do you ever feel as if people seem to drop hints about you or say things with a double meaning?' and 'do you ever feel as if you are being persecuted in some way?' The PDI provides a total score – the number of unusual beliefs the person is said to hold – and, for each belief, ratings of the conviction with which it is held, the level of preoccupation the person has with the belief, and the level of distress they feel it causes. Whilst this method takes a cognitive approach to beliefs (which can themselves be seen as both structures of feeling and components of thinking – Cromby, 2012), it nevertheless provides a useful perspective.

Peters et al. (2004), using a 21-item version of the PDI, compared the scores of a large general population sample with the scores of people who were psychiatric patients and diagnosed as having delusions. The authors used the shorthand labels of 'healthy' and 'deluded' for the two samples. In Figure 1 we can see how many beliefs were held by people in each of the samples. If we look at the general population ('healthy') sample we can see that relatively few people endorsed none of the beliefs – indeed, the vast majority of this sample endorsed at least some of the beliefs. The authors reported that the difference between the two samples was not the existence of unusual beliefs per se, but the levels of conviction, preoccupation and distress associated with them. Another study compared members of New Religious Movements (NRMs: Druids and Hare Krishnas), non-religious people, Christians and 'deluded people' (their term for the same inpatient sample), and reported no differences between NRMs and 'deluded people' in numbers of beliefs or the conviction with which they were held. Rather, the key differences were in the preoccupation and distress associated with them (Peters et al., 1999).

In the Netherlands, van Os, Hanssen, Bijl and Ravelli (2000) conducted a survey of 7,076 Dutch people from the general population using a structured interview schedule with follow-up telephone interviews by psychiatrists for anyone where there was at least one rating on an item relating to psychosis. They reported that 3.3 per cent had 'true' delusions (i.e., beliefs which met the diagnostic criteria for delusional belief), whilst an additional 8.7 per cent had delusions that were 'not clinically relevant' – that is, they were 'not bothered by it and not seeking help for it' (van Os et al., 2000, p. 13). This raises the intriguing possibility that, in addition to mental health service users, there may be twice that number of people in the wider population who have unusual experiences or beliefs, but who are not in distress or causing distress to others, and are living outwardly conventional everyday lives.

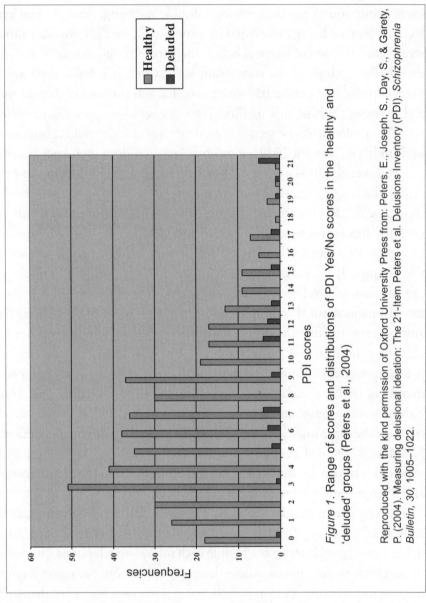

Figure 1. Range of scores and distributions of PDI Yes/No scores in the 'healthy' and 'deluded' groups (Peters et al., 2004)

Reproduced with the kind permission of Oxford University Press from: Peters, E., Joseph, S., Day, S., & Garety, P. (2004). Measuring delusional ideation: The 21-Item Peters et al. Delusions Inventory (PDI). *Schizophrenia Bulletin, 30,* 1005–1022.

Whilst it can be hard for us to fully accept this, there are numerous accounts of people living with extraordinary experiences (Romme, Escher, Dillon, Corstens & Morris, 2009). There are also high-profile people who might not have been given psychiatric diagnoses who live apparently functional lives, who do not appear to have either experienced distress because of their beliefs or to have received mental health services. Harper (2011a) discusses Sun Ra (a black American avant garde jazz musician) and David Icke: here, we will briefly consider David Icke's views.

Icke was a professional footballer who became a BBC TV sports presenter in the 1980s. He was involved in the Green Party in the late 1980s, but parted company with them following a number of spiritual experiences. A week after resigning from the Green Party he held a press conference to announce that he had become a 'channel for the Christ spirit' and predicted that the world would end in 1997 after a series of natural disasters. Icke subsequently began wearing only turquoise because he considered it a conduit of positive energy. Although the audience on Terry Wogan's BBC chat show appeared to laugh when they heard his views, according to journalist Jon Ronson, Icke is 'a global sensation' who 'lectures to packed houses all over the world, riveting his audiences for six hours at a time with extraordinary revelations' (Ronson, 2001, p. 151). He has a website (www.davidicke.com) which announced a second live date at the O2 Brixton academy in London in September 2010 to meet excess demand following a previous sell-out lecture in May 2010, and has written numerous books about his ideas, in particular that the world is run by a race of shape-shifting alien lizards who have interbred with humans.

Thus it would seem that unusual beliefs, or experiences like hearing voices and seeing visions, are not necessarily associated with distress: other kinds of feelings can be implicated. Indeed, the category of eccentric is frequently ascribed to those who are open about these experiences (Weeks & James, 1997). Whilst people are usually described as eccentric when their views are idiosyncratic, sometimes whole groups of people profess beliefs that many consider unusual. Shaw (1995) describes his experiences with a number of new religious groups, including the Aetherius Society which believes that their founder was in telepathic communication with UFOs. Of course, particularly when discussing religious, philosophical, political or moral claims, assertions about whether a belief is unusual can be problematic (Harper, 2011a). It seems that it is the *fit* between particular beliefs and experiences and other aspects of people's lives that powerfully influences whether distress (their own, or that of others) is associated with them.

Clinical implications

We have suggested that intensely distressing episodes of paranoia should be seen as habits of felt thinking and action acquired in response to events in the social world. We have also argued that it is the context of beliefs and experiences and their 'fit' in a person's life that may be important in determining whether they might cause problems for them. How might these observations be of use to those and those seeking to help people referred to mental health services? First, it is important to consider the wider context within which distress is identified (for either the person or others). Second, it is important to consider how the person's biographical context may give metaphorical meaning to the belief or experience, since this may suggest how habits of felt thinking and action are linked to prior adverse experiences.

Wider context

It is important not to assume that the experience or belief is necessarily distressing. One needs to consider the source of the referral: did it come from the person, a relative, or an agency as a result of requests by neighbours etc.? If the person is not in distress then maybe, rather than trying to change the person's relationship with their experience (e.g., through trying to alter their appraisal of it), what may be needed is help with relating that experience to the wider world, devising practical strategies to manage and negotiate their feelings in a world which may find them disturbing. There could be a range of tacit skills deployed by those in the general population with similar experiences – for example, people might carefully consider those with whom to discuss their unusual beliefs.

If the person is not distressed it may help to direct them to groups who share similar beliefs or experiences, since social isolation seems to accentuate distress (Read & Bentall, 2013). These groups may also offer protocols, practices and rituals that enable even a person preoccupied with a belief to set it in a context, reducing its immediacy and personal salience by sharing with the group, and locating it within a narrative with broader meanings. Thus, Hearing Voices Network groups embrace an agnostic approach to causality, enabling people to develop their own conceptual frameworks. Similarly, UFO abduction groups have developed complex belief systems setting these experiences in a wider historical and cultural context of the possibilities of human–alien communication (Clancy, 2005).

If the person themselves is not distressed by their experience or belief, but their family (for example) are disturbed or concerned, it may help to closely examine how this concern arises. It may be that simply talking to their family less about their beliefs and/or experiences will be helpful. Indeed, this is a common strategy deployed by those in hospital who wish to be discharged (Dillon, 2011). Frequently, a person's ability to talk less to those close to them is facilitated by engagement with a group – like those mentioned above – where experiences *can* be freely discussed.

Equally, it is important not to assume that these experiences or beliefs aren't distressing. Indeed, it is easy to romanticise those who hold beliefs that are seen as unusual as cognitive dissidents, to view their experiences in solely libertarian terms. If the person *is* distressed it is still important to investigate the context in which these feelings arise. Is it the belief or experience per se, the nature of their relationship with it, or the way they negotiate it with the wider world? It may help to clarify criteria by which the person would judge whether their relationship with – and negotiation of – the belief or experience had improved. Following Michael White's approach to helping service users clarify their position in relation to psychiatric medication (Stewart, 1995), therapists could consider how they might help service users determine whether their relationship with their beliefs contributes to – or subtracts from – their quality of life, ways in which their beliefs might be enabling and disabling, and how their effects (on themselves, and others) might best be monitored.

Biographical context

It may also help to explore the metaphorical meaning of a person's feelings in relation to their biography – for example, does it convey something about how they have made sense of aversive events earlier in life? Read and Bentall (2013) provide various examples of such links from the mental health literature, including this from Heins, Gray and Tennant (1990):

> A woman, who had been sexually assaulted by her father from a very young age and raped as a teenager, had the delusion that 'people were watching her as they thought she was a sexual pervert and auditory hallucinations accusing her of doing "dirty sexy things"'.
> (Cited in Read & Bentall, 2013, p. 270)

Of course, such explorations need to be conducted in a therapeutically safe and containing manner, setting problematic feelings in a meaningful context.

Even if a service user does not wish or is not able to leave their belief behind, it may be important to discuss how they might revise their relationship with it or its role in their life. Recently, cognitive behavioural approaches have begun to move in this direction, particularly concerning beliefs that seem hard to shift. Tamasin Knight, who received cognitive behavioural therapy but did not find that approach a good fit for her, explains how this kind of revision might occur:

> Some years ago I became very distressed as I believed I had a physical illness that would kill me in the not too distant future. I later became able to cope with this by thinking that if this was the case, then I should do the things I felt were important and enjoyed right away, rather than leave them to the future. By getting involved in activities I felt were important and worthwhile and building up my social network, the unpleasant beliefs I experienced became less central and troublesome in my life. (Knight, 2004, p. 13)

This is a pragmatic approach, focusing on a person's life goals rather than whether their beliefs are true. Given that final and convincing proof in relation to some beliefs may be impossible to acquire, the question becomes: how do we move forward? This might involve activities with which the person wishes to be involved but which fear has prevented. Such involvement might increase self-confidence and reduce social isolation, both factors which appear to be implicated in the development of unusual beliefs and experiences (Read & Bentall, 2013). In the next section we discuss a range of interventions that are consistent with the approach we have outlined.

Alternative interventions

Interventions from a range of theoretical traditions would be consistent with our approach. However, given the dominance of individual psychotherapeutic approaches and the relative neglect of a more collective and contextualised approach, here we will focus mainly on interventions with groups and wider networks. We will begin by focusing on the Hearing Voices Movement as it has led the way in developing collective alternatives, but we will then look at paranoia self-help groups, the Open Dialogue approach and, finally, community psychology. Following reports that many in the general population heard voices, the Hearing Voices Movement attempted to de-pathologise this experience. In the UK, the Hearing Voices Network follows this approach, welcoming a diversity of causal explanations, and voice hearers are encouraged to find their own ways of understanding and managing their experiences (Romme et al., 2009). Often this involves meeting with others who have similar experiences. How might such groups be helpful? One important factor may be that they help people develop explanations for their experiences that make sense to them *and* fit with the way they and others see the world. Of course, some explanations may be distressing, so groups might also help people to develop explanations that do not unduly distress them. Groups may also put people in contact with communities of others who share similar meanings – for example, Spiritualist church groups which see voices as having religious significance: this can help reduce social isolation. In addition, groups often engage in routine collective activities which ground the person in a community, for example, the regular meetings of Hearing Voices groups or the rituals and services of religious groups (Clarke, 2010).

In recent years, these insights have led to the development of paranoia support groups (Bullimore, 2010; James, 2003). Knight (2009) describes the process of setting up the 'Better believe it!' support group at the Joan of Arc project in Exeter and also includes the findings of an evaluation after the group had been meeting for two years. The founding conference of the Paranoia Network in Manchester in 2004 was attended by over 100 people; accounts of it can be found in Hornstein (2012) and Jacobson and Zavos (2007), whilst the Romme et al. (2009) volume includes accounts by some of the presenters.

The family is an important social context for some service users, but a continual challenge in psychotherapeutic work is to avoid colonising service users' experience with a monological interpretation (e.g., biomedical, cognitive, etc.). Seikkula, Alakare and Aaltonen's (2001a, b) 'Open Dialogue' approach explicitly involves the elaboration of multiple perspectives on distress, utilising the reflecting team tradition within systemic therapy. Here a small team of professionals meet with service users and their families with the specific aim of generating a range of explanations in a safe and containing manner, with the aim of placing problematic feelings in a meaningful context, rather than simply offering one explanation and one treatment.

Community psychology is another approach to engaging with the social context. May (2007) has discussed the development of community-based approaches for people having experiences considered psychotic – for example, the work of Evolving Minds in Yorkshire. Holland's (1991) White City project is also a useful model. Holland adopted a social action psychotherapy approach focused on women in West London's White City area, offering sessions of individual therapy that led into group work and then into collective social action. One issue that is often neglected is the need for societal changes, since environments are consistently shown to be strong causal factors in the development and maintenance of distress. Consequently, policy recommendations also flow from our approach, and these may become especially important in a so-called 'Age of Austerity' that seems likely to fuel increased social fragmentation and decreased trust in communities (Harper, 2011a, b).

Conclusion

Paranoia, like other terms used to describe mental health difficulties, is contested. In this chapter, we have tried to show how this term need not be understood in the context of a disease. Instead, we have argued, paranoia can be understood in the multiple contexts of everyday life and the unique contexts of personal biographies. This understanding of paranoia begins to distance it from the stigma that is inevitably associated with biomedical explanations for such experiences. It directs our attention to social and material circumstances, to the fit between beliefs, experiences and their contexts; it also directs our attention to personal biographies, and the habits of feeling they produce. Various research questions flow from our approach, and we have elaborated these elsewhere (Cromby & Harper, 2009). Here, we have explored some ways in which clinicians might help people who experience paranoia, and examined some of the ways in which people who experience paranoia are already helping themselves. However, since paranoia is a socially and materially constituted embodied experience, a way of being in the world, it necessarily reflects the circumstances and contingencies *of* that world. Consequently, its amelioration will always be a matter of political, economic and social policy, as well as therapeutic intervention.

References

Andreasen, N. (2000). Schizophrenia: The fundamental questions. *Brain Research Reviews, 31,* 106–112.

Athanasiou, A., Hantzaroula, P., & Yannakopoulos, Y. (2008). Towards a new epistemology: The 'affective turn'. *Historein, 8,* 5–16.

Bennett, M. R., & Hacker, P. M. S. (2003). *Philosophical Foundations of Neuroscience.* Oxford: Blackwells.

Bentall, R. P. (2004). *Madness Explained: Psychosis and human nature.* London: Allen Lane/Penguin.

Bentall, R. P., Corcoran, R., Howard, R., Blackwood, R., & Kinderman, P. (2001). Persecutory delusions: A review and theoretical integration. *Clinical Psychology Review, 21,* 1143–1192.

Bentall, R. P., Kinderman, P., & Kaney, S. (1994). The self, attributional processes and abnormal beliefs: Towards a model of persecutory delusions. *Behaviour Research and Therapy, 32,* 331–341.

Bleuler, E. (1912). *Affectivity, Suggestibility, Paranoia* (C. Ricksher, Trans.). Utica, NY: State Hospitals Press.

Bleuler, E. (1950). *Dementia Praecox or the Group of Schizophrenias* (J. Zitkin, Trans.). New York: International Universities Press. (Original work published 1911)

Boyle, M. (2002). *Schizophrenia: A scientific delusion?* (2nd ed.). London: Routledge.

Bullimore, P. (2010). 'The paranoia group.' *Asylum: The Magazine for Democratic Psychiatry, 1*(1), 26.

Burton, N. (2006). *Psychiatry.* Oxford: Blackwells.

Clancy, S. A. (2005). *Abducted: How people come to believe they were kidnapped by aliens.* London: Harvard University Press.

Clarke, I. (Ed.). (2010). *Psychosis and Spirituality: Consolidating the new paradigm* (2nd ed.). Chichester: Wiley.

Clough, P., & Halley, J. (Eds.). (2007). *The Affective Turn: Theorising the social.* Durham, NC: Duke University Press.

Cromby, J. (2007). Toward a psychology of feeling. *International Journal of Critical Psychology, 21,* 94–118. Retrieved 12 June 2012 from http://www-staff.lboro.ac.uk/~hujc4/

Cromby, J. (2012). Beyond belief. *Journal of Health Psychology, 17,* 943–957.

Cromby, J., & Harper, D. (2009). Paranoia: A social account. *Theory and Psychology, 19*(3), 335–361.

Damasio, A. R. (1999). *The Feeling of What Happens: Body, emotion and the making of consciousness.* London: William Heinemann.

Dillon, J. (2011). The personal *is* the political. In M. Rapley, J. Dillon & J. Moncrieff (Eds.), *De-medicalising Misery.* Basingstoke: Palgrave Macmillan.

Harper, D. (2011a). The social context of 'paranoia'. In M. Rapley, J. Dillon & J. Moncrieff (Eds.), *De-medicalising Misery.* Basingstoke: Palgrave Macmillan.

Harper, D. (2011b). Social inequality and the diagnosis of paranoia. *Health Sociology Review, 20,* 420–433.

Heins, T., Gray, A., & Tennant, M. (1990). Persisting hallucinations following childhood sexual abuse. *Australian and New Zealand Journal of Psychiatry, 24,* 561–565.

Holland, S. (1991). From private symptom to public action. *Feminism & Psychology, 1,* 58–62.

Hornstein, G. A. (2012). *Agnes's Jacket: A psychologist's search for the meanings of madness.* Ross-on-Wye: PCCS Books.

Jacobson, M., & Zavos, A. (2007). Paranoia Network and conference: Alternative communities and the disruption of pathology. *Journal of Critical Psychology, Counselling and Psychotherapy, 7*(1), 28–39.

James, A. (2003). Voices of reason. *The Guardian* 10 December. Retrieved 8 February 2010 from: http://society.guardian.co.uk/societyguardian/story/0,7843,1103141,00.html

Johnson, M. (2007). *The Meaning of the Body: Aesthetics of human understanding.* Chicago: University of Chicago Press.

Kendler, K. (2005). Towards a philosophical structure for psychiatry. *American Journal of Psychiatry, 162,* 433–440.

Knight, T. (2004). You'd better believe it. *Open Mind,128,* 12–13.

Knight, T. (2009). *Beyond Belief: Alternative ways of working with delusions, obsessions and unusual experiences.* Peter Lehmann Publishing: Berlin. Retrieved 15 January 2010 from: http://www.peter-lehmann-publishing.com/beyond-belief.htm

Kraus, M., & Keefe, R. (2007). Cognition as an outcome measure in schizophrenia. *British Journal of Psychiatry, 191*(Suppl. 50), s46–51.

Langer, S. (1967). *Mind: An essay on human feeling* (Vol. 1). Baltimore, MD: The Johns Hopkins University Press.

LeDoux, J. (1999). *The Emotional Brain.* London: Phoenix.

Lewis, H. B. (1971). *Shame and Guilt in Neurosis.* New York: International Universities Press.

May, R. (2007). Working outside the diagnostic frame. *The Psychologist, 20,* 300–301.

Panksepp, J. (1998). *Affective Neuroscience.* Oxford: Oxford University Press.

Park, S., & Thakkar, K. (2010). 'Splitting of the Mind' revisited: Recent neuroimaging evidence for functional dysconnection in schizophrenia and its relation to symptoms. *American Journal of Psychiatry, 174*(4), 366–368.

Peters, E., Day, S., McKenna, J., & Orbach, G. (1999). Delusional ideation in religious and psychotic populations. *British Journal of Clinical Psychology, 38,* 83–96.

Peters, E., Joseph, S., Day, S., & Garety, P. (2004). Measuring delusional ideation: The 21-item Peters et al. Delusions Inventory (PDI). *Schizophrenia Bulletin, 30,* 1005–1022.

Pilgrim, D. (2001). Disordered personalities and disordered concepts. *Journal of Mental Health, 10,* 253–265.

Read, J., & Bentall, R. P. (2013). Madness. In J. Cromby, D. Harper & P. Reavey, *Psychology, Mental Health and Distress.* London: Palgrave.

Romme, M., Escher, S., Dillon, J., Corstens, D., & Morris, M. (Eds.). (2009). *Living with Voices: 50 stories of recovery.* Ross-on-Wye: PCCS Books.

Ronson, J. (2001). *Them: Adventures with extremists.* London: Picador.

Scheff, T. (2003). Male emotions/relations and violence: A case study. *Human Relations, 56*(6), 727–749.

Seikkula, J., Alakare, B., & Aaltonen, J. (2001a). Open dialogue in psychosis I: An introduction and case illustration. *Journal of Constructivist Psychology, 14,* 247–265.

Seikkula, J., Alakare, B., & Aaltonen, J. (2001b). Open dialogue in psychosis II: A comparison of good and poor outcome cases. *Journal of Constructivist Psychology, 14,* 267–284.

Shaw, W. (1995). *Spying in Guru Land: Inside Britain's cults.* London: Fourth Estate.

Stewart, K. (1995). On pathologising discourse and psychiatric illness: An interview within an interview. In M. White, *Re-authoring Lives: Interviews and essays.* Adelaide, Australia: Dulwich Centre Publications.

Van Os, J., Hanssen, M., Bijl, R. V., & Ravelli, A. (2000). Strauss (1969) revisited: A psychosis continuum in the general population? *Schizophrenia Research, 45,* 11–20.

Vygotsky, L. S. (1962). *Thought and Language* (E. Hanfmann & G. Vakar, Trans.). Cambridge, MA: MIT Press.

Weeks, D., & James, J. (1997). *Eccentrics.* London: Phoenix.

Chapter 3

Meaning, Madness and Marginalisation

Steven Coles

Finding meaning in our life experiences and social world appears fundamental to being human (Bruner, 1990). We make sense of ourselves and our life through our connections to others, either proximally through our family, friends and associates, or through more distal influences such as the media, culture and political structures. The culture we grow up in shapes our way of being and viewing the world (Bourdieu, 1984; Cole, 1996); whilst there will be nuances at a family and microsocial level, currently, the broad thrust of Western cultures is to understand ourselves in individualistic terms (see Smail, 2001; Bauman, 2008). Individualism is perhaps positive for those who are successful in life as they garner the acclaim for what they achieve, though such achievement is somewhat empty without being connected to a wider social purpose, but it is far more problematic for those who are less well resourced and struggling in life. The norms and values of society lead people to view their difficulties as stemming from personal deficits and they are discouraged from making sense of their life in social terms. The process of finding meaning and making sense of experience is particularly important in relation to madness. Those deemed mad have often had a variety of experiences that they find overwhelming, confusing and frightening (e.g., hearing voices and difficult life experiences) and Western societies appear to have very limited ways of helping people make sense of unusual experiences. Such experiences are usually understood to be the result of individual deficits.

In Western societies the definition of a person as mad is a social negotiation conducted in a culture that encourages individualistic ways of understanding the world. At a micro level the label of madness is first bestowed upon a person by those in society who are in closest proximity to the person to be classified as mad (see Coulter, 1973, 1979). The mad are defined by family, friends, neighbours, perhaps the police, or educators. The person's articulations or behaviour are interpreted as breaking current norms of behaviour or expression and deemed not to make sense within their current cultural context; furthermore, the person is unable to articulate a culturally acceptable rationale for their behaviour (see Rogers and Pilgrim, 2010, for further discussion). Psychiatry then reaffirms and sanctions a person as mad and redefines madness through the process of diagnosis, usually attaching a diagnostic label of schizophrenia, bipolar disorder or such like. This process takes a lay judgment of what is considered unacceptable and makes it a technical and professional matter. Currently psychiatry is gripped by a reductionist biological paradigm; it therefore declares a diagnosis such as schizophrenia to be a disease with a strong genetic aetiology, and reaffirms the problem as an individual deficit and the content of a person's madness as lacking meaning. It should be noted that psychiatry not only rubber stamps what has already been deemed unacceptable by society; it has shaped and restricted what society judges as normal and has limited how such diversity is understood and made sense of (see Conrad, 2007, for a discussion of processes of medicalisation).

The following will question whether madness can be assumed to be meaningless and best understood as an individual deficit and, in particular, will look at theory and research that highlights the importance of disempowerment to understanding madness. The chapter will then focus on psychiatric diagnosis and how it understands madness, more specifically it will consider the ideological characteristics of diagnosis and how it conceals, reaffirms and initiates relationships of domination and submission. The final section looks at how professionals could use their power to criticise the status quo and create space to find meaning in madness. The chapter will focus on the diagnosis of schizophrenia, as it is prototypical of medicalised notions of madness (see Rogers and Pilgrim, 2010, for further discussion of lay and professional perspectives on madness).

Madness and disempowerment

Madness holds meaning and issues of power often lie at its heart. Those who are eventually considered mad by society have suffered some form of marginalisation and disempowerment in their trajectory to madness, either relationally, socially, materially, or culturally. Within psychological and psychiatric theory power has often misleadingly been conceived as an internal construct or individual characteristic (Coles, 2010). Instead the notion of power expounded here follows the writings of Smail (2001) and Foucault (1980, 1982/1994). Smail (2001) conceives power as the ability of a social group or individual to influence others in accordance with their interests, and considers the main sources of power as flowing downwards from distal sources such as politics, economics, and media. These distal forces are then felt through more proximal influences, such as family, work, education, relationships, and housing. Furthermore, there will be chains of influence, so whilst parents might have a significant impact on the development of their children, there will be a flow of powerful forces currently and historically running through and shaping these parents for good and ill. Whilst power can be conceived as flowing downward from distal sources, Foucault (1980, 1982/1994) highlights how power acts between individuals – power being an action that shapes another's action. Foucault considers people to be caught within a web or net of power relations. The key points are that power acts between people, it is multi-levelled and multi-directional, and whilst an individual might have some influence, the main sources of power are through people acting in coordination with others. These coordinated groups might include private companies, media organisations, governmental departments, community groups and so forth, each having varying levels of influence.

From a developmental perspective a child has very limited power over their environment and is reliant on the benign care of adults. Childhood abuse is an obvious example of the damaging act of a relatively powerful adult on a child. However, until very recently, the case of physical and sexual violence has been given little prominence in relation to experiences labelled as psychotic symptoms. This is despite research relating such violence to a range of other forms of psychological distress (e.g,. Mullen, Martin, Anderson, Romans & Herbison, 1993; Read, Hammersley & Rudgeair, 2007; Tyler, 2002). This appears due to madness being assumed as having a genetic/biological cause. This is unfortunate as many of these biological beliefs and genetic arguments are now criticised, including the methodology and assumptions of the 'schizophrenia' genetic twin and adoption studies (e.g., Joseph, 2004). However, there is a growing body of research highlighting a link between childhood abuse and experiences labelled as symptoms of psychosis, particularly that of hearing voices (e.g., Read, Rudgeair & Farrelly, 2006). Johnstone (2007) also highlights that the content and themes of people's unusual beliefs and experiences, such as hearing voices, are often obviously related to experiences of sexual and physical violence. Only a mental health system that pays little attention to, or gives little credence to, the meaningfulness of people's beliefs and experiences could be quite so myopic.

Unusual and suspicious beliefs are one of the defining features of professional notions of madness, and themes of marginalisation and powerlessness often run through such beliefs. There is a body of research highlighting that people deemed to be paranoid have good reason to be suspicious of others, as the environments that they have grown up in have been threatening, intrusive and/or overwhelming. Cromby and Harper (2009) give an overview of this research and highlight how paranoia can be understood if viewed from the perspective of complex blends of feeling, which are tied to aversive social worlds and material circumstances (see also Chapter 2, this volume, by Cromby and Harper). At a developmental and proximal level Rankin, Bentall, Hill and Kinderman (2005) found that people, described as experiencing or who had previously experienced paranoid beliefs, had recollections of '… parents who frequently disagree with them, who try to influence them without negotiation, who are overcritical and unsupportive, and with whom patients have intense, involved relationships' (p. 22). A large community study looking at sociodemographic factors found experiences of discrimination, victimisation and low socioeconomic status to be related to mistrust and paranoia (Mirowsky & Ross, 1983). From research conducted from a diagnostic framework a causal link has been found between experiences of discrimination and beliefs others have found unusual ('delusional ideation') (Janssen et al., 2003; see also Bentall & Fernyhough, 2008). This research suggests that people growing up in environments with few resources or little ability to influence their world are understandably more likely to feel suspicious of others. Furthermore, qualitative research highlights that such beliefs, which are deemed unusual by some, share characteristics with beliefs that are more generally accepted, and are shaped by our personal history and cultural context (Roberts, 1991). Rhodes and Jakes (2000) found the underlying themes of such beliefs were often linked to desires for attachment, a sense of disconnection from others or the need for a sense of power.

Another defining feature of the diagnosis of mental illness has been the presence of auditory hallucinations or hearing voices that others cannot perceive. Research into voice hearers' relationship with their voices has highlighted the importance of power (e.g., Romme & Escher, 1993;

Birchwood et al., 2004). Birchwood et al. (2004) highlight that feeling disempowered in relationship to others and society appears to mirror and drive a negative relationship with a person's voice. The experience of hearing voices also highlights the cultural dearth of meaningful explanations for people to understand this experience; this is despite the fact that this experience is far more common than is openly discussed (Romme & Escher, 1993). The lack of meaningful ways to understand this experience also compounds a person's disempowerment and confusion, and can lead to isolation and a greater sense of disconnection from local support networks and communities. The types of explanations offered to those who hear voices will shape their experience of hearing voices. Currently the dominant explanation available for this experience in Western societies is 'mental illness'. The lack of alternative explanatory frameworks can push individuals into one of two positions, either for individuals to accept the medical model and subservience to the psychiatric system, or rejection of this viewpoint. Acceptance of the medical model is problematic as it has many negative associations and notions such as the assumption of chronic and negative outcome, societal stigma, a blinkered view of psychiatric medication and the need for expert and often coercive treatment. Whereas rejection of the medical model leaves the voice hearer the considerable task of making sense of their experiences without the support of a more positive and accepted societal framework, as well as the risk of being coerced into services where a person's viewpoint will be rejected and seen as meaningless. Organisations such as the Hearing Voices Network have attempted to offer a wider and more humane range of explanations, but they are often running against the grain of statutory services (see Chapter 10, this volume, by Longden, Corstens and Dillon).

In summary, the above shows that madness is explicable at the level of people's social, interpersonal and material world. A key theme for understanding madness is power or powerlessness in different realms of a person's world. The lack of, and limited endorsement of, meaningful explanations of madness creates further marginalisation. The following will critically analyse the dominant professional explanation for madness – psychiatric diagnosis.

Diagnosis and ideology: Initiating and sustaining relations of domination

Diagnosis is currently the dominant way to conceptualise madness within professional circles and mental health services. Furthermore, psychiatry has made repeated attempts at 'psychoeducation' to spread a diagnostic framework to the general population, so that lay concepts and experiences of misery, fear and madness are respectively relabelled and transformed into the medical entities 'depression', 'anxiety' and 'schizophrenia'. These labels come packaged with biological assumptions of causation and the need for technical cures. Moreover, the number of diagnostic categories increase with each new edition of the diagnostic manuals, as do the number of people diagnosed as suffering mental disorder (see Kutchins and Kirk, 1997, for an overview). As well as being ubiquitous, diagnosis sits at the nexus of power and meaning. The concept of ideology is useful for understanding the roles and functions of diagnosis, due to its connection of meaning and power. Thompson (1990) has reformulated the notion of ideology and defined it as all the ways in which concepts, symbols and ideas are used so to establish and sustain relations of domination. The following will consider the characteristics and processes in which the application of medical concepts and ideas (diagnosis) to certain behaviours and utterances (e.g., expressing unusual beliefs, hearing voices) initiate and reinforce power relations.

The previous section has highlighted the complex web of power and powerlessness that might play out in a person's pathway to madness before they reach the attentions of mental health services, such as familial relationships, employment (or lack of), discrimination, lack of control or access to resources. Whilst the person deemed mad is already entrenched in a web of power relations (usually in a subordinate position), the professional bestowal of the diagnosis of schizophrenia gives legitimacy to the idea that the person deemed mad is the problematic piece in a complex social-relational web, and that others can be exonerated. The diagnosis seals off and pays attention to the one supposedly disordered element of an otherwise well-ordered web of relationships. Diagnosis conceals the problematic nature of power relations that led a person to madness and justifies the status quo. Attempts at criticism of diagnosis and its biological assumptions can often raise intense emotional reactions. These reactions are not due to the rigors of an academic/scientific debate (diagnosis can claim no weight in this realm), but arise because denouncement of diagnosis risks revealing relations of domination and could mean the spotlight is swung from a single problematic individual to a complex web of agents and interests (see Johnstone, 1999, 2007).

Diagnosis not only reinforces, sustains and legitimates existing hierarchies, it also establishes new relationships, such as relationships with mental health professionals. It is important for the maintenance of the status quo that a new power relation is established, as the social crisis that brought the person into mental health services means that the current hierarchy is in jeopardy. A new relationship is established where one party (the professional) has certain legal powers within the Mental Health Act over the other party (the one labelled mentally disordered). In turn these 'disordered citizens' lose certain civil liberties entitled to all other citizens. The righteousness of the legal powers of the mental health professional over parts of society is argued via the status and technical expertise of the professional. However, the position of the medical professional has been insecure, particularly following high profile attacks from 'anti-psychiatrists'. Diagnosis has played its role in psychiatry's attempt to secure its position and status, by advocating diagnosis to be a scientific enterprise. During the 1980s diagnosis came to be no longer just related to medical technical skill or training, but required the narrative of science to be embedded within its symbolic characteristics. In sum, diagnosis helps to initiate a new power relation of the mad with the medical professional and has utilised the narrative of science to ward off criticism (see Pilgrim, 2007, for a discussion of the role of professionals' interests in the survival of psychiatric diagnosis).

As well as diagnosis purporting itself to be a scientific enterprise (fascinated with research on reliability at the expense of meaning), it has other characteristics that help psychiatry maintain its position. One of these characteristics is the dual narrative that diagnosis contains; it has an explicit narrative of theoretical and scientific neutrality, and an implicit narrative of biological reductionism and causation (see Boyle, 2002, for further discussion). Diagnosticians conceal diagnoses' biological reductionism in claims to be atheoretical and not imputing causation, but then utilise a classification system designed to study body parts (using the language of illness, symptoms and disorder) to understand behaviour and experience. Diagnosticians can use this dual narrative to stymie critique, whilst continuing to reduce people's experience and behaviour to biological causes. This biological reductionism obscures the power relations that led a person to madness in the first place.

Diagnosis is a powerful practice that *sanitises* a range of complex human interactions, interpretations, feelings and a rich range of subjectivities. Diagnosis transforms this complexity into a clean and orderly object – a medical problem that can be acted upon with a medical solution. This solves a number of problems for a range of interest groups and actors, but the creation of a medical object legitimises a number of direct acts of physical power that would otherwise be difficult to justify and would raise difficult ethical problems for society. This includes incarceration without trial or defence counsel; it allows people to be physically restrained in order to be injected with psychiatric drugs against their will; and allows people, who have the capacity to weigh up the costs and benefits of their psychiatric drugs, to be conveyed back to hospital so as to enforce medication compliance (community treatment orders). These acts of direct and physical power are only made legitimate by the sanitisation process of diagnosis that transforms a person into an object. This process not only cleanses people's lives of their meaning but removes their civil liberties under the guise of a medical procedure. This procedure circumvents the usual protections afforded other citizens, for example, only those deemed mentally disordered or suspected terrorists can be detained without trial (Vassilev & Pilgrim, 2007).

By stripping madness from its context (diagnosis being a key process), it protects the powerful who caused harm in the first place, such as the small minority owning the majority of resources, governmental policies, people committing domestic violence, and so forth. Diagnosis also establishes and reinforces the status and privilege of the mental health professional, a key being psychiatry, but includes other professionals and interest groups such as the pharmaceutical industry (see Chapter 6, this volume, by Busfield). A decontextualised madness also allows society as whole to wash its hands of problematic ethical dilemmas (see Chapter 5, this volume, by Pilgrim and Tomasini) by placing madness in the hands of those deemed experts of biologically disordered individuals. However, for the person deemed mad the stripping away of context removes any chance of the person being able to make sense of their experiences and the power relations they are linked to.

Utilising professional power critically

The following will briefly look at some initial and tentative ways for practitioners to utilise their power more critically. Professional power could be used to create space to find meaning in madness, which would necessitate highlighting the acts of power in a person's path to madness. Professionals could also reflect critically on their own practices in mental health services. The section will focus on ideas for practitioners at an individual and group/ professional level; however, it is often not in the interests of professionals to be critical of the status quo. Therefore, they should not be the sole, or even most important, interest group locating meaning in madness. Significant change in mental health services will require actions far wider than those documented here; fundamentally it will necessitate alterations at a social and cultural level.

Individual practitioner level

For individual practitioners a first step to creating space so as to make madness meaningful involves informing people within services and their families that the professional conceptualisation of madness is contested. It is not ethically justifiable, even for those who are in favour of psychiatric diagnosis, to bestow upon people a diagnostic label as if it were a straightforward, robust scientific and technical entity. Those continuing to diagnose, some perhaps coerced into doing so by organisational systems and pressures, at the very minimum need to provide people with information regarding the difficulties inherent in diagnosis, its uncertain status and an outline of alternatives. This would create space for alternative explanations of madness to be heard and acted upon.

At root, madness is about disempowerment, and psychiatric diagnosis is a means to quieten, or at worst silence, a person's perspective and experience. Therefore practitioners need, first, to reflect upon all the ways in which they are disempowering people so as to minimise these negative actions, and second, to consider ways in which they can support people to have a greater voice within mental health services and get access to positive resources in their world. This might include supporting a person in their articulation of the negative effects of psychiatric drugs and/or linking such a person with others who have similar difficulties in order to enable a collective response to such difficulties (see Chapters 16 and 17, this volume, by Nottingham and Leicester Medication groups, respectively). It is also important that a critical practitioner questions dominant knowledge such as psychiatric diagnosis at a team level and within multidisciplinary meetings, and gives voice to subordinated perspectives; this may also encourage other staff with doubts about the status quo to speak up.

For those more questioning of diagnosis, several authors (e.g., Johnstone, 2006) have put the case forward for collaboratively working with people who use services to negotiate a shared meaning of their difficulties and, wherever possible, a way forward. This would often involve understanding people's experiences in relation to their social world and life history. Pilgrim (2000) notes that an understanding of a person's context and world is more likely to help us understand their needs than the label of schizophrenia. The Division of Clinical Psychology has produced guidelines regarding one way of making sense of people's experience in the form of psychological formulations (DCP, 2011). Whilst such guidelines run the risk of professionalising the act of meaning-making that is open to all, formulation does have utility in creating space to form a shared understanding of madness and highlight acts of power. However, formulation can be problematic; some forms can: pathologise the individual and ignore their context; impose an 'expert' perspective and undermine the views of the distressed individual; and at worst can be little better than psychiatric diagnosis (Harper & Moss, 2003; Johnstone, 2006). Johnstone (2006) has outlined ideas to caution against such difficulties when formulating, such as: workers should reflect on their values and assumptions; formulations need to be flexible and tentative; they should be conducted sensitively, collaboratively and give significant weight to the perspective of the person they are focused on; and the necessity of including social context within each formulation. Beyond this, it is essential that power and resources are placed at the centre of any formulation; Hagan and Smail (1997) have devised a power-mapping tool which is a flexible format that looks outward to the positive and negative influences and resources in a person's world.

Forming a shared meaning of madness is important, either through formulation or other means, because, by definition, those deemed mad lack a shared narrative with those around them. Furthermore, the act of diagnosis further disconnects people deemed mad from others and from finding the meaning in their experiences, as diagnosis officially confirms and portrays the content of madness as meaningless. It is therefore important for a practitioner to support and negotiate a shared explanation of people's experiences. However, there are likely to be difficulties in creating a shared narrative that is acceptable to other parties. Giving some legitimacy to those deemed mad and their life experiences potentially presents a challenge to the narratives of those around the person, such as the family system. Family members' sense of who they are and their role in the person's life is potentially challenged and brought into question if the person deemed mad is seen as a product of their social environment. Highlighting the meaningfulness of madness also challenges the narratives of psychiatric professionals, in terms of their biological reductionism and expertise. Finding the meaning in madness requires linking a person's social world and environment with their distress and behaviour; in Western societies this challenges a cultural narrative of the self-managing and autonomous individual.

Group and professional level: Speaking up

Critical practitioners are more likely to have influence as a group if they can form a collective position and act on this. In doing this, practitioners need to be cognisant of the risk of colonising the arena and sidelining survivor and service user perspectives, as well as dominating a political role which should belong to all citizens. However, there are topics critical practitioners can legitimately comment on, including psychiatric diagnosis. Psychiatric diagnosis has become embedded within multiple systems inside and outside of mental health services and there are a variety of interest groups supporting its continuation (Pilgrim, 2007). It is therefore essential that there is a collective critique and espousal of alternatives, both from professionals, survivors and other interest groups, if a more humane and meaningful framework is to be applied to madness.

In the area of psychology, despite anxiety and ambivalence (see Boyle, 2011), there are signs that the profession is perhaps beginning to find its voice on psychiatric diagnosis. At a grass roots' level a group of clinical psychologists in the East Midlands formed a critical position paper on diagnosis (Coles & SPIG, 2010). Furthermore, the British Psychological Society (BPS, 2011) has commented critically on proposals for the new *Diagnostic and Statistical Manual of Mental Disorders* (*DSM-5*), which noted that the 'Society is concerned that clients and the general public are negatively affected by the continued and continuous medicalisation of their natural and normal responses to their experiences …'. This inspired the Society for Humanistic Psychology (a division of the American

Psychological Association [APA]) to write an open letter to *DSM-5* Task Force, which constructively critiques *DSM-5* proposals, particularly its biological reductionism and deficits in its empirical underpinnings. The letter is supported by numerous other APA divisions, the BPS and other psychological organisations. The open letter is now a petition (www.ipetitions.com/petition/dsm5/) with over 12,500 signatures at the time of writing. It is important for such collective and questioning voices to persist and work alongside other interest groups critical of the status quo.

Final comments

The roots of madness lie in marginalisation; diagnosis conceals this disempowerment and initiates and maintains relations of domination. It is the responsibility of questioning practitioners to find their voice and speak out on such misuses of power. Finding meaning in madness also speaks to the need for all of us in society to reclaim a richer and healthier meaning of ourselves and our society, to move away from the atomised, isolated consumer to realise that an individual only has real meaning in connection and in concert with others.

References
Bauman, Z. (2008). *The Art of Life*. Cambridge: Polity Press.
Bentall, R. P., & Fernyhough, C. (2008). Social predictors of psychotic experiences: Specificity and psychological mechanisms. *Schizophrenia Bulletin, 34,* 1012–1020.
Birchwood, M., Gilbert, P., Gilbert, J., Trower, P., Meaden, A., Hay, J., Murray, E., & Miles, J. N. V. (2004). Interpersonal and role-related schema influence the relationship with the dominant 'voice' in schizophrenia: A comparison of three models. *Psychological Medicine, 34,* 1571–1580.
Bourdieu, P. (1984). *Distinction: A social critique of the judgement of taste*. Cambridge, MA: Harvard University Press.
Boyle, M. (2002). *Schizophrenia: A scientific delusion?* (2nd ed.). London: Routledge.
Boyle, M. (2011). Making the world go away, and how psychology and psychiatry benefit. In M. Rapley, J. Moncrieff & J. Dillon (Eds.), *De-medicalizing Misery: Psychiatry, psychology and the human condition*. Basingstoke: Palgrave Macmillan.
British Psychological Society (BPS). (2011). *Response to the American Psychiatric Association: DSM-5 development*. Leicester: BPS.
Bruner, J. (1990). *Acts of Meaning*. Cambridge, MA: Harvard University Press.

Cole, M. (1996). *Cultural Psychology.* Cambridge, MA: Harvard University Press.

Coles, S. (2010). Clinical psychology's interest in the conceptualisation and use of power. *Clinical Psychology Forum, 212,* 22–26.

Coles, S., & SPIG. (2010). *Position on Psychiatric Diagnosis.* East Midlands: Psychosis and Complex Mental Health Special Interest Group. Retrieved 12 June 2012 from, http://dcp-sigpr.bps.org.uk/dcp-sigpr/publications-%26-documents/publications_home.cfm

Conrad, P. (2007). *The Medicalization of Society.* Baltimore, MD: The Johns Hopkins University Press.

Coulter, J. (1973). *Approaches to Insanity.* New York: John Wiley.

Coulter, J. (1979). *The Social Construction of Mind: Studies in ethnomethodology and linguistic philosophy.* London: Macmillan.

Cromby, J., & Harper, D. (2009). Paranoia: A social account. *Theory & Psychology, 19*(3), 335–361.

Division of Clinical Psychology (DCP). (2011). *Good Practice Guidelines on the Use of Psychological Formulation.* Leicester: British Psychological Society.

Foucault, M. (1980). *Power/Knowledge: Selected interviews and other writings 1972–1977* (C. Gordon, Ed.). New York: Pantheon Books.

Foucault, M. (1994). The subject and power. In J. D. Faubion (Ed.), *Power: Essential works of Foucault – Vol. 3.* London: Penguin Books. (Original work published 1982)

Hagan, T., & Smail, D. (1997). Power-mapping – I: Background and basic methodology. *Journal of Community and Applied Social Psychology, 7,* 257–267.

Harper, D., & Moss, D. (2003). A different kind of chemistry? Reformulating 'formulation'. *Clinical Psychology, 25,* 6–10.

Janssen, I., Hanssen, M., Bak, M., Bijl, R. V., de Graaf, R., Vollebergh, W., et al. (2003). Discrimination and delusional ideation. *British Journal of Psychiatry, 182,* 71–76.

Johnstone, L. (1999). Do families cause 'schizophrenia'? Revisiting a taboo subject. In C. Newnes, G. Holmes, & C. Dunn (Eds.), *This is Madness* (pp. 119–134). Ross-on-Wye: PCCS Books.

Johnstone, L. (2006). Controversies and debates about formulation. In L. Johnstone & R. Dallos (Eds.), *Formulation in Psychology and Psychotherapy: Making sense of people's problems.* Hove: Routledge.

Johnstone, L. (2007). Can trauma cause psychosis? Revisiting (another) taboo subject. *Journal of Critical Psychology, Counselling and Psychotherapy, 7*(4), 211–220.

Joseph, J. (2004). Schizophrenia and heredity: Why the emperor has no genes. In J. Read, L. R. Mosher & R. P. Bentall (Eds.), *Models of Madness* (pp. 67–84). Hove: Brunner-Routledge.

Kutchins, H., & Kirk, S. A. (1997). *Making Us Crazy.* London: Constable.

Mirowsky, J., & Ross, C. E. (1983). Paranoia and the structure of powerlessness. *American Sociological Review, 48,* 228–239.

Mullen, P. E., Martin, J. L., Anderson, J. C., Romans, S. E., & Herbison, G. P. (1993). Childhood sexual abuse and mental health in adult life. *British Journal of Psychiatry, 163,* 721–732.

Pilgrim, D. (2000). Psychiatric diagnosis: More questions than answers. *The Psychologist, 13,* 302–305.

Pilgrim, D. (2007). The survival of psychiatric diagnosis. *Social Science and Medicine, 65,* 536–544.

Rankin, P., Bentall, R. P., Hill, J., & Kinderman, P. (2005). Perceived relationships with parents and paranoid delusions: Comparisons of currently ill, remitted and normal participants. *Psychopathology, 38,* 16–25.

Read, J., Hammersley, P., & Rudgeair, T. (2007). Why, when and how to ask about childhood abuse. *Advances in Psychiatric Treatment, 13,* 101–110.

Read, J., Rudgeair, T., & Farrelly, S. (2006). The relationship between child abuse and psychosis: Public opinion, evidence, pathways and implications. In W. Larkin & A. P. Morrison (Eds.), *Trauma and Psychosis.* London: Routledge.

Rhodes, J. E., & Jakes, S. (2000). Correspondence between delusions and personal goals: A qualitative analysis. *British Journal of Medical Psychology, 73,* 211–225.

Roberts, G. (1991). Delusional belief systems and meaning in life: A preferred reality. *British Journal of Psychiatry, 159*(Suppl. 14), s19–28.

Rogers, A., & Pilgrim, D. (2010). *A Sociology of Mental Health and Illness* (4th ed.). Maidenhead: Open University Press.

Romme, M., & Escher, S. (1993). *Accepting Voices.* London: Mind Publications.

Smail, D. (2001). *The Nature of Unhappiness.* London: Robinson.

Society for Humanistic Psychology. (2011). *Open Letter to DSM-5 Taskforce.* Retrieved 12 June 2012 from, http://dsm5-reform.com/the-open-letter-to-dsm-5-task-force/

Thompson, J. B. (1990). *Ideology and Modern Culture.* Cambridge: Polity Press.

Tyler, K. A. (2002). Social and emotional outcomes of childhood sexual abuse: A review of recent research. *Aggression and Violent Behavior, 7,* 567–589.

Vassilev, I., & Pilgrim, D. (2007). Risk, trust and the myth of mental health services. *Journal of Mental Health, 16,* 347–357.

Chapter 4

From Constructive Engagement to Coerced Recovery

Alastair Morgan & Anne Felton

People with direct experience of mental distress have for many years demanded increased involvement in mental health services, their own care and ultimately their own lives. This is in part a response to the pervasive and potentially disempowering experience of being diagnosed with a mental health problem and using mental health services. A 'Recovery' approach dominates in contemporary mental health practice and espouses a focus on hope, growth, self-adaptation and discovery providing a real opportunity for people to make choices about their own lives and to challenge the controlling influence of mental health services.

Recovery has received increasing emphasis within mental health policy and literature (Department of Health [DH], 2004, 2006). This requires professionals to look beyond people as 'the patient' to help enable them to realise their goals, recognising the many other roles that people occupy within society. According to Repper and Perkins (2009), supporting recovery means prioritising the individual, their wishes and goals. It requires an understanding of the relationship between health and social factors and a need to recognise the significance of choice and control for that person within their own life. Such a position has been echoed in health policy of recent years as health services are encouraged to work in partnership with people using services (DH, 2000, 2001, 2005). However, there is a central paradox at the heart of contemporary mental health care. At the time when the principles of recovery based on choice and respect are central within service provision, there is an increasing emphasis on coercion. Why, when recovery is everywhere as a badge of services, is coercion increasing?

We can objectively claim that the mental health system is more coercive due to the changes brought about in the Mental Health Act 2007, with the introduction of Supervised Community Treatment. Supervised Community Treatment was introduced on 3rd November 2008 in England

and Wales. Under the powers granted by Supervised Community Treatment, certain people detained under specific sections of the Mental Health Act can be discharged under a community treatment order that contains conditions with which they have to comply, including taking their medication (Lawton-Smith, 2010). Latest figures from the Care Quality Commission indicate that a total of 10,171 community treatment orders (CTOs) have been put in place in the period between November 2008 to March 2011, although some 41 per cent of those have been revoked at the time of writing (Health and Social Care Information Centre, 2011). The overall number of people subject to formal coercion under the Mental Health Act in England and Wales increased by 5 per cent in 2010–2011 (Health and Social Care Information Centre, 2011).

In this chapter, we want to focus on a developing discourse that attempts to justify this increasing coercion with a specific group of so-called 'revolving door' people. These people are those with diagnoses of severe mental illness (often psychosis) who have a history of multiple formal admissions to hospital, difficulties in engagement and social vulnerabilities (including housing insecurity and substance misuse). This is the group who are purportedly targeted by CTOs (see Churchill, Owen, Singh & Hotopf, 2007). They are also the group who were at the heart of a recovery agenda initiated at the end of the 1990s to attempt to constructively engage people who had previously disengaged (Sainsbury Centre for Mental Health [SCMH], 1998). This agenda, based around constructive engagement, started from the position that it is services that need to change in order to provide a more inclusive, social and recovery-oriented approach. The contention of this chapter is that this emphasis on constructive engagement, with its attendant balancing of mutual rights and responsibilities, is rapidly being replaced by an agenda of coerced recovery for a defined group of 'difficult to engage' people. In this agenda coercion is conceptualised as the first step on the road to recovery (Davidson & Roe, 2007; Priebe et al., 2009; Molodynski, Rugkåsa & Burns, 2010).

We will explore three areas of this discourse on coerced recovery here; a discourse on risk, a discourse around 'treatment pressures' that explores different uses and meanings of coercion, and a discourse that argues that community treatment orders are ethically justifiable. It is our contention that this growing body of literature tips the balance too far towards coercion, and that we need to return to a model of true recovery-oriented practice based around constructive engagement, choice and respect.

Before beginning to explore these three areas, it is important to define some of the central terms we are using. First, it is important to try to delineate the central themes of a recovery approach. As many commentators have noted, the concept of recovery in mental health care is often vague and masks a number of disagreements and conflicts (Social Care Institute for Excellence, 2007; Davidson & Roe, 2007; Pilgrim, 2008; Stickley & Wright, 2011). Pilgrim (2008) has neatly encapsulated this conceptual confusion by disentangling three concepts of recovery in the literature. First, there is the concept of recovery as 'biomedical treatment'. This concept emphasises the importance of medication for recovery and defines recovery in accordance with insight into a diagnosed illness and responsiveness to medical treatment. Pilgrim (2008, p. 296) writes of this as 'old wine in new bottles'. Second, there is a concept of recovery that is concerned with developing a repertoire of social skills and resources that will support coping with the effects of distress and enable the person to live the fullest life possible. The emphasis here is on an improvement in wellbeing. This approach was at the heart of the constructive engagement agenda (SCMH, 1998, Pilgrim, 2008). Finally, there is the more rights-based model that views recovery as freedom from coercion, labelling and the invalidation caused by psychiatric diagnosis and societal discrimination. This concept of recovery is closely tied to a discourse based around surviving the damage wrought by psychiatry, and creating meaning from your own experience (Turner-Crowson & Wallcraft, 2002; Crossley, 2006; Pilgrim, 2008). Clearly, and as Pilgrim identifies, there is a great deal of scope for conflict between these three concepts of recovery, and without a clear definition, we might wonder whether there is a usable concept of recovery in mental health.

Whilst acknowledging this conceptual confusion and conflict, Stickley and Wright (2011) have attempted to draw together some central themes for a definition of recovery from a systematic review of the peer-reviewed literature. Although they accept that there is no universal definition of recovery, they construct some prerequisites from the literature that could be termed core components of any recovery approach. These core components are first, an emphasis on working in a manner that respects choices, fosters hope and is broadly informed by what they term a 'humanistic philosophy'. Second, there is a strong emphasis on recognising the centrality of individual accounts or narratives of people's experience of mental distress. Third, there is a foregrounding of the importance of people developing meaning based on their mental distress. Fourth, there is the importance of 'meaningful occupation' (Stickley & Wright, 2011, p. 253). They do acknowledge the tensions that are concerned with a balance between risk and working in a recovery-oriented manner that is evident from their survey of the literature.

We now have a working framework for recovery that acknowledges the diversity of its meaning but nevertheless identifies its core constitutive components. What of coercion? Is there a commonly agreed definition of coercion? Anderson (2011) writes that coercion would always be concerned with identifying a particular way in which one agent (or structure) forces another agent to do something that is against their will. In this way, coercion normally always involves a violation of rights. Anderson (2011) picks out two ethical elements to coercion. First, there is an ethical concern with the coercer and the means by which they coerce. Second, there is a focus on the coerced, and how coerced people may respond to forms of coercion. These two elements are framed by a larger ethical discussion on the justifications for coercion. Similarly, these justifications are usually twofold; based on a paternalistic justification for a violation of autonomy in the name of a greater good (one thinks of the enforcement of wearing seatbelts in cars here), or a capacity-based justification that overrides autonomy in the best interests of the person.

This philosophical debate is mirrored in the literature on coercion in psychiatry. Szmukler and Appelbaum (2008) focus on the acts of coercion and define a range of different pressures that exist in mental health care, some of which can be termed coercive and some of which are not. They also differentiate between threats and offers in coercive situations. This is an important idea drawn from an influential paper on coercion by Robert Nozick. Nozick (1969) argues that in any coercive situation it is important to identify a baseline prior to the situation of coercion. For Nozick a baseline refers to a 'normal course of events' (Nozick, 1969, p. 447). Coercion can be broken down into a threat or an offer dependent on the way in which it is communicated against a background of the normal course of events. In discussing this, Anderson (2011) gives the following example. An armed robber issues the following proposal to a victim: he must hand over his goods and remain unharmed or keep them and receive harm. In the normal course of events one enjoys one's goods unmolested so the armed robber's proposal is a threat not an offer. On the other hand a salesman offers a customer a free holiday if they sign up to an insurance package, and as a free holiday is not a normal course of events, this can be construed as an offer not a threat. As Anderson (2011) acknowledges, the level of background power involved here is also significant. This might seem an abstruse discussion, but we will later see how this distinction between offers and threats is being used in psychiatry (Molodynski et al., 2010).

Szmukler and Appelbaum (2008) also note the distinction between objectivist and subjectivist accounts of coercion. An objectivist account will attempt to justify coercion through a recourse to ethical principles either through the invocation of a paternalistic justification of an infringement of rights on the basis of better consequences, or on the basis of a 'best-interests' capacity approach. A subjectivist account will explore the perception of the person being coerced, and there is an important literature on perceived coercion within psychiatry (Lidz et al., 1995). The subjectivist idea of a perceived coercion, though, is a double-edged sword. One could argue that if the person perceives they are being coerced then they are, regardless of the objective background, but also if they do not perceive they are being coerced then objective levels of coercion do not need to be taken into account. Szmukler and Appelbaum (2008) sensibly argue for a combination of subjective and objective accounts of coercion.

We have outlined some initial debates around concepts of recovery and coercion, and before we move to exploring the three discourses that contribute to a move from a constructive engagement agenda towards a coerced recovery framework, we need to identify what is meant by constructive engagement. The most important document here was published in 1998 by the Centre for Mental Health (then termed Sainsbury Centre for Mental Health). Keys to Engagement (SCMH, 1998) outlined the blueprint for an approach to working with people who had difficulties engaging with psychiatric services that was to become increasingly influential in the decade following its publication and with the setting up of functional teams in mental health services with the National Service Framework for Mental Health published in 1999. Although the document was initially part of the impetus for the setting up of Assertive Outreach services in the UK, the approach laid out within it soon spread across a range of community mental health services. An emphasis on practical help, a holistic focus on care not limited to medical treatment alone, alongside an intensive team approach to working and persistent efforts to engage marked a new attempt to re-orientate mental health services towards the needs of service users (Davidson & Campbell, 2007). Reading some of the early documents, it is clear how this emphasis on engagement was inspired by a recognition of the failure of services to provide accessible and respectful care for their client group (e.g., Bryant, 2001).

It would be excessively revisionist, however, to argue that this was the only agenda behind constructive engagement. Even the definition of engagement within the formative documents from the Sainsbury Centre involves a conflict between a risk agenda and an agenda around supportive care. Keys to Engagement (SCMH, 1998) emphasises that engagement should be constructive and not coercive, but even its definition acknowledges the need to 'keep track of people'. At the heart of the constructive agenda was the old conflict between respecting autonomy and a duty of care. As Davidson and Campbell (2007) note, the background to the development of assertive outreach services was equally marked by a discourse on public safety, and a perception of increasing risks to the community at large from people with mental health problems. This coercive background was mirrored by a service user reaction to the constructive engagement process as itself coercive. MacMillan (2005, p. 6) famously wrote of the assertive outreach approach as a form of 'therapeutic stalking'. Rose (2001) wrote of the dangers of assertive outreach becoming a form of inducing and bribing service users to partake in a traditional model of medical mental health care.

Constructive engagement was hardly an ethical nirvana. However, there was a balance between an attempt to engage and work constructively with people and at the same time to respect their rights. This balance could be upheld due to the lack of community mandatory treatment, which meant that negotiation and working to the agenda of the person at the receiving end of services was a model of care even if it was framed by the always present possibility of a coercive use of the Mental Health Act. Williamson (2004) writes interestingly about the ethical balancing act involved here of respecting the person's right to define their own mental distress whilst at the same time reserving the right to disagree, ultimately to the point of a coercive Mental Health Act assessment. However, there can only be a creative tension here, if the dice are not loaded from the start. The reality that the service user was able to assert a right not to take medication, not to frame their distress in terms of illness, not to see a psychiatrist, can all enable the possibility for different ways of working and being. It is these ways of working and being that are being closed down as we tip the balance too far towards a coercive agenda that is framed through the culture of risk in mental health care.

Mental health care: A culture of risk

Risk management has been described as being at the heart of effective mental health practice with Care Programme Approach policy making a clear commitment to standards for the regular assessment and management of risk (DH, 1999, 2008b). Yet clinical risk assessment based on professionals' judgements alone has been criticised for its inconsistency and lack of accuracy of prediction (Morgan, 2007; Witterman, 2004). Evidence has also been proposed to suggest risk predictions made by mental health professionals are only slightly more accurate than those created by chance (Doyle & Dolan, 2002).

Essentially this reflects a positivistic position in which risk is perceived as a phenomenon that can be identified and quantified, and in which statistical calculations are privileged (Smith, 2004). Risk calculations are consequently treated as objective facts, even when the influence of subjectivity in judgements is acknowledged. Debate within these scientific and technical approaches is mostly concerned with accuracy of prediction (Lupton, 1999). This is reflected within the mental health literature as research continues to seek more effective standardised tools and an improved evidence base for the assessment of risk (Royal College of Psychiatrists, 2008) revealing an assumption that accuracy of prediction can actually be improved. Crucially, definitions of risk as a quantifiable concept extend to claims that it can, consequently, be managed (McDonald, Waring & Harrison, 2005). Risk therefore serves as a process to reduce uncertainty and enhance control. Within this approach the risk predictions of experts are presented as value free and unbiased (Lupton, 1999).

Context of risk

The growth of risk assessment and management within government policy occurred at a time of deinstitutionalisation, perceived failures in community care and high profile incidents of violence perpetrated by people with mental health problems, fuelling public fears about the dangers posed. These concerns are reinforced throughout proposals to amend the Mental Health Act (Harper, 2004) enhancing an association between risk, danger and mental illness and a need for control through containment. Authorities are required to develop effective measures to predict such incidences of danger and act accordingly to reduce their occurrence, cementing risk management as a central part of mental health services' function (Freshwater & Westwood, 2006).

Douglas (1992) emphasises the need to view risk in its social and political situation and suggests that such objective perspectives on risk are impossible. Douglas also claims that risk is inherently political, though is rarely understood this way. This political agenda is manifested through its use to apportion blame for a risk of danger to certain social groups. The focus on risk management in mental health services therefore, has to be recognised in this context in which it developed. The incidence of homicides committed by people with mental health problems is rare, 5–10 per cent of all homicides (James, 2006; Szmukler, 2000). Even the research from the perspective that risk is quantifiable, linking mental illness and violence provides contradictory and ambiguous information on the nature of this relationship and the factors that are implicated (Appelbaum, Robbins & Monahan, 2000; Douglas, Guy & Hart, 2009; Rogers & Pilgrim, 2010). Yet people with mental health problems are subject to controls based on their perceived dangerousness in ways that others who may pose more of a danger and be equally 'treatable' (such as drink drivers) are not (Pilgrim, 2007; Szmukler & Holloway, 2000). This reflects Douglas's ideas regarding the use of risk as a blaming system directed towards certain groups within society. Additionally, Jasanoff (1999) claims that risk arbitrates between knowledge and power, proposing that in accordance with Foucault's power/knowledge construct risk analysis forms a discourse; one which positions some as experts and others as 'inarticulate, irrelevant or incompetent' (Jasanoff, 1999, p. 137). 'Expertise' in risk tends to be most visible when harm occurs and therefore is most associated with failure, which is a product of the great paradox of risk. Risk is most evident when things go wrong and therefore when expertise has failed to manage that risk (Horlick-Jones, 2004). In this respect the discourse of scientific risk analysis contributes to the 'blame' culture of health care in which adverse events are constructed as failures in risk management resulting from problems in professional assessment, communication or understanding of risk. In accordance with these arguments it is health professionals who have the power to define risks. Service users are constructed as the perpetrators of risk consequently lacking the expertise to participate in the risk assessment and management process.

The culture of risk and the power embedded within it provides the frame for the current discourse around working with people who have difficulties engaging with services. This discourse consists of a logic of containment and treatment which has replaced that of participation and engagement. An interesting example of such a discourse that is becoming highly pertinent and prominent within the assertive outreach literature is the discussion on uses of treatment pressures and leverage in mental health. It is to this discourse that we now turn.

You will recover whether you like it or not

Szmukler and Appelbaum (2008) outline a number of treatment pressures, uses of interpersonal leverage and coercion. They articulate this range of pressures through an example of a community psychiatric nurse (CPN) communicating with a person who is refusing their medication. It is no coincidence that the issue of engagement here is reduced to a matter of compliance with medication as we will see that this becomes the sole test of recovery for many people engaged in this debate. Szmukler and Appelbaum (2008) outline a hierarchy of pressures from the lowest to the highest beginning with persuasion and moving through interpersonal leverage to inducements, threats and full-blown coercion. The CPN responds to the refusal of medication with persuasion if she listens to the reasons and then attempts to lay out the possible issues with stopping medication and alerts the person to previous patterns around medication use. Rightly, Szmukler and Appelbaum see this as relatively unproblematic. However, the notion of persuasion rather than education or negotiation already seems to put into place a particular power relationship. When we move on to interpersonal leverage things get murkier. The CPN responds by looking sad and disappointed by the person's decision. Inducement occurs when the CPN offers a ticket for a football game if the person takes their medication (an offer not a threat if we remember Nozick's account earlier). A threat occurs when the CPN says she will not fill out a benefits claim form unless the person takes medication. Full coercion occurs with a Mental Health Act assessment followed by possible forced treatment. Szmukler and Appelbaum are admirably concerned about all of these pressures and quite rightly argue that one should aim for a minimum necessary use of any pressure in a therapeutic relationship.

However, others have taken this argument further. Molodynski et al. (2010) outline the same series of pressures applied to a hypothetical CPN (Tom) and client (Debbie). However their conclusion is far more concerning. They write that:

Interactions such as these between Tom and Debbie occur every day in clinical practice. The lower levels of pressure may be helpful and appropriate in our relationships with patients. After all pressure is ubiquitous in human relationships and likely to be particularly pertinent in challenging and difficult ones. (Molodynski et al., 2010, p. 110)

This statement can best be described as a form of therapeutic nihilism. If interactions such as these do occur every day then they should be fought against not accepted. Everything from interpersonal leverage upwards to formal coercion is unacceptable unless the formal coercion is framed through its legal safeguards. The fact that pressures are ubiquitous in society does not make them acceptable or ethical, and we should be even more scrupulous when faced with vulnerable people to demonstrate that we are working in a respectful and sensitive manner.

However, Molodynski et al. (2010) go further by arguing that a rights-based approach abandons clients and that the use of compulsion and leverage should be viewed as consistent with recovery. They argue if we allow people to make their own choices, particularly this group of 'revolving door patients', we are not enabling them to improve their lives. A flourishing and satisfying life and a recovery from mental illness begins with coercion.

These arguments about the necessity to take a responsibility for your own recovery are mirrored by Davidson and Roe (2007, p. 467) who argue in the following manner that '… a person's recovery is something that he or she needs to pursue actively, and there are individuals who have yet to take up this challenge'. Later they write that there are people who choose not to recover, and compare them with 'people with lung cancer who continue to smoke' (Davidson & Roe, 2007, p. 468). The challenge of recovery is taken up only by those who accept they have an illness, take their medication and agree to live their lives in accordance with the ways in which the psychiatric system thinks they should. If they take up this challenge, then later down the line they can make choices and live meaningful lives. If they refuse to take up this challenge, in some circumstances, we might coerce them to do so for their own good.

You will recover, and we have ways of making you recover. One of these ways that is being increasingly written about and researched in relation to the 'revolving door population' is the Money for Medication approach (Claasen, 2007; Priebe et al., 2009). Classen (2007) writes about a project in East London where assertive outreach clients were given £5 to £10 for each depot injection they received. Again, if we remember Nozick's argument, this is considered to be an offer not a threat, as something that they would normally expect is not being withdrawn. Of course, this ignores the larger power background to these issues, particularly the social vulnerabilities that are cynically being manipulated in such cases. Claasen (2007) accepts that this is a form of inducement, but doesn't worry too unduly about the issue of informed consent and how it might be compromised by systematic bribery. He writes that 'consent to any treatment decision is a complex issue' (Claasen, 2007, p. 191). He later claims that the bribe is merely a matter of 'tilting the balance of an individual's informed decision making' (Claasen, 2007, p. 192). There is no acknowledgement that being treated with antipsychotic depot medication has numerous costs as well as benefits, but Claasen writes about it as an unmitigated good, similar to the act of giving up smoking.

Priebe et al. (2009) also write of Money for Medication as a positive option for facilitating recovery. They do worry about some drawbacks, but their listing of the drawbacks only betrays their inability to understand the abuse of power involved. The concerns they list involve the person becoming financially dependent, demanding more money over time, that the person will not want to terminate the scheme, and that they will squander their additional income on drugs (Priebe et al., 2009). There is no concern about what such a transaction means to the person at the receiving end, and how they might feel by 'accepting' such a bargain. Research into the experiences of clients who are subject to community treatment orders has shown how it affects their own self-image and identity (Gibbs, Dawson, Ansley & Mullen, 2005), but there seems little concern for that here.

This kind of therapeutic nihilism tips the balance away from a tension of rights and responsibilities encapsulated by the constructive engagement agenda towards an emphasis on adherence to medication as the key goal in mental health care that can be achieved without consideration of service user autonomy.

The extension of coercion into the community

The most significant development in mental health services in the UK in the past 10 years has been the legal sanction for an element of community treatment brought in with the amendments to the Mental Health Act 2007. Those people who have been detained under Section 3 or some forensic sections can be put on CTOs, and the CTO enables the person to be recalled to hospital for up to 72 hours if they are not complying with the conditions of their order (DH, 2008a). The formal conditions that are placed on a person within a CTO are that they must make themselves available for treatment, although they cannot be forcibly treated in the community. However, a number of adjunct conditions can be applied, the most significant of which is usually that the person must take their medication as prescribed, although other conditions related to where a person lives and use of illegal drugs can be applied at the discretion of the Responsible Clinician (DH, 2008a).

Supervised community treatment was introduced in England and Wales against a background of much controversy and a united opposition amongst health care professionals and service users organised through the Mental Health Alliance (Mental Health Alliance, 2005). The background evidence for the effectiveness of CTOs was extensively reviewed by Churchill et al. (2007) and found to be lacking. Churchill et al. (2007) found that there was no evidence for any reduction in re-admission rates or length of hospital stay and on a range of patient satisfaction measures CTOs were found to be negative. As Burns and Dawson (2009) write, there are serious questions about how ethical such a treatment can be when it is implemented without any evidence base at all. This leads us to conclude that the background discourse on the risk culture of mental health meant that CTOs were an inevitability and would be introduced in England and Wales regardless of evidence. In fact, the clamour for CTOs was already embedded within the discourse around constructive engagement at the end of the 1990s (DH, 1998).

However, what is of concern is the readiness with which CTOs have become an established and extensive part of the armoury of mental health services and are rapidly becoming an unquestioned part of the picture. In a survey of 533 psychiatrists in England and Wales most found CTOs useful (Lawton-Smith, 2010). This subjective survey is backed up by the extensive use of CTOs in practice as we have noted earlier (Health and Social Care Information Centre, 2011). However, we shouldn't be fooled into thinking that larger societal pressures and forces do not continue to play a role within the implementation of such legislation. One of the most concerning aspects of the implementation of CTOs has been the acknowledged overuse with people from a black and minority ethnic background (Care Quality Commission, 2011).

It is unlikely that this acceptance of CTOs as a natural fact of contemporary mental health practice will be changed soon. The research agenda around CTOs in the UK is currently dominated by an ongoing randomised controlled trial comparing CTOs with Section 17 leave (a granted leave of absence from hospital for people subject to compulsory admission) which is known as the OCTET trial (Oxford Community Treatment Order Evaluation Trial). This randomised comparison claims to be able to demonstrate the benefits or otherwise of CTOs in a properly conducted randomised trial (OCTET, 2011), but these benefits will only be demonstrated by a comparison of two forms of coercion; either CTOs or Section 17 leave. As Burns and Dawson (2009) highlight, a proper comparison of community coercion versus intensive assertive outreach is not ethical once CTO legislation has been passed, so we are left with evidence that is already weighted towards coercion.

Given the lack of evidence for CTOs and the flawed arguments put forward for their justification, it is difficult to conclude otherwise than that their implementation is wholly political in nature. Kisely and Campbell (2007) write that there is little evidence that CTOs will address the needs of 'revolving door' clients and that the introduction of CTOs demonstrates how 'health policy remains determined by social or political factors as much as evidence' (Kisely & Campbell, 2007, p. 374). What is of even more concern is the manner in which CTOs are now accepted as natural fact, and not even questioned within advocates of recovery in mental health. In one of the few published documents offering a critical perspective on the recovery paradigm, there is no mention of CTOs (MindThink Report, 2007). It is now more important than ever to question the effectiveness and morality of CTOs and to argue that there can be no such thing as recovery alongside community coercion.

There is no alternative

A pragmatic response to the analysis of this increasing movement towards coercion in community mental health care might argue that there is no alternative to this. Indeed Gert, Culver and Clouser (2006) argue that paternalism is acceptable if there is no alternative. However, the existence of CTOs should not replace everything we have learned positively about constructively engaging with vulnerable people, and working with risk in therapeutic ways.

The way in which we view risk in contemporary society according to Douglas (1992) suggests avoiding risk and therefore loss of liberties is the accepted norm. Consequently, acting outside of this norm and deliberately risk taking is seen as abnormal and pathological. An example of how this may operate in mental health services is perhaps the response to service users who want to come off their medication: why decide not to take medication and risk relapse? However, risk taking has the potential to both support individuals' recovery and challenge the narrow and limiting conceptualisation of risk in mental health services. Positive or therapeutic risk taking is about individuals having the opportunity to make choices, decide and follow different options. Positive risk taking is characterised by a process of enabling the person to make decisions about the level of risk they are prepared to take with their health and safety (DH, 2004). Morgan (2000) argues that it is vital to support service users taking chances and learning from their experiences yet it requires recognition that in the short term certain risks may be increased for the benefit of long-term gains. The need for a more positive and collaborative approach to working with risk is recognised (DH, 2004, 2007). Furthermore a number of positives have been noted for voluntary risk taking such as self-improvement, emotional engagement, control and social recognition (e.g., Lupton & Tulloch, 2002; Parker & Stanworth, 2005).

Yet for people using mental health services, as we have seen in this chapter, their opportunity to make choices and take risks is bound by their relationships with mental health services and the professionals working in them. Organisational culture and a fear of being blamed is recognised as a barrier for staff to supporting individuals to take therapeutic risks (Godin, 2004), creating tensions for promoting risk taking and ultimately recovery. This challenge comes as no surprise in the face of the coercive practices examined here. Robertson and Collinson's (2011) research emphasises the complex process for professionals negotiating risk taking with service users. For the participants in their study the influence of the social and organisational context on the level of risk taking was significant. There is a tension for the professionals in terms of managing their own anxiety and making choices about the level of positive risk that can be taken whilst striving for a balance between gains for the individual and the maintenance of safety in the face of uncertainty. These constraining influences on attempting to manage risk are well recognised, yet if we accept these constraints rather than seek opportunity to overcome them, there is danger that recovery remains a rhetoric or even justification for doing what has always been done and maintaining the status quo, leaving no alternative but to be coerced into recovery.

References

Anderson, S. (2011). Coercion. In *Stanford Encyclopedia of Philosophy.* Retrieved 2 February 2012 from, http://plato.stanford.edu/entries/coercion/

Appelbaum, P., Robbins, P., & Monahan, J. (2000). Violence and delusions: Data from the MacArthur Violence Risk Assessment Study. *American Journal Psychiatry, 157*(4), 566–572.

Bryant, M. (2001). *Introduction to User Involvement – Engagement or co-option.* London: Sainsbury Centre for Mental Health.

Burns, T., & Dawson, J. (2009). Community treatment orders: How ethical without experimental evidence? *Psychological Medicine, 39,* 1583–1586.

Care Quality Commission. (2011). *Monitoring the Mental Health Act in 2010/ 2011.* Retrieved 2 February 2012 from, http://www.cqc.org.uk/sites/default/files/media/documents/cqc_mha_report_2011_main_final.pdf

Churchill, R., Owen, G., Singh, S., & Hotopf, M. (2007). *International Experiences of Using Community Treatment Orders.* Institute of Psychiatry: London.

Claasen, D. (2007). Financial incentives for antipsychotic depot medication: Ethical issues. *Journal of Medical Ethics, 33,* 189–193.

Crossley, N. (2006). *Contesting Psychiatry: Social movements in mental health.* London: Routledge.

Davidson, G., & Campbell, J. (2007). An examination of the use of coercion by assertive outreach and community mental health teams in Northern Ireland. *British Journal of Social Work, 37*(3), 537–555.

Davidson, L., & Roe, D. (2007). Recovery from versus recovery in serious mental illness: One strategy for lessening confusion plaguing recovery. *Journal of Mental Health, 16*(4), 459–470.

Department of Health. (1998). *Modernising Mental Health Services.* Retrieved 2 February 2012 from, http://webarchive.nationalarchives.gov.uk/+/www.dh.gov.uk/en/Publicationsandstatistics/Publications/PublicationsPolicyAndGuidance/DH_4003105

Department of Health. (1999). *Effective Care Co-ordination in Mental Health Services: Modernising the care programme approach – A policy booklet.* London: HMSO.

Department of Health. (2000). *The NHS Plan: A plan for investment, a plan for reform.* London: DH.

Department of Health. (2001). *Involving Patients and the Public.* London: HMSO.

Department of Health. (2004). *Essential Shared Capabilities: A framework for the whole of the mental health workforce.* London: HMSO.

Department of Health. (2005). *Creating a Patient-led NHS: Delivering the NHS Improvement Plan.* London: HMSO.

Department of Health. (2006). *From Values to Action: The Chief Nursing Officer's review of mental health nursing.* London: HMSO.

Department of Health. (2007). *Best Practice in Managing Risk.* London: HMSO.

Department of Health. (2008a). *Mental Health Act Code of Practice.* Retrieved 2 February 2012 from, http://www.dh.gov.uk/en/Publicationsandstatistics/Publications/PublicationsPolicyAndGuidance/DH_084597

Department of Health. (2008b). *Refocusing the Care Programme Approach: A policy and positive practice guidance.* London: HMSO.

Douglas, K., Guy, L., & Hart, S. (2009). Psychosis as a risk factor for violence to others: A meta-analysis. *Psychological Bulletin, 135,* 679–706.

Douglas, M. (1992). *Risk and Blame Essays in Cultural Theory.* London: Routledge.

Doyle, M., & Dolan, M. (2002). Violence risk assessment: Combining actuarial and clinical information to structure clinical judgements for the formulation and management of risk. *Journal of Psychiatric and Mental Health Nursing, 9*(6), 649–657.

Freshwater, D., & Westwood, T. (2006). Risk, detention and evidence: Humanizing mental health reform (editorial). *Journal of Psychiatric and Mental Health Nursing, 13,* 257–259.

Gert, B., Culver, C., & Clouser, K. (2006). *Bioethics: A systematic approach.* New York: Oxford University Press.

Gibbs, A., Dawson, J., Ansley, C., & Mullen, R. (2005). How patients in New Zealand view community treatment orders. *Journal of Mental Health, 14,* 357–368.

Godin, A. (2004). 'You don't tick boxes on a form': A study of how community mental health nurses assess and manage risk. *Health, Risk & Society, 6,* 347–360.

Harper, D. (2004). Storying policy: Constructions of risk in proposals to reform UK mental health legislation. In B. Hurwitz, V. Skultans & T. Greenhalgh (Eds.), *Narrative Research in Health and Illness.* London: BMA Books.

Health and Social Care Information Centre. (2011). *In-patients formally detained in hospitals under the Mental Health Act, 1983 and patients subject to supervised community treatment, Annual figures, England, 2010/11.* NHS Information Centre, Community and Mental Health Team. Retrieved 2 February 2012 from, http://www.ic.nhs.uk/pubs/inpatientdetmha1011

Horlick-Jones, T. (2004). 'Experts in risk ... do they exist?' (editorial). *Health, Risk and Society, 6*(2), 107–114.

James, A. (2006). Mind the gaps. *Mental Health Today,* November, 8–9.

Jasanoff, S. (1999). The songlines of risk. *Environmental Values, 8*(1), 135–152.

Kisely, S., & Campbell, L. (2007). Does compulsory or supervised community treatment reduce 'revolving door' care? Legislation is inconsistent with recent evidence. *British Journal of Psychiatry, 191,* 373–374.

Lawton-Smith, S. (2010). *Supervised Community Treatment, Briefing Paper 2.* Mental Health Alliance. Retrieved 2 February 2012 from, http://www.mentalhealthalliance.org.uk/resources/SCT_briefing_paper.pdf

Lidz, C., Hoge, S., Gardner, W., Bennett, N., Monahan, J., Mulvey, E., & Roth, L. (1995). Perceived coercion in mental hospital admission. Pressures and process. *Archives of General Psychiatry, 52,* 1034–1039.

Lupton, D. (1999). *Risk.* London: Routledge.

Lupton, D., & Tulloch, J. (2002). 'Life would be pretty dull without risk': Voluntary risk-taking and its pleasures. *Health, Risk and Society, 4*(2), 113–124.

Macmillan, I. (2005). Targeting clients in community could amount to 'therapeutic stalking'. *Mental Health Practice*, September, *9*(1), 6.

McDonald, R., Waring, J., & Harrison, S. (2005). 'Balancing risk, that is my life': The politics of risk in a hospital operating theatre department. *Health, Risk and Society, 7*(4), 397–411.

Mental Health Alliance. (2005). *Towards a Better Mental Health Act: The Mental Health Alliance Policy Agenda.* Mental Health Alliance. Retrieved 2 February 2012 from, http://www.mentalhealthalliance.org.uk/policy/documents/AGENDA2.pdf

MindThink Report. (2007). *Life and Times of a Supermodel – The recovery paradigm for mental health.* London: Mind. Retrieved 2 February 2012 from, http://www.mind.org.uk/campaigns_and_issues/report_and_resources/911_mindthink_report_3_life_and_times_of_a_supermodel

Molodynski, A., Rugkåsa, J., & Burns, T. (2010). Coercion and compulsion in community mental health care. *British Medical Bulletin, 95,* 105–119.

Morgan, J. (2007). *'Giving Up the Culture of Blame'. Risk assessment and risk management in psychiatric practice.* London: Royal College of Psychiatrists.

Morgan, S. (2000). *Clinical Risk Management: A clinical tool and practitioner manual.* London: Sainsbury Centre for Mental Health.

Nozick, R. (1969) Coercion. In S. Morgenbesser, P. Suppes & M. White (Eds.), *Philosophy, Science and Method: Essays in honour of Ernest Nagel.* New York: St. Martin's Press.

Oxford Community Treatment Order Evaluation Trial. (2011). Retrieved 2 February 2012 from, http://www.justice.gov.uk/ajtc/adjust/articles/OxfordCommunityTreatmentOrderEvaluationTrial.pdf

Parker, J., & Stanworth, H. (2005). Go for it! Towards a critical realist approach to voluntary risk-taking. *Health, Risk and Society, 7*(4), 319–336.

Pilgrim, D. (2007). New 'mental health' legislation for England and Wales: Some aspects of consensus and conflict. *Journal of Social Policy, 36,* 79–95.

Pilgrim, D. (2008). 'Recovery' and current mental health policy. *Chronic Illness, 4,* 295–304.

Priebe, S., Burton, A., Ashby, D., Ashcroft, R., Burns, T., David, A., et al. (2009). Financial incentives to improve adherence to anti-psychotic maintenance medication in non-adherent patients – A cluster randomised controlled trial (FIAT). *BMC Psychiatry, 9,* 61.

Repper, J., & Perkins, R. (2009). Recovery and social inclusion. In I. Norman & I. Ryrie (Eds.), *The Art and Science of Mental Health Nursing*. Maidenhead: Open University Press/McGraw-Hill Education.

Robertson, J., & Collinson, C. (2011). Positive risk taking: Whose risk is it? An exploration of community outreach teams in mental health and learning disability services. *Health, Risk and Society, 13*(2), 147–164.

Rogers, A., & Pilgrim, D. (2010). *A Sociology of Mental Health and Illness* (4th ed.). Maidenhead: Open University Press/McGraw-Hill Education.

Rose, D. (2001). *Users' Voices. The perspectives of mental health service users on community and hospital care.* London: Sainsbury Centre for Mental Health.

Royal College of Psychiatrists. (2008). *Rethinking Risk to Others in Mental Health Services: Final report of scoping group.* London: Royal College of Psychiatrists.

Sainsbury Centre for Mental Health. (1998). *Keys to Engagement. Review of care for people with severe mental illness who are hard to engage with services.* London: Sainsbury Centre for Mental Health.

Smith, M. (2004). Mad cows and mad money: Problems of risk in the making and understanding of policy. *British Journal of Politics and International Relations, 6,* 312–332.

Social Care Institute for Excellence. (2007). *A Common Purpose: Recovery in future mental health services* (joint position paper). London: Social Care Institute for Excellence. Retrieved 2 February 2012 from, www.scie.org.uk/publications/positionpapers/pp08.asp

Stickley, T., & Wright, N. (2011). The British research evidence for recovery, papers published between 2006 and 2009 (inclusive). Part One: A review of the peer-reviewed literature using a systematic approach. *Journal of Psychiatric and Mental Health Nursing, 18,* 247–256.

Szmukler, G. (2000). Homicide inquiries: What sense do they make? *Psychiatric Bulletin, 24,* 6–10.

Szmukler, G., & Appelbaum, P. (2008). Treatment pressures, leverage, coercion and compulsion in mental health care. *Journal of Mental Health, 17*(3), 233–244.

Szmukler, G., & Holloway, F. (2000). Reform of the Mental Health Act. Health or safety? *British Journal of Psychiatry, 177,* 196–200.

Turner-Crowson, J., & Wallcraft, J. (2002). The recovery vision for mental health services and research: A British perspective. *Psychiatric Rehabilitation Journal, 25,* 245–254.

Williamson, T. (2004). Can two wrongs make a right? *Philosophy, Psychiatry and Psychology, 11*(2), 159–163.

Witterman, C. (2004). Violent figures; risky stories. *Advances in Psychiatric Treatment, 10,* 275–276.

Chapter 5

Mental Disorder and the Socio-ethical Challenge of Reasonableness

David Pilgrim & Floris Tomasini

Introduction

Outside of the biomedical orthodoxy of neo-Kraepelinian psychiatry a number of topics have pre-occupied its critics. This chapter will touch upon two of these: the social context of diagnosis, and the emergence of a new social movement opposing psychiatric theory and practice. However, this exploration is not used to illuminate the failings of psychiatry, which is a well-trodden path, but the failure of radicalised and disaffected patients to find common cause with the disability movement. Our thesis at the outset, to be demonstrated below, is that this common cause has floundered over the matter of reasonableness.

During the 1970s new social movements emerged on diverse fronts about women's rights, race, age, sexuality, disability, animal rights and ecology. Early social theorists of this wide-ranging trend, taking social analysis beyond the traditional labour movement emphasis of Marxism, were divided from the outset about its political potential. Some, such as Touraine (1981), envisaged that there would be a convergence of interest and campaigns and we would witness these movements coalescing. However, others were more doubtful and suggested that, by their very nature, the movements would co-exist in parallel about separate aspirations and a pre-occupation with 'single issue politics' (Melucci, 1989; Offe, 1984).

We would argue that the latter authors have been correct about their predictions and this outcome has particular relevance for debates about social progress in mental health campaigns, which focus on matters such as recovery, social inclusion and coercion. By the 1980s, with the emergence

This is an abridged version of an article that appeared in *Disability and Society* (Pilgrim, D., & Tomasini, F. (2012). On being unreasonable in modern society: Are mental health problems special? *Disability and Society, 27,* 631–646) and a presentation at the Symposium on 'Distress or Disability?' at Lancaster University, 17th November 2011.

of the disability movement, the notion of 'disablism' prompted the variant of 'mentalism'. Since then some (but not all) psychiatric survivors have argued that the social model of disability by activists with physical impairments can and should be adopted about mental health problems. The broad logic here is that disabling social attitudes and environmental forms of organisation construct disability and therefore are open to political challenge and rectification.

But if a social model of disability were applied to mental health problems in the same way that it has to physical health problems, what would be the implications? In particular if contexts can be 'disabling', what would a social context look like that was 'enabling' in relation to people with diagnoses of mental disorder? Beresford (2000, 2002) welcomes an ongoing dialogue between psychiatric survivor activists and representatives of the disabled people's movement in order to develop a 'social model of madness and distress'. This 'suggests a different lexicon to mental health service users, based on ideas of support, personal assistance and non-medicalised provision' (Beresford, 2002, p. 583).

Beresford (2000) outlines three areas of overlapping sets of concerns between survivors and disabled people:

- Psychiatric system survivors are constructed as disabled, by state legislation and policy makers in the health and social care services. (Sometimes the term 'mental disabilities' is heard in these circles to cover those with mental health problems and learning disabilities.)

- It is not uncommon for survivors to have physical impairments, sometimes directly related to clinical iatrogenesis from biomedical psychiatry (e.g., obesity and its complications and movement disorders).

- Both disabled people and psychiatric system survivors are subject to discrimination and oppression.

Despite this aspirational logic about a convergence of interest, the empirical reality has been that in the past 20 years the physical disability movement and the survivors movement, by and large, have *not* found common cause. We now offer an explanation for this failure and we can start with the obvious ambivalence in the two groups about one another. There has been an unwillingness of many psychiatric survivors to personally identify themselves as being 'disabled' or 'impaired', and there has been a recalcitrance among some disabled people to include people with mental health problems in their ranks (Beresford, Gifford & Harrison, 1996; Mulvany, 2000).

On being unreasonable in its social context

Someone with a physical impairment may face a range of emotional reactions in others, such as pity, guilt, embarrassment and occasionally disgust. In the case of mental health problems, especially with the attribution of madness, we find a different range of emotional reactions, especially fear and distrust (though depression and anxiety can invoke pity). Physically disabled people are disadvantaged in society but this is not about an attributed loss or lack of reason. Instead it has largely been about their expressed needs being ignored within a disabling environment. By contrast, that loss or lack of reason is *at the centre* of the social reaction typically evoked by mental health problems. In the case of mental health problems, social exclusion is actively justified on grounds of people's inability to reason. Furthermore, a whole legislative apparatus has been constructed to ensure such exclusion, which is deemed to be socially progressive (World Health Organization, 2005). Whereas with the growth of urbanisation under industrial capitalism, most physically disabled people lived at home with their families, a complex and expensive asylum system was developed to sequestrate mental disorder. Thus physically disabled people were by and large tolerated *but ignored,* but this was not the case with madness: it was not tolerated and it was not ignored.

Mental health policy has not then been an expression of political ignorance and neglect (as has been the case often in relation to physical disability) but a deliberate and highly considered point in modern polity. Most of us take for granted in contemporary cultures that a loss or lack of reason actively warrants lawful paternalistic social control. This is an example of what Bourdieu (1977) following Aristotle calls 'doxa', which refers to common assumptions that operate without reflection in particular times and places.

For example, the British Secretary of State for Health in 1998, Frank Dobson, lamented that 'care in the community has failed' and that more beds were needed of 'the right kind in the right place' (Dobson, 1998). He was particularly concerned about patients who were 'a nuisance' or a 'danger to themselves or others'. Politicians only look to what they judge to be expedient, in the public imagination. In this case what Dobson had in mind, and what he thought would resonate with the consciousness of others, was a conflation of 'nuisance' and 'danger', with the latter subsuming risk to self and others.

Dobson was simply reflecting a discourse about post-Enlightenment normative expectations. We now expect people we encounter privately and publicly to act reasonably (unless they are drunk). When they do not we will then tend to ascribe mental abnormality to them. Whereas in pre-modern times madness retained an ambiguous cultural quality, since the eighteenth century it has been increasingly conceptualised as meaningless pathology, only worthy of paternalistic containment and suppression. For example, in antiquity madness was seen as being given by the gods and so had virtuous qualities – it was not merely dismissed as pathology as it is today. In the past 200 years state-endorsed social control (*parens patrie*) was justified philosophically by J. S. Mill in his views on emerging citizenship. For Mill, children, idiots and lunatics were in need of care because of their ill-formed or *lost* reason. In the past 200 years in Western industrialised societies, to be unreasonable has been a focus of interest for state-sanctioned medical authority. It has also been grounds for seemingly legitimate suspicion and rejection from those who were sane by common consent. Mayer (1985) notes that the history of social control is not merely about the state and its agents; ordinary people exercise their own forms of powerful informal labelling and control. The desire to control mental health problems occurs in the lay arena of the family (Coulter, 1973) and the street (Rogers, 1990). Psychiatric professionals rubber-stamp decisions *made already* by significant others or the general public respectively. Thus, Dobson was playing to a well-established and well-populated public gallery. The relationship between professionals and lay people about the ascription of mental disorder is complex. For example, in societies *that lack* a professional psychiatric presence, lay people still socially control and socially exclude mad people in their midst (Rogers & Pilgrim, 2010). This is a caution against blaming the psychiatric profession for the control and exclusion of some forms of psychological difference in society. At the same time, some forms of immoral conduct were indeed medicalised in the twentieth century, such as substance misuse (see below). Another example is how unhappiness is often now converted in the minds of lay people into a medical condition ('depression') (Pilgrim & Bentall, 1999). The influence of professionals over lay people about framing socio-ethical transgressions as forms of mental disorder is called 'protoprofessionalisation' by de Swaan (1990).

With this trend of medicalisation came an overlaying mystification: that mental health problems *were the same* as physical health problems and that state provision of care should be developed extensively and access to it welcomed by all. However, if 'access' to mental health care is so desirable, why do we need legislation to enforce it and protect us against the deprivations and risks in its wake? Physical disorders are linked with the 'inverse care law' (Tudor-Hart, 1971) but this is not the case in relation to mental disorders. This 'law' tells us that those in most need of health care (the poor) receive it the least. Contrast this with the socio-economic status of chronic psychiatric patients. Poor patients are *over-represented* in 'mental health services', they are not under-represented. Psychiatric patients are typically unemployed and they live in poor neighbourhoods, where they are overly exposed to the 'ambient hazards' of crime, poor housing conditions, noise and road traffic risks (Stockdale et al., 2007; Hiday, 1995). 'Modern mental health services' then remain part of an apparatus of social control to regulate one part of the 'underclass'.

As Scull (1979) noted, whereas the poor might come to depend on the state for relief in the workhouses of the nineteenth century, pauper lunatics were disruptive and would refuse the routines demanded of them. For Scull, the policy challenge for the emerging capitalist state was not just those who were unemployed, but at times it was specifically about those who were also *unemployable because they lacked or had lost their reason* ('idiots and lunatics'). It became evident during the twentieth century that male deviance in this disruptive part of the underclass was particularly a focus for the state's apparatus of control.

Now women are admitted to acute psychiatric units at the same rate as men but the latter are twice as likely to be present at any particular moment in time (Mental Health Act Commission, 2009). Posing less average threat to others, women are discharged sooner. Women have now virtually disappeared from high secure psychiatric environments and their access to the norms of childcare responsibility is probably one driver in this gender separation, alongside the actual risk that men pose compared to women on average.

The point about higher detention rates generally for men is shown in Figure 1 and in particular relation to security levels in Figure 2.

Thus norms of rationality shape the character of the state control of psychological deviance. The age distribution of coerced population reinforces this point. The greatest incidence of mental health problems

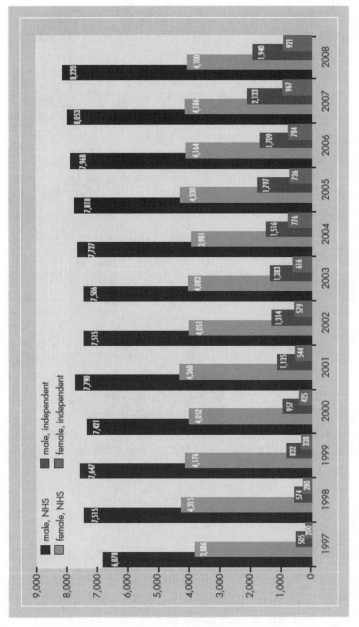

Figure 1. Patients detained in psychiatric units in England and Wales (Mental Health Act Commission, 2009)

occurs in very old age and in those of schooling age, but actual state investment in 'mental health services' is concentrated on the risky action of those of *working and child-rearing age* (SCMH, 2003) (see Figure 3). This suggests that it is not the expressed needs of people who are distressed that is being prioritised in services but the requirement to limit risk and enforce rules – a normative imperative about rationality.

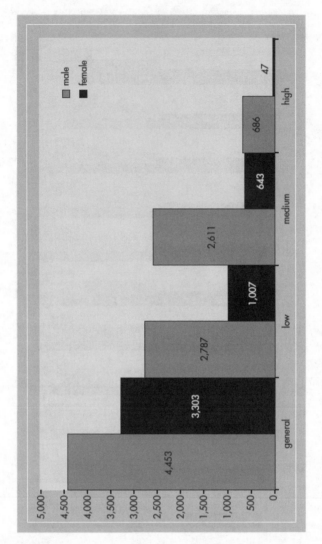

Figure 2. Patient sex differences in levels of psychiatric security in England and Wales (Mental Health Act Commission, 2009)

This data summarises the structural and historical context of being unreasonable. We now turn to the political implications of mental disorder, especially if the latter become a focus for campaigning to improve citizenship or to protest against human rights infringements.

Transactional nuances of being unreasonable in everyday modern life

The implications of being unreasonable in modern society are nuanced, not simple. As Szasz (1963) noted, it is not being dangerous that is at issue here but 'the manner in which one is dangerous'. Thus to appreciate the

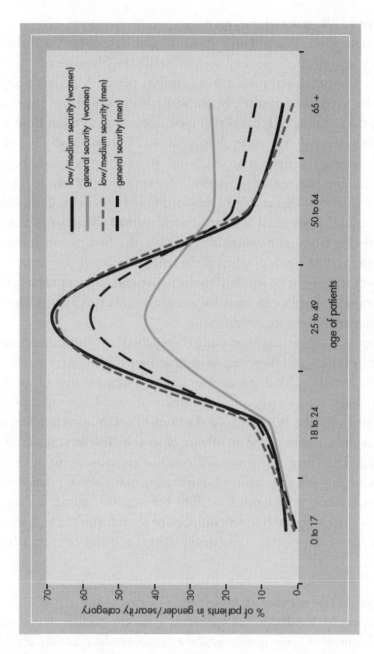

Figure 3. Detained patients by age in England and Wales (Mental Health Act Commission, 2009)

different ways that being unreasonable invoke first the lay desire for social control and then the professional willingness to provide it, we can make certain nuanced distinctions.

Nuance 1: Nuisance and danger

The implications of conflating nuisance and danger (as Frank Dobson did) are serious, because they are potentially highly misleading and an offence against natural justice. For example, person X pesters people on the street to tell them insistently, but with a warm smile, that he or she has found the meaning of life and that God is speaking to them from all the televisions arrayed in a nearby shop window. They are friendly and excited about sharing the news with everyone. In another example, person Y threatens others aggressively with a knife (as a pre-emptive warning) because he or she believes that strangers are plotting to harm them. Both of these people could be described as being 'severely mentally ill', 'frankly psychotic' or 'suffering from schizophrenia'. However, the first person is harmless (though maybe irritating) whereas the latter is an active danger to others. Both of them might be reported to the police and both could be detained and removed to a place of safety for assessment by a psychiatrist. However, their rule transgressions are different.

Person X is insisting on making claims about the world which are not shared by others, and they are pestering and probably unnerving strangers with these claims. Madness arouses fear in others because of its lack of intelligibility and stereotypical culturally acquired assumptions about associated violence. Person Y is on the brink of committing a violent crime and has already committed an offence of sorts by threatening others with violence. Thus mad, like non-mad, conduct contains forms of antisocial action ranging from the benign but irritating to the actively dangerous. In non-psychiatric populations we find cold-callers selling replacement windows or 'chuggers' enlisting support for charities on the high street are at one end of this spectrum and drunk drivers and violent criminals are at the other.

Nuance 2: The manner in which one is a risk to self

'Mental health legislation' is a misnomer and a euphemism. It is about the lawful control of some people who are deemed to be mentally disordered but not others, rather than being about improving mental health. Preventing risk to self is one important aspect of this arrangement but it reveals a double standard about human rights. The state can intervene to prevent self-harm and suicide even though the latter in most countries is not illegal. Moreover, people who are *not* considered to be mentally disordered might be obese, smoke cigarettes, drink alcohol excessively and indulge in unprotected sex. Racing car drivers have high social status and mountaineers are admired for their courage even though they are putting their lives at risk. Young people habitually pierce and tattoo their bodies but it is not called self-harm. We control some people who injure or mutilate their bodies or act in a way which endangers their wellbeing but not others.

Nuance 3: The manner in which one is a risk to others

Boxers and mercenary soldiers set out to inflict harm on others but they are deemed to be sane. Others called 'mentally disordered', who may act in a harmless but unintelligible way, may lose their liberty without trial because they are a 'nuisance' and frightening to those present. They are not physically violent though like the boxer or mercenary. Again there seems to be inconsistency here in public policy. For example, a good case could be made for a curfew for all under 30s to be off the streets between dusk on Fridays and dawn on Mondays. This would save many lives from the reduction in road traffic accidents, rates of sexually transmitted diseases and unwanted pregnancies would drop, as would the rate of sexual offences and violence against people on the streets and in domestic settings. All of this violence perpetrated by sane citizens is replayed every weekend in town centres and urban homes. But legislation that enforced such a curfew would, understandably, be met with derision and scorn by most of us. However, for those deemed mentally disordered the law warrants intrusions of this sort on their freedom of action, and is simply accepted as being justifiable and even claimed to be a form of social progress (World Health Organization, 2005).

Nuance 4: Self-centredness and the impaired recognition of others

We are all *to some extent* self-centred, but some of us are substantially more self-centred than others. When the latter emerges to such a degree that it offends or troubles others then this can be codified by medical personnel as a form of 'personality disorder'. But madness in its acute manifestation also reflects gross self-preoccupation (this is why mad people are frightening and infuriating). This is about the infringement of what Thoits (1985) calls 'emotion rules': we learn how to conduct ourselves appropriately in different social contexts, while constantly bearing in mind the expectations and rights of others.

Goffman (1959/1990, 1963) noted that we are all expected to make sense of our actions to others in the context of rule transgressions in order to respect the rights of others to go about their daily business untroubled. Following Goffman's lead, Shotter (1981) notes that this meta-rule of mutual accountability underpins our right to citizenship and is necessary for public life to flow uninterrupted:

> Along with this right however goes a duty to be accounted competent members of their society, people are also expected to act responsibly … they *must be ready to answer for what they do* and evaluate their actions in terms they share with others in their community … Without such abilities, and without the rights and duties, the enablements and constraints in society carefully constructed (it seems) to nurture such abilities and maintain them in existence, *social life as we know it would be impossible*. (Shotter, 1981, pp. 173–174, emphasis added)

Mentally disordered patients offend the meta-rule, where rule infractions warrant accounts to others that he/she is being socially disruptive, irritating and unnerving. To use Dobson's phrase, they are being a 'nuisance': they pose a serious threat to the very possibility of a *minimal* sense of a social life, where implicit rules of social functioning involve a sense of reasonableness towards others and their needs. If we were all recurrently self-centred or unintelligibly idiosyncratic then there could be no functioning society because there would be no implicit social contract that warranted any recurrent mutual accountability. This would also subvert the success of any sustained social role achievement upon which the cohesion of any society depends.

Those who are acutely psychotic will not or cannot provide an account of their behaviour as being socially intelligible and/or reasonable. This potentially makes their rule infractions the most serious, as it arouses the prospect of (real or imagined) risks to self or others. Although neurotic patients provide intelligible accounts of their behaviour they still break other rules, especially around adult obligations to others at home or at work. For example, the agoraphobic may be quite intelligible and highly insightful about their fears, but they still resist conforming to what may reasonably be considered the duty of an adult citizen: leaving their house and readily fulfilling their duties as a citizen, worker, spouse or parent.

In the case of those deemed to be 'personality disordered', then their self-centredness is not merely a by-product of their mental state (say of madness or extreme fear) but actually *constitutes* that state on a regular basis. They use others as a means to gratify their personal needs. Occasionally this type of habitual self-centredness is socially tolerated as a form of 'blindness' to reasonable behaviour at the expense of full role achievement, as in the successful business man who manipulates others to acquire success, fame, power or remuneration. This trend in public and commercial life has been described as 'snakes in suits' by Babiak and Hare (2000).

Discussion

If this focus on reasonableness is fair comment and has explanatory value then a number of implications flow from it. All people with mental health problems in some way or other are deemed to be conducting themselves in an unreasonable way, but this is not the end of the matter. They are rarely unreasonable about everything all of the time and some unreasonable people are not deemed to have a mental health problem at all. Thus social contingencies and specific social norms define when unreasonableness is deemed to be pathological, is sometimes ignored, and sometimes even socially valued.

Where does all of this leave people with mental health problems? At the individual level, to lose one's reason can have profound and long-term implications. So strong is the stigma about lay labelling and professional diagnoses, it is not surprising that many people will 'cover' their label from others (Goffman called this 'passing'). It is noteworthy that the capacity to 'come out' about mental health problems is also shaped by the type of label implied. A number of celebrities now are willing to share their psychiatric experiences (Ruby Wax, Stephen Fry, Alastair Campbell are recent examples in the UK). Depressive difficulties are easier to use in such acts of self-disclosure, intended at helping a process of de-stigmatisation, compared to those with a diagnosis of psychosis.

This point about the hierarchy of stigma in relation to mental disorder is important. For those without mental health problems, sadness is an emotion that is readily available as a source of pity or empathy. By contrast, voice-hearing or some fixed and rigid beliefs may be completely outside of their experience. All of this makes the acceptance of individual people with mental health problems variable. It is of little surprise that those with 'common mental health problems' or fear and sadness are attracted to passing (hence 'phobics anonymous', 'depressives anonymous' and related organisations) in order to avoid the stereotyping and stigma traditionally linked to mental illness. By contrast, those willing to 'come out' and be at the core of an oppositional social movement to psychiatric orthodoxy tend to be those who have suffered recurrently at the hands of the coercive wing of the state apparatus of social control, i.e., those with 'severe and enduring mental health problems'. Thus a case for *collective reasonableness* is constructed by a group of people, within this new social movement, who individually are largely discreditable for their lack of reason linked to their severe mental disorder. In other words, if people with a diagnosis of mental disorder lack credibility *as individuals*, this does not mean that their consensus points about their sense of oppression are not open to reasonable consideration when expressed by them collectively. This has been the achievement of the psychiatric survivors movement.

The resistance of the physical disability movement to this logic about collective credibility may have arisen for two main reasons. First, those with physical disabilities who are sane and not highly self-centred in their approach to life may simply reject the oddity and narcissism of those with mental health problems, as much as would any non-disabled person with no history of mental health problems. Second, the implied social changes from one group have a radically different focus to that of the other. Whereas disablism is very environmentally focused, it is difficult to see what a psychologically enabling environment would look like. The main focus of psychiatric survivors has not been about their environment (apart from the poor living conditions they share with all of those in poverty) but about their discriminatory treatment. The latter includes dedicated legislation, not applicable to others, which warrants coercive assaults and detention by agents of the state. However, given that this is affirmed by the voting public as socially progressive and desirable, we are reminded that the identification and control of psychological difference in society starts in the lay not the professional arena. It is in the family, on the streets, or at the workplace. Thus a critical preoccupation with the psychiatric profession can easily miss this important point.

Given this synergy between those who are sane by common consent and so-called 'mental health work', to what degree should madness and misery be simply tolerated? What are the best ways to use unhappiness constructively? What should any of us do when faced with people who recurrently act in ways that we consider unreasonably self-centred? When should risk to self and others be a concern and when should it be ignored? Should coercive solutions to risk be abandoned and what would be the consequences? If they are retained what are the consequences? These sorts of questions would then go beyond our current taken-for-granted routines based upon the combination of medicalised routines and legal measures of maintaining social order.

By discussing 'mental disorder' in such socio-ethical terms we are also forced to address philosophical questions about social accountability and moral agency, whether that is about the tolerance and compassion of non-patients or the extent of required accountability of patients themselves. These have been little addressed to date because of the doxa of paternalism on one side and the narrative of victimhood on the other. The latter is quite understandable (psychiatric patients *have* been victimised). However, that true-enough empirical picture can divert us from these deeper questions about agency and accountability.

If society considers that patients are avoiding their adult responsibilities, fail to account for their actions or are significantly self-centred, then in most forms of social organisations (however tolerant and compassionate) there will be negative consequences for those failures. At the same time, taken-for-granted paternalism also diverts us from questions of discrimination and hypocrisy. There is a 'wilful blindness' (Heffernan, 2011) about these matters in mental health debates from professionals and policy makers. That is we do not habitually reflect on the injustice and violence inflicted on psychiatric patients in daily routines of 'mental health care'.

There are multiple groups in a post-enlightenment society defining and responding to what is unreasonable; neither does it seem feasible to envision a society, however compassionate, that would tolerate certain forms of behaviour. It is therefore not helpful to only critique psychiatry. Furthermore, as the psychiatrists Bracken and Thomas (1998) note, their own profession can 'no longer claim any privileged understanding of madness, alienation or distress' (p. 17). And an implication of this confession is that any such understanding should now be the responsibility of us all. Such a responsibility will require a more open, accessible and equitable discussion regarding how society defines and responds to what is reasonable.

References

Babiak, P., & Hare, R. (2000). *Snakes in Suits: When psychopaths go to work.* New York: HarperCollins.

Beresford, P. (2000). What have madness and psychiatric system survivors got to do with disability and disability studies? *Disability and Society, 15*(1), 162–172.

Beresford, P. (2002). Thinking about 'mental health': Towards a social model. *Journal of Mental Health, 11*(6), 581–584.

Beresford, P., Gifford, G., & Harrison, C. (1996). What has disability got to do with psychiatric survivors? In J. Reynolds & J. Read (Eds.), *Speaking Our Minds: Personal experience of mental distress and its consequences.* Buckingham: Open University Press.

Bourdieu, P. (1977). *Outline of a Theory of Practice.* Cambridge: Cambridge University Press.

Bracken, P., & Thomas, P. (1998). A new debate in mental health. *OpenMind, 89,* 17.

Coulter, J. (1973). *Approaches to Insanity.* New York: Wiley.

De Swaan, A. (1990). *The Management of Normality.* London: Routledge.

Dobson, F. (1998). *Frank Dobson Outlines Third Way for Mental Health.* Press release, Department of Health.

Goffman, E. (1963). *Stigma: Some notes on the management of spoiled identity.* Harmondsworth: Penguin.

Goffman, E. (1990). *The Presentation of Self in Everyday Life.* London: Penguin. (Original work published 1959)

Heffernan, M. (2011). *Wilful Blindness.* London: Simon & Schuster.

Hiday, V. (1995). The social context of mental illness and violence. *Journal of Health and Social Behaviour, 36,* 122–137.

Mayer, J. A. (1985). Notes towards a working definition of social control in historical analysis. In S. Cohen & A. Scull (Eds.), *Social Control and the State.* Oxford: Basil Blackwell.

Melucci, A. (1989). *Nomads of the Present: Social movements and individual needs in contemporary society.* Philadelphia, PA: Temple University Press.

Mental Health Act Commission. (2009). *Coercion and Consent: Monitoring the Mental Health Act 2007–2009* (13th Biennial Report). London: The Stationery Office.

Mulvany, J. (2000). Disability, impairment or illness? The relevance of the social model of disability to the study of mental disorder. *Sociology of Health and Illness, 22*(5), 582–601.

Offe, C. (1984). Reflections on the welfare state and the future of socialism (Interviewed in 1982 by David Held and John Keane). In J. Keane (Ed.), *Contradictions of the Welfare State.* London: Hutchinson.

Pilgrim, D., & Bentall, R. P. (1999). The medicalisation of misery: A critical realist analysis of the concept of depression. *Journal of Mental Health, 8,* 261–274.

Rogers, A. (1990). Policing mental disorder: Controversies, myths and realities. *Social Policy and Administration, 24*(3), 226–236.

Rogers, A., & Pilgrim, D. (2010). *A Sociology of Mental Health and Illness* (4th ed.). Maidenhead: Open University Press.

Sainsbury Centre for Mental Health. (2003). *Money for Mental Health: A review of public spending on mental health care.* London: SCMH.

Scull, A. (1979). *Museums of Madness.* Harmondsworth: Penguin.

Shotter, J. (1981). Telling and reporting: Prospective and retrospective uses of self-ascriptions. In C. Antaki (Ed.), *The Psychology of Ordinary Explanations of Social Behaviour.* London: Academic Press.

Stockdale, S. E., Wells, K. B., Tang, L., Belin, T. R., Zhang, L. & Sherbourne, C. D. (2007). The importance of social context: Neighbourhood stressors, stress buffering mechanisms and alcohol, drug and mental disorders. *Social Science & Medicine, 65,* 1867–1881.

Szasz, T. S. (1963). *Law, Liberty and Psychiatry.* New York: Macmillan.

Thoits, P. (1985). Self-labeling processes in mental illness: The role of emotional deviance. *American Journal of Sociology, 91,* 221–249.

Touraine, A. (1981). *The Voice and the Eye: An analysis of social movements.* Cambridge: Cambridge University Press.

Tudor-Hart, J. (1971). The inverse care law. *The Lancet, 1*(7696)(Feb 27), 405–412.

World Health Organization. (2005). *Assessment Instrument for Mental Health Systems.* Geneva: World Health Organization.

Chapter 6

The Pharmaceutical Industry
and Mental Disorder

Joan Busfield

My aim in this chapter is to examine the part played by the pharmaceutical industry in shaping professional understandings and practices in relation to mental disorder. Of course such understandings and practices are influenced by a range of actors, including the ideas and interests of psychiatrists and other mental health professionals themselves, the activities of government, of health providers and insurance companies, both private and charitable, and of the lay public. In this chapter, however, I focus on the part played by the pharmaceutical industry while making reference to its relation with other actors. In order to examine the industry's impact I start by considering some of its key features, concentrating on the interlinked issues of commercialisation and power. I then look at some of the ways the industry's activities affect understandings and practices in relation to mental disorder.

The pharmaceutical industry

The pharmaceutical industry is now a major global industry with worldwide sales from prescribed drugs of $856 billion in 2010 (IMS Health, 2011). It is dominated by a small number of large, multinational companies – companies that also often have animal health and/or consumer product divisions covering areas such as dental care, nutritional products and 'health' drinks. The 10 largest, measured in terms of pharmaceutical sales revenue, all have headquarters in either the United States or Europe (some Japanese companies feature in the top 20), although their manufacturing activity is more widely distributed. For example, the British-based GlaxoSmithKline, which accounts for 5 per cent of the world market, manufactures its products in 32 countries (GlaxoSmithKline, 2010). Together the top 10 account for well over a third of world pharmaceutical sales revenue. A list of the top 10 in 2010 is given in Table 1.

Table 1. *Top Ten Companies by Pharmaceutical Sales Value, 2010*

	Company	Headquarters	Sales $ billion
1	Pfizer	US	55,602
2	Novartis	Switzerland	46,806
3	Merck & Co	US	38,468
4	Sanofi-Aventis	France	35,875
5	AstraZeneca	UK	35,535
6	GlaxoSmithKline	UK	33,664
7	Roche	Switzerland	32,693
8	Johnson & Johnson	US	26,773
9	Abbott	US	23,833
10	Eli Lilly	US	22,113

Source: IMS Health Midas, December 2010

The ranking of the top companies changes over time, partly because of new product developments and partly because of mergers and acquisitions. Moreover companies in countries like China, India and Brazil are beginning to play a more important role in the pharmaceutical market and the Western dominance may not remain. In addition to having manufacturing plants for Western companies, such countries also have their own indigenous pharmaceutical industry, largely made up of numerous small and medium-sized enterprises. Some of the largest of these companies are beginning to invest in their own research and development (R&D) facilities and are exporting drugs to Western countries. For example, the Indian companies, Ranbaxy and Dr Reddy's, export medicines to the US as well as Russia and Brazil.

Pharmaceutical products are designed as treatments for health problems, and have an important role in promoting health and wellbeing, sometimes very successfully. Nonetheless the industry is a highly commercial one that seeks to maintain or increase profits and the market for its products. The commercial character of its practices is manifest in a number of ways. First, in order to increase profitability the major companies make extensive use of patents and brand names. A patent grants a monopoly, usually for a period of 20 years, on the specific product or process so a higher price can be charged, since exclusive ownership restricts (though it does not eliminate) competition for the period of the patent's life. (The fact that a patent is usually taken out well before approval is obtained reduces the period when the monopoly can be exploited, though there are ways patents can be extended and even when the patent ends the brand name can help to sustain sales and revenue.)

Patented drugs generate the bulk of the revenue and profits of the leading companies with a small number of patented drugs termed 'blockbusters' proving highly profitable.[1] The industry typically justifies the use of patenting and the high prices of such drugs in terms of the cost of the R&D involved, though the oft-quoted figure of $800 billion to develop a new drug that is approved for release onto the market is contested (Goozner, 2005). However, in order to maintain and enhance profitability companies need to develop new products to replace those that go off patent. The creation of a 'pipeline' of drugs, one or two of which might become the next generation blockbusters, is important for major companies and a key reason for their investment in R&D. It is also frequently a motive for mergers and acquisitions, with major companies taking over smaller, more innovative ones, including biotechnology companies. However, in the last 20 years fewer new compounds of therapeutic value have been identified and this poses a threat to profits (Abraham, 2010).

The commercial character of the industry is also manifest in the companies' frequent pursuit of 'me-too' drugs – that is medications that are similar to ones already approved, but sufficiently distinct for a separate patent to be granted. These are often little different in terms of efficacy but if the market for a product looks strong then other companies will want to join in – as is the case with the market for smart phones. As a result, patented products do typically face some competition. For example, there are at least 10 types of SSRIs (selective serotonin reuptake inhibitors) for the treatment of depression (see below).

The third feature demonstrating the industry's commercial character is the focus on products that can be used to treat common conditions over a long period of time, since both aspects increase the potential market for a drug. Common health problems, such as depression, that are held to require long-term medication, are ideal from the commercial point of view as they push up sales. We can see the attraction of, and bias towards,

---

1 Blockbuster drugs have sales of $1 billion or more.

products requiring long-term use if we examine the top product classes across the world in terms of sales value. These are given in Table 2.

Table 2. *Top Five Product Classes by Sales Value, 2010*

	Product group
1	Cholesterol and tryglyceride regulators (statins)
2	Antiulcerants
3	Antipsychotics
4	Antidepressants and mood stabilisers
5	Angiotensin-II antagonists (for hypertension)

Source: IMS Health (2011)

It is noteworthy that two of the top five classes are for psychoactive medications: antipsychotics and antidepressants, which I consider further below, indicating the significant role they have played in pharmaceutical sales.[2] These drug classes are not of course the top-selling drug classes worldwide by volume – antibiotics and analgesics almost certainly head the list – but many of these are out of patent and do not generate the same level of revenue.

Fourth, the highly commercial character of the industry is manifest in its concentration on Western markets where the level of affluence is such that they can be afforded, and on diseases common in these countries. As the data in Table 2 suggest, the top product classes by sales are treatments for conditions more frequently identified in richer countries where infectious illnesses have largely been controlled. This is shown very clearly by the fact that 90 per cent of the industry's R&D spending goes on health problems that account for only 10 per cent of the global burden of disease (WHO, 2004). Perhaps not surprisingly the US, currently the richest country in the world, is by far the largest market for pharmaceutical products, accounting for nearly a half of world sales by value, though this also reflects the fact that it hosts 5 of the 10 largest companies, and that US drug prices are high.

---

2 Leading companies have recently been withdrawing investment in psychopharmacology research because of the costs and difficulties (Nutt & Goodwin, 2011).

Finally, the industry's commercial character is also demonstrated by the effort some companies make to identify conditions that might benefit from drug treatments and in the process broaden the boundaries of what is deemed to require medical intervention. Drugs are increasingly used for conditions not previously considered illnesses, as with high cholesterol, now considered a risk factor for heart problems and to require treatment by taking cholesterol-lowering statins. Indeed, as Table 2 shows, in 2010 cholesterol-lowering drugs were the top product class is terms of sales revenue. One consequence is that alternative forms of action, like marked changes in diet or increases in exercise, are largely sidelined. And since such conditions are often judged to require long-term medical treatment, the medicines are potentially highly profitable for companies. Yet their value for the broad range of patients for whom they are prescribed is often contested. For example, there is debate as to whether statins are being used for too broad a range of patients, with evidence suggesting that, despite frequent claims to the contrary, they may not be useful for the purposes of primary prevention in patients *without* cardiovascular disease (Curtiss & Fairman, 2010). This boundary expansion is particularly problematic in the case of mental disorders where it has been extensive, not least because there is evidence, discussed later, that many psychoactive drugs are largely ineffective and used too widely.

It is clear that the current concentration of the industry in the hands of a relatively small number of large multinational companies helps to increase the industry's power – power that is economic, ideological and political.[3] We can see the way in which the industry exerts its power if we look at its relation to some other key actors in the field. First, there is the medical profession. Since many of the industry's products, especially those in patent, need to be medically prescribed, it is essential for the industry to secure the support of the profession. At the same time, the profession needs the industry since medicines provide a major weapon in the medical armoury for trying to fight illness and maintain health. In that respect the relationship between industry and profession is symbiotic. Yet clinicians' need for the industry increases the industry's power over the profession, which is the object of much of its marketing activity (marketing accounts for over 20 per cent of the industry's budgets, Gagnon & Lexchin, 2008).

---

3 I use here Mann's (1993) framework of four types of power: ideological, economic, military and political.

New medicines are advertised in medical journals, often intensively, and industry salesmen (detailers) visit doctors' surgeries with information about their products, leaving samples and small gifts to remind them of brand names (often far easier to remember than generic chemical names – compare 'sildenafil' with Viagra) and to encourage prescribing, the evidence indicating that even small gifts influence prescribing, though this is denied by many doctors (Katz, Caplan & Merz, 2003). Medical support for new drugs is also secured by targeting opinion leaders in the profession, particularly those in academia, with financial support for conferences, acting as consultants, carrying out research, finding research participants, as well as the ghosting of papers.

The control the industry exercises over the science that underpins drug development and approval further limits medicine's power in resisting the blandishments of the industry. The bulk of the scientific work underlying drug development and studies of efficacy that precede approval is funded by the industry, with studies of efficacy carried out by the industry tending to overstate a drug's value (Kjaegard & Als-Nielsen, 2002). And doctors working in clinical contexts usually do not have the time or ready access to the data to evaluate companies' claims. Instead they have largely to rely on information companies provide about products and their effectiveness (Busfield, 2006).

The public is another actor in the field and the second target of the industry's marketing activity. In most countries including Britain (the exceptions are the US and New Zealand) direct-to-consumer advertising is not legally permitted. However pharmaceutical companies provide publicity about drugs in other ways. For instance, company press releases are often the source of articles in newspapers and magazines describing new products with strong claims as to their value. Companies also frequently provide data on the extent of particular health problems for which they offer drugs, arguing that they are trying to increase awareness of the problem for the public good and not to increase sales. Yet at the same time they are of course generating markets for their products. They also help to fund user groups that campaign for improved access to particular treatments. All this encourages individuals, if they identify themselves as having a particular problem, to request a specific medicine. Only rarely do public pressure groups emerge that are critical of particular products.

Governments are also key actors in the field since they have responsibility for regulating the industry, particularly in relation to ensuring the safety of drugs, and also may have to pay for medicines as part of their funding of health services, and so have an incentive to keep their prices down. Indeed governments are potentially more powerful than the industry. However they often have a strong economic interest in supporting the industry since it can constitute an important productive activity within the country, contributing to GDP and providing a source of employment and exports. They may also want to persuade the industry to sell its products to them at reasonable prices. Not surprisingly we find the industry actively engaged in lobbying governments to support the industry (Angell, 2005) and, as with other corporations, companies may even threaten to move their activities elsewhere if they do not receive what they consider sufficient support, for instance in the form of reduced corporation tax or the ability to offset R&D costs.

Some of the drugs developed by the pharmaceutical industry have undoubtedly been of enormous value (antibiotics, analgesics, antihistamines, and treatments for AIDS are obvious examples). It is nonetheless a highly commercial industry which primarily pursues its own interests and seeks to maximise profits – something often masked by the fact that it operates in the healthcare field where the focus is on providing help and reducing pain and distress. And as a large, profitable industry it exercises considerable power – power that, for the reasons I have suggested, is not curtailed to any great extent by other actors such as the medical profession or governments. What then is the impact of the industry in the mental health field? How has it contributed to the shaping of understandings and practices in relation to mental illness?

The impact of the pharmaceutical industry

We can see the industry's impact on mental health thinking and practice in three main areas: in the increasing predominance of pharmaceutical treatments; in encouraging and sustaining biological understandings of mental illness; and in helping to expand the boundaries of mental illness.

In exploring its impact we need to bear in mind some features of psychiatry, the senior mental health profession. Psychiatry is a specialty of medicine and training in natural sciences predominates; yet its activities were long-separated from the rest of medicine, based as they were largely in mental hospitals, and its ideas and practices have often been seen as unscientific. Moreover its core client group are individuals with acute mental health problems, often from deprived social backgrounds, with many social difficulties such as poverty, unemployment and homelessness, whose behaviour is often regarded as difficult and dangerous – all characteristics that further lower its prestige within medicine. Psychiatry's standing was also further threatened when its ideas and practices were widely attacked in the 1960s by a diverse group of 'anti-psychiatrists' including psychiatrists such as Thomas Szasz (1961) and R. D. Laing (1967), and sociologists Erving Goffman (1961) and Thomas Scheff (1966). Such attacks received widespread attention in the media at a time when the reliability of psychiatric diagnosis was also being questioned. Faced with such criticisms, many psychiatrists were determined to strengthen the scientific foundations of their practice and to achieve greater integration with the rest of medicine – a context that, I suggest, particularly exposed the profession to the influence of an increasingly powerful pharmaceutical industry.

Pharmaceutical treatments
One area of psychiatric practice where the industry's impact is highly visible is in the increasing use of psychoactive drugs. When considering this area it is helpful to divide these drugs into three broad groups – antipsychotics, minor tranquillisers and antidepressants.

a. Antipsychotics
The first use of chlorpromazine on psychiatric patients in France in 1952 was a turning point in psychiatry's history. It was not, of course, the first drug to be used to treat psychiatric problems. In the early twentieth century sedatives and barbiturates were used to calm and control individuals both inside and outside the asylum. However, chlorpromazine, synthesised by the French company Rhone-Poulenc, was quickly seen as having a more marked effect, particularly on inpatients given a diagnosis of schizophrenia, helping to reduce the symptoms, though there were severe side effects including involuntary (extrapyramidal) movements, which patients not surprisingly disliked. Its calming effects were first noted by a surgeon, Henri Laborit, who saw the drug's potential psychiatric value. Smith Kline & French secured the licence for its sale in the US not fully aware of its psychiatric potential. It was, however, soon being marketed across the country – sales representatives providing information and samples to psychiatrists, and

meeting with mental hospital administrators, making the case that the drug was highly cost-effective. The drug, branded as Largactil in Europe and Thorazine in the US, was soon widely used, despite its unpleasant side effects. Initially termed a 'neuroleptic' or 'major tranquilliser' in the 1960s, when other products like reserpine and haloperidol had come onto the market, the label 'antipsychotic' became common. The evidence indicated, however, that the drugs controlled symptoms but did not cure (Warner, 1985). Nonetheless, their use almost certainly facilitated the implementation of the major policy shift, envisaged in the 1950s, of moving psychiatric services away from mental hospitals.

In the mid-1990s when the earlier psychotics were out of patent, a new generation of 'atypical' antipsychotics without the same degree of extrapyramidal effects, but more expensive and profitable, began to be used. These included olanzapine (marketed as Zyprexa by Eli Lilly). Initially hailed as more effective than earlier antipsychotics and with fewer side effects, they require close monitoring of blood levels and any greater effectiveness is now highly contested (Jones et al., 2006). Antipsychotics, especially the atypical antipsychotics, though not approved for this purpose, are also widely prescribed off-licence for elderly patients with dementia (Haw, Yorston & Stubbs, 2009) – a controversial practice, that in the case of Zyprexa, Eli Lilly encouraged (Abraham, 2010). The extension of the market for antipsychotics in this way had clear commercial advantages and is one reason why they were one of the top product classes by revenue in 2010, despite the fact that epidemiological data show very clearly that psychotic disorders are not very common, though they are typically held to require long-term medication (see Robins & Regier, 1991; McManus et al., 2009). However, in Britain following a 2009 report for the Department of Health (Banerjee, 2009) there has been some effort to reduce the use of antipsychotics to subdue those with dementia.

b. Minor tranquillisers

In the 1950s, alongside chlorpromazine, new drugs to treat anxiety were also being introduced – a time when under the impact of Freudian ideas, anxiety neurosis was a frequent diagnosis for those with less severe mental health problems who came to medical attention. The first was meprobamate, whose calming properties were initially identified in 1950 by Frank Berger, a researcher at Wallace Laboratories in New Jersey, established by Carter Products, a small company previously concentrating on proprietary medicines. Testing of the drug on humans began in 1951 and after further trials approval was secured from the Food and Drug Agency (FDA) in 1955, and the drug was launched as a 'minor tranquilliser' (in contrast to the major tranquillisers like chlorpromazine) under the brand name Miltown. Wyeth, a far larger company with expertise in marketing, obtained a licence to sell it under the name Equanil. Miltown quickly and unexpectedly became fashionable (it gave a sense of subjective wellbeing and became known as the 'happy pill'), with Hollywood stars taking a lead (prescribed and illicit drugs were widely used in the film world) and for a while Miltown and Equanil were generating more profits than any other drug (Tone, 2009).

Two equally successful drugs soon followed, both developed by Leo Sternbach when working in the US laboratories of the Swiss company, Hoffman La Roche, who were keen to find a drug to match the success of Miltown. The first was a new chemical marketed as Librium (named from the last syllables of equilibrium), a benzodiazepine that had similar effects to meprobamate, but was more potent though less toxic and less of a sedative. Approved by the Food and Drug Administration in 1960, it quickly replaced Miltown and Equanil as the most frequently prescribed anxiolytic. The second was Valium, another benzodiazepine, released in 1963. It was more potent than Librium but without its unpleasant aftertaste; by 1968 its sales had overtaken those of Librium and until 1981 it generated more revenue than any other medication. Yet Librium still sold well and the total market for tranquillisers was increased (Tone, 2009). Initially the minor tranquillisers and other psychoactive drugs were often seen as facilitating psychotherapy, but the conflict model of psychological dynamics underpinning this view was increasingly replaced by a deficit model in which medication alone was regarded as sufficient treatment and there was no need to explore any psychodynamics (Ehrenberg, 2010). Some evidence of the addictive properties of minor tranquillisers had emerged in the early years (those of barbiturates were by then well known), but these were not systematically explored, and it was not until the 1970s that their habit-forming properties came to be well-recognised, and by the early 1980s sales had levelled.

c. Antidepressants

Severe depression in inpatients, then usually termed 'endogenous depression', was the target of the early drugs for depression. One, was imipramine, a tricyclic drug (reflecting its three-ringed chemical structure) produced by the Swiss company, Geigy, and initially tried out on patients who had been given a diagnosis of schizophrenia, as it had some similarities to the phenothiazines. Its antidepressant action was first noted by Roland Kuhn in Germany in 1955. However Geigy were hesitant about marketing it to treat depression, but when in 1961 three companies, Merck, Roche and Lundbeck, identified a similar triclyclic, amitryptaline, Merck marketed it heavily as an antidepressant. Another compound, iproniazid, developed by Hoffman la Roche and described as a 'psychic energiser', also began to be used to treat depressed patients from 1957. It was shown to inhibit the production of the enzyme monoamine oxidase and termed a MAOI to reflect its chemical action. In the late 1980s these drugs were joined by a new group of selective serotonin reuptake inhibitors for less severe depression, of which the best known is Prozac, developed by Eli Lilly. Prozac, like the earlier Librium and Valium, attracted enormous attention and came to be viewed as another 'happiness pill'. The SSRIs are very extensively used, yet the evidence suggests that antidepressants, irrespective of type, are only marginally more effective than placebos (Kirsch, 2009).

Psychoactive medications are now widely prescribed and play a dominant role in psychiatric practice. As early as the 1990s a study of mental health service users in Britain found some 98.6 per cent reported having been treated with psychoactive drugs, and 85 per cent had had continuous drug treatment for at least a year (Rogers, Pilgrim & Lacey, 1993). Their widespread use is reflected in the fact that antipsychotics and antidepressants feature in the classes of medicines that generate the highest global revenues, and their use is still increasing. In England, for example, some 8.5 million prescriptions for antipsychotics were issued outside hospital in 2009 compared with 5.6 million 10 years previously – a 52 per cent increase. The corresponding figures for antidepressants were 39.1 million in 2009 and 20.1 million in 1999 – a near doubling in 10 years (NHS Information Centre, 2010; Department of Health, 2000). It is hard to avoid the conclusion that the pharmaceutical industry has played a major role in making psychoactive drugs *the* standard treatment for mental disorder, even though other treatments are also used and sometimes emphasised – for instance, the British Department of Health's policy, introduced in 2007, to improve access to psychological therapies.

Biochemical understandings
The second area where the pharmaceutical industry has had a major impact on psychiatry is in contributing to the dominance of biological explanations

of mental disorder, and the frequent exclusion of alternatives. Psychiatry has a long history of asserting both that insanity is inherited and that the causes of mental disorders are to be found in brain processes, though such ideas have often co-existed with a strong emphasis on the role of social or psychological processes. However, the increasing use of psychoactive medications from the mid-1950s onwards strengthened the search for biochemical causes and contributed to the biological turn in psychiatry in the 1970s. This biological focus was reflected in, and reinforced by, the third edition of the American Psychiatric Association's *Diagnostic and Statistical Manual of Mental Disorders (DSM-III)* (APA, 1980), which largely eschewed the psychoanalytic thinking that had been dominant, with responsiveness to specific drugs serving as one factor determining whether a condition was included (Lane, 2007, p. 75). Indeed, the effect of specific drugs on particular mental states was increasingly treated as the main evidence for the view that biochemical factors were the key causes of that disorder. Consequently the task was to determine how individual drugs affect brain processes, and to use this understanding as the basis for identifying the causes of each disorder.

As Joanna Moncrieff (2009) has argued, this involved an important shift in thinking about the drugs themselves. Initially psychoactive medicines tended to be viewed in terms of their general effects – so, for example, they were grouped together as sedatives, or major or minor tranquillisers. The focus was on the general effects of the drug – a drug-specific model. However, a more disease-specific model became common in which psychoactive drugs were seen as acting on particular disorders, reflected in the increasing use of the disease-specific terms – antidepressant and antipsychotic. We can see this change in the case of chlorpromazine, where the view that the drug inhibited dopamine production – dopamine is an important neurotransmitter carrying nerve signals within the brain – underpinned the theory that schizophrenia resulted from the over-stimulation of dopamine receptors in the brain. The thinking is captured in Figure 1.

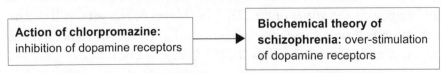

Figure 1. Chlorpromazine and the dopamine theory of schizophrenia

A number of authors have argued, however, that the evidence supporting the dopamine theory is poor, consisting of little more than the fact that the drugs act on dopamine receptors (Moncrieff, 2009). There has been a similar trajectory in relation to the SSRIs used to treat depression. Here the description of the mode of action incorporated in the label for the drugs rapidly becomes the explanation of the condition, even though some antidepressants *enhance* the reuptake of serotonin (Kirsch, 2009).

In a similar way that alternative treatments to drugs have often been sidelined, so too have alternative explanations, and since the introduction of the 1980 *DSM-III* there has been far less research on the role of social and psychological factors than on biochemical processes. The extent to which the widespread use of psychoactive treatments has encouraged the focus on brain processes is reflected in the changes in the language used in the field. There is increasing talk of neuropsychiatry and neuropsychopharmacology, and even depression, long considered largely to have social and psychological causes, being described as a brain disease (Nutt & Goodwin, 2011). This 'neuromania' (Tallis, 2011) results from the primacy given to biological processes even though it is clear that explanatory pluralism (Kendler, 2005) is needed, and that biological factors are often not the key causes – the factors that make a difference. Clearly neurochemical processes are involved, but mostly they do not adequately explain the occurrence of the mental states and behaviour in question such as sadness, fear, anxiety or being deluded. For that we need to turn to psychological and above all social factors, including the social conditions and events in people's lives.

Expanding the boundaries of mental disorder

The third way in which the pharmaceutical industry has influenced ideas and practices is by encouraging the extension of the boundaries of mental disorder. We can see the expansion most clearly in the number of diagnostic categories, in 1952 there were 109 in the *DSM-I*, by 1980 this figure had risen to 265 diagnostic categories in the *DSM-III* and by 1994 there were 297 diagnostic categories in the *DSM-IV* (Mayes & Horwitz, 2005). The expansion will almost certainly be continued in the *DSM-5* since a range of new disorders is already proposed (APA, 2011). The industry is not the only influence on the expansion – for example, psychoanalytic ideas emphasising the continuity of the normal and abnormal have played a part. Equally, US health insurance companies have helped to widen the boundaries by insisting on a clear psychiatric diagnosis if mental health care is to be covered by their policy. Further, clinicians have been keen to ensure that the categories extend to the full range of mental health problems they encounter in their everyday practice. However, pharmaceutical companies have also played a major role. We can see this if we examine some of the additions to the *DSM* in the later editions. These largely arise from the process of subdivision that creates new disorders, and from the inclusion of entirely new disorders.

One example is the differentiation of panic disorder from anxiety. In the first two editions of the *DSM* there was a single category, anxiety neurosis, which could include panic symptoms. The 1968 *DSM-II* delineated the condition like this:

> This neurosis is characterized by anxious over-concern extending to panic and frequently associated with somatic symptoms. Unlike *Phobic neurosis* (q.v.), anxiety may occur under any circumstances and is not restricted to specific situations or objects. This disorder must be distinguished from normal apprehension or fear, which occurs in realistically dangerous situations. (APA, 1968, p. 39)

The closest *DSM-III* equivalent is generalized anxiety disorder (GAD), described as follows:

> The essential feature is generalized, persistent anxiety of at least one month's duration without the specific symptoms that characterize Phobic Disorders (phobias), Panic Disorder (panic attacks), or Obsessive-Compulsive Disorder (obsessions or compulsions). The diagnosis is not made if the disturbance is due to another physical or mental disorder, such as hyperthyroidism or Major Depression.
>
> Although the specific manifestations of the anxiety vary from individual to individual, generally there are signs of motor tension, autonomic hyperactivity, apprehensive expectation, and vigilance and scanning. (APA, 1980, p. 232)

Here panic is not included in the symptom list, having become a disorder in its own right. The description of panic disorder begins:

> The essential features are recurrent panic (anxiety) attacks that occur at times unpredictably, though certain situations, e.g., driving a car, may become associated with a panic attack. The same clinical picture

occurring during marked physical exertion or a life-threatening
situation is not termed a panic attack. (APA, 1980, p. 230)

After then describing the character of panic attacks, the next paragraph
ends 'Attacks usually last minutes; more rarely hours' (ibid.). The *DSM*
accepts therefore that panic is a form of anxiety, contrasting the two
disorders largely in terms of the duration and intensity of anxiety. GAD
requires generalised, persistent anxiety, whereas, panic attacks are more
intense but episodic, though the criteria for panic disorder require at least
three attacks within a three-week period.

But why was panic separated out from more diffuse anxiety creating
two disorders instead of one? The first paper arguing for the existence of a
distinct group of patients with severe panic attacks was published by US
psychiatrist, Donald Klein, in 1964. It put pharmaceuticals centre stage,
focusing on the responses of a group of hospitalised patients with panic
attacks to drugs – in particular the antidepressant, imipramine. The study
was supported by two companies, Geigy which had developed imipramine,
and Smith Kline & French which had the US licence for chlorpromazine.
Klein argued that whereas patients with panic attacks had not responded
to psychotherapy, electroconvulsive therapy (ECT) or sedatives, and did
not respond to phenothiazines like chlorpromazine, they did show
improvement when treated with imipramine. He further argued that the
varying responses to drugs were valuable as 'dissecting tools' within
psychiatric subpopulations, though he distinguished two subgroups in his
sample on the basis of precipitating factors.

Klein's concentration on drug responses was clearly valuable to the
industry looking for new markets for their drugs. Moreover, he argued
that 'chronic use of "antidepressant medication" may be of prophylactic
value and that medication termination is often followed by symptomatic
exacerbation' (1964, p. 407), so indicating the potential need for long-
term treatment. His results were further supported by research at Harvard
in the 1970s that helped to legitimise the idea of panic disorder (Healy,
1997). Importantly, Klein later became a member of both the *DSM-III*
task force and the subgroup working on anxiety disorders and so was in a
position to help secure the disorder's inclusion. The pharmaceutical
company, Upjohn (later part of Pharmacia and then Pfizer), which had
developed a new benzodiazepine, Xanax, that had some antidepressant
properties, and was seeking to identify a market for it, then proceeded to

publicise it specifically as a treatment for panic disorder. This was at a time when the market for benzodiazepines was declining because of the problems of dependence and addiction. The company also funded trials to establish that panic disorder was a distinct disorder that could be treated by Xanax. However, though 'The results were not entirely convincing', the new disorder was widely identified and Xanax frequently prescribed: 'Among insiders, panic jokingly became "the Upjohn illness"' (Shorter, 1997, p. 320).

Of course it could be argued that the differentiation of panic disorder and GAD simply added a greater degree of precision to psychiatric classification, but that there was no overall extension of boundaries. However, not only is the empirical evidence for such distinctions often weak (Kirk & Kutchins, 1992), but adding new categories makes it more likely that particular psychological states will be viewed as pathological. In this case, for instance, panic was no longer a symptom of other anxiety disorders, and GAD was constructed rather broadly and loosely.

The impact of differentiation on diagnostic boundaries can be seen especially clearly with the addition in the 1980 *DSM-III* of social phobia as a separate disorder, given a further label, social anxiety disorder, in the 1994 *DSM-IV*. In the *DSM-II* a single category of phobic neurosis was described like this:

> This condition is characterized by intense fear of an object or situation which the patient consciously recognizes as no real danger to him. His apprehension may be experienced as faintness, fatigue, palpitations, perspiration, nausea, tremor, and even panic. Phobias are generally attributed to fears displaced to the phobic object or situation from some other object of which the patient is unaware. A wide range of phobias have been described. (APA, 1968, p. 40)

However, Isaac Marks, a Maudsley psychiatrist, had begun to categorise the phobias he encountered, suggesting that those prompted by external stimuli fell into four groups: agoraphobia, social phobias, animal phobias, and other specific phobias (Marks & Gelder, 1964; Marks, 1970). Yet he also asserted 'We need to know more about social phobics before definitely classifying them on their own' (1970, p. 383), adding 'evidence is lacking that this is a coherent group' (1970, p. 386).

Other psychiatrists supported this important qualification; nonetheless the idea of subdividing phobias was picked up by the *DSM* task force, apparently to Marks' consternation (Lane, 2007, p. 79). One reason was that Robert Spitzer, the psychiatrist who headed the task force, was keen to abandon the concept of anxiety neurosis because of its psychoanalytic connotations, and breaking it up into several disorders provided a means of doing this. And adding social phobia as a distinct disorder was also easier once it was decided to include panic disorder as a separate condition. The *DSM-III* description of social phobia began:

> The essential feature is a persistent, irrational fear of, and compelling desire to avoid, situations in which the individual may be exposed to scrutiny by others. There is also a persistent, irrational fear that the individual may behave in a manner that will be humiliating or embarrassing. (APA, 1980, p. 227)

Once social phobia was included there began to be reports that a MAOI antidepressant, phenelzine (Nardil), developed by Parke-Davis, was useful for its treatment, and having a treatment for the new disorder encouraged psychiatrists to diagnose it more frequently and its boundaries expanded. Indeed the 1987 revision of the *DSM-III* specifically loosened the criteria by cutting out the key term 'irrational'. Not surprisingly whereas social phobia was initially seen as a rare condition, by 2000 it was being described as very common (Lane, 1997, p. 100). This type of loosening of diagnostic criteria has occurred elsewhere – most obviously with post-traumatic stress disorder where the 1994 *DSM-IV* no longer required an individual to have directly experienced a traumatic event, but need only have been 'confronted' with one (Rosen, Spitzer & McHugh, 2008). The result is the potential domain of psychiatry is expanded.

An example of the introduction of a group of new disorders is provided by the inclusion in the 1980 *DSM-III* of a set of sexual dysfunctions. The first *DSM* in 1952 had a single category of sexual deviation mentioning a number of types such as homosexuality, transvestism and paedophilia. The 1968 *DSM-II* listed each separately – eight plus a residual 'other' category – an instance of subdivision. However the *DSM-III*, under the broader heading of psychosexual disorders, added an entirely new group of seven sexual dysfunctions, such as 'inhibited sexual desire' and 'inhibited sexual excitement', plus a residual 'atypical' category. Such atypical or 'not otherwise specified' (NOS) categories usually have looser criteria and so further broaden the boundaries of mental disorder. A number of factors underpinned the addition of sexual dysfunctions to the *DSM*, including

Masters and Johnson's (1970) work on sexual inadequacy and the growth of sex therapy – an instance of how clinicians' interests have helped to expand the range of disorders. However, while initially the typical treatment was some form of psychotherapy, since the late 1990s the pharmaceutical industry has responded with new drugs, notably Pfizer's Viagra in 1998, and in so doing have increased the use of the new categories and widened their boundaries (Moynihan, 2003).

Whilst it can be argued that this widening of the boundaries of mental illness helps to enable those with mental health problems to get the treatment they may need, equally it can be argued that it facilitates the pathologisation of individuals, locating the problem within them, and helping to ensure that the social and environmental factors that often give rise to their mental states and behaviour are largely ignored.

Conclusion

I have argued in this chapter that the pharmaceutical industry has had a profound, but highly questionable effect on the understandings and practices of mental health professionals. The industry has had an impact in three related areas: in the increased use of pharmaceutical treatments for mental health problems and the sidelining of alternatives; in the increased emphasis on biological understandings of mental disorder to the exclusion of other accounts; and in the widening of the boundaries of disorder so that an ever-increasing number of individuals are held to be mentally ill, and their social problems disregarded. By these means the industry has supported and strengthened the biological bias of psychiatry, pushing alternative treatments and explanations aside, and has also helped to widen the boundaries of mental disorder, so expanding psychiatry's potential domain. These changes have undoubtedly helped to sustain psychiatry's position as the leading profession within the mental health field. Nonetheless its position is by no means entirely secure (Pilgrim & Rogers, 2009), and it faces attacks both on the value of its ideas and practices, including the effectiveness of its treatments, and competition from other mental health professionals, often with very different approaches.

References

Abraham, J. (2010). Pharmaceuticalization of society in context: Theoretical, empirical and health dimensions. *Sociology, 44,* 603–622.

Angell, M. (2005). *The Truth about the Drug Companies.* New York: Random House.

APA. (1968). *Diagnostic and Statistical Manual of Mental Disorders* (2nd ed.) (*DSM-II*). Washington, DC: American Psychiatric Association.

APA. (1980). *Diagnostic and Statistical Manual of Mental Disorders* (3rd ed.) (*DSM-III*). Washington, DC: American Psychiatric Association.

APA. (2011). DSM-5: The future of psychiatric diagnosis. Retrieved 11 August 2011 from, www.dsm5.org/Pages/Default.aspx

Banerjee, S. (2009). *The Use of Antipsychotic Medication for People with Dementia: Time for action.* London: Department of Health.

Busfield, J. (2006). Pills, power, people: Sociological understandings of the pharmaceutical industry. *Sociology, 40,* 297–314.

Curtiss, F. R., & Fairman, K. A. (2010). Tough questions about the value of statin therapy for primary prevention. *Journal of Managed Care Pharmacy, 16,* 417–423.

Department of Health. (2000). Prescriptions dispensed in the community, statistics for 1989 to 2000: England. *Statistical Bulletin 2000/20.* London: Department of Health.

Ehrenberg, A. (2010). *The Weariness of Self.* Montreal: McGill-Queens University Press.

Gagnon, M-A., & Lexchin, J. (2008). The cost of pushing pills. *PLoS Medicine 5,* 29–33.

GlaxoSmithKline (2010). *Annual Report 2010.* Retrieved 31 October 2011 from, www.gsk.com/investors/reps10/GSK-Annual-Report-2010.pdf

Goffman, E. (1961). *Asylums.* New York: Doubleday.

Goozner, M. (2004). *The $800 Million Pill: The truth behind the cost of new drugs.* Berkeley, CA: University of California Press.

Haw, C., Yorston, G., & Stubbs, J. (2009). Guidelines on antipsychotics for dementia: Are we losing our minds? *Psychiatric Bulletin, 33,* 57–60.

Healy, D. (1997). *The Anti-depressant Era.* Cambridge, MA: Harvard University Press.

IMS Health. (2011). *World Pharmaceutical Market Summary, June 2011.* Norwalk, CT: IMS Health.

IMS Health Midas. (2010). *Top 20 Global Corporations, 2010, Total Audited Markets.* Retrieved 6 July 2011 from, www.imshealth.com/.../imshealth/Global/.../Top_20_Global_Companies.pdf

Jones, P. B., Barnes, T. R. E., Davies, L., et al. (2006). Randomized controlled trial of the effect on quality of life of second- vs first-generation antipsychotic drugs in schizophrenia. *Archives of General Psychiatry, 63,* 1079–1087.

Katz, D., Caplan, A. L., & Merz, J. F. (2003). All gifts large and small: Towards an understanding of the ethics of pharmaceutical industry gift giving. *American Journal of Bioethics, 3,* 39–46.

Kendler, K. S. (2005). Toward a philosophical structure for psychiatry. *American Journal of Psychiatry, 162,* 433–440.

Kirk, S. A., & Kutchins, H. (1992). *The Selling of DSM.* New York: Aldine.

Kirsch, I. (2009). *The Emperor's New Drugs: Exploding the antidepressant myth.* London: Bodley Head.

Kjaegard, L. L., & Als-Nielson, B. (2002). Association between competing interests and authors' conclusions. *BMJ, 325,* 249–252.

Klein, D. (1964). Delineation of two drug-responsive anxiety syndromes. *Psychopharmacologia, 5,* 397–408.

Laing, R. D. (1967). *The Politics of Experience and the Bird of Paradise.* Harmondsworth: Penguin.

Lane, C. (2007). *Shyness: How normal behavior became a sickness.* New Haven, CT: Yale University Press.

Mann, M. (1993). *The Sources of Social Power* (Vol. II). Cambridge: Cambridge University Press.

Marks, I. M. (1970). The classification of phobic disorders. *British Journal of Psychiatry, 116,* 377–386.

Marks, I. M., & Gelder, M. G. (1964). Different ages of onset in varieties of phobia. *American Journal of Psychiatry, 123,* 218–221.

Masters, W., & Johnson, V. (1970). *Human Sexual Inadequacy.* New York: Little Brown.

Mayes, R., & Horwitz, A. V. (2005). *DSM-III* and the revolution in the classification of mental illness. *Journal of the History of the Behavioral Sciences, 41,* 249–267.

McManus, S., Meltzer, H., Brudh, T., et al. (2009). *Adult Psychiatric Morbidity in England, 2007.* London: NHS Information Centre.

Moncrieff, J. (2009). *The Myth of the Chemical Cure* (rev. ed.). London: Palgrave.

Moynihan, R. (2003). The making of a disease: Female sexual dysfunction. *BMJ, 326,* 45–47.

NHS Information Centre. (2010). *Prescriptions Dispensed in the Community: England, statistics for 1999 to 2009.* London: Health and Social Care Information Centre.

Nutt, D., & Goodwin, G. (2011). ECNP summit on the future of CNS drug research in Europe 2011. *European Neuropsychopharmacology, 21,* 495–499.

Pilgrim, D., & Rogers, A. (2009). Survival and its discontents: The case of British psychiatry. *Sociology of Health and Illness, 31,* 947–961.

Robins, L. N., & Regier, D. A. (Eds.). (1991). *Psychiatric Disorders in America: The epidemiologic catchment area study.* New York: Free Press.

Rogers, A., Pilgrim, D., & Lacey, R. (1993). *Experiencing Psychiatry.* London: Macmillan.

Rosen, G. M., Spitzer, R. L., & McHugh, P. R. (2008). Problems with the post-traumatic disorder diagnosis and its future in the *DSM-V*. *British Journal of Psychiatry, 192,* 3–4.

Scheff, T. J. (1966). *Being Mentally Ill.* London: Weidenfeld & Nicholson.

Shorter, E. (1997). *A History of Psychiatry.* New York: John Wiley.

Szasz, T. S. (1961). The myth of mental illness. *American Psychologist. 15,* 113–118.

Tallis, R. (2011). *Aping Mankind: Neuromania, Darwinitis and the misrepresentation of humanity.* Durham: Acumen.

Tone, A. (2009). *The Age of Anxiety: A history of America's turbulent affair with tranquilizers.* New York: Basic Books.

Warner, R. (1985). *Recovery from Schizophrenia.* London: Routledge & Kegan Paul.

WHO. (2004). *The World Medicines Situation.* Geneva: World Health Organization.

Chapter 7

Clinical Psychology in Psychiatric Services: The magician's assistant?

Steven Coles, Bob Diamond & Sarah Keenan

… there is a point at which dissenters from the orthodoxy are told not only that they are wrong, but that such views should not be held or expressed at all. (Johnstone, 1993, p. 32)

As clinical psychologists working in what are predominantly psychiatric services, we observe the obscuring of people's history and context behind psychiatric taxonomies and labels such as 'schizophrenia'. We've witnessed the massive investments by the Department of Health in psychological therapies (DH, 2001) and there are plans to extend cognitive behavioural-oriented therapies to all groups from 2011/12, including people being labelled with diagnoses such as psychosis, bipolar and personality disorders (DH, 2011). Despite our concerns over the efficacy of therapy (Epstein, 2006; Hubble, Duncan & Miller, 2005; Moloney, 2006), we have wondered whether additional investment in talking approaches could go some way to counter the present preoccupation with individual pathology and help reveal the real difficulties people face? Unfortunately, our analysis highlights how clinical psychology and therapy can equally mask the importance of context in people's distress. This chapter explores how psychiatry uses the biogenetic model to attempt to vanish the social, material and historical causes of distress. We also consider how psychology's preoccupation with individualistic explanations and cognitive behavioural approaches assist this enchantment. This leaves us with the crucial question: If we are far from convinced about the usefulness of therapy and do not wish to partake in the magic show, what should clinical psychologists be doing and advocating? The latter part of the chapter details some practical attempts to answer this question.

This chapter is a revised and updated version of the article: Coles, S., Diamond, B., & Keenan, S. (2009). Clinical psychology in psychiatric services: The magician's assistant? *Clinical Psychology Forum, 198,* 5–10.

Obscuring the context in the psychiatric system

Within psychiatric services the people we work with often live within difficult social and economic contexts and it is those difficult historical and current circumstances that are causally related to their distress (Meltzer et al., 2002; Miller & McClelland, 2006). People who use services usually have little power and few resources in their immediate world. We believe that supporting people to access these proximal powers and resources is essential to their wellbeing (Hagan & Smail, 1997). However, the services we work within view these difficult social circumstances as the consequence of a genetic, biological and diagnosable illness. This is despite the fact that psychiatric diagnoses, such as schizophrenia, are meaningless constructs (Boyle, 1999) and genetic adoption and twin research have multiple flaws in terms of methodology and assumptions (Joseph, 2003; Marshall, 1990). Therefore these difficult circumstances and lack of power are obscured from view from the general public, the minds of mental health professionals and even the people who come into contact with services (whether intentional or not is another matter). The social circumstances of the individual might be acknowledged, but often as a secondary concern.

Boyle (2007) and Pilgrim (2007) have raised the point that the question of whether or not the diagnosis of 'schizophrenia' is meaningful or 'exists' no longer needs to be answered – it doesn't; the question we should be asking is why does the concept persist? Boyle (2002) has perceptively detailed some of the rhetoric and discourse that privileges biology and helps create the illusion of 'schizophrenia' as a brain disorder. Another and related type of answer is to consider in whose *interest* it is for the individualised explanations and treatments of distress to flourish? Perhaps the answer is too easy, but it seems the proximal winners to an individualised notion of distress are the professional 'experts' in mental illness. Pilgrim (1991) has noted that clinical psychology and psychiatry need to have individualised causes and treatments to help justify their role, status and related financial rewards. Pilgrim (2007) highlights a complex web of interests that have helped maintain the survival of psychiatric diagnosis, such as politicians, media, the pharmaceutical industry, recipients of services, their relatives, the professional interest of psychiatry and the growth business of clinical psychology. This is not to deny 'critical' elements in these groups, but emphasises that concepts do not persist simply because of their scientific integrity or virtue (Smail, 2005). The perpetuation of such unsubstantiated concepts and practices are important in creating an illusion of a mysterious expertise that is carefully controlled, maintained and performed by mental health professionals.

Within psychiatric services it is often considered vital to work against the common-sense view of the world, which has always told us that distress occurs because people have difficult lives, and instead mystifies the process by turning people's experiences into a disease process. Indeed it seems that this ability to turn experiences into disease is often seen as a sign of successful professional training. This process leads to a system which neatly justifies enforcing major tranquillisers to the point where people can no longer think or feel, and it denies them their liberty as a part of a cure for their 'mental illness'. Harper (2001) summarises the limitations of the biomedical model as too narrow, individualistic, self-serving and impoverished of meaningful information. He advocates us to 'have the courage of our convictions and refuse to traffic in these terms' (p. 25).

Beyond maintenance of professional interest, there are other forces that perhaps help maintain the individualised explanation of distress and behaviour. For example, currently, in a highly individualistic Western society with an ever-increasing gap between richest and poorest (Wilkinson & Pickett, 2009) and a neo-liberal culture of 'people obtain what they deserve' (by implication the undeserving get what they 'deserve'), societal explanations are not being sown on fertile ground. It seems it is more comfortable for professionals to understand distress as relating to faulty individuals, rather than accepting the implication that the society we are part of is at the root of people's distress and difficulties. Services often genuinely want to help those they witness as distressed; however a societal understanding may leave them feeling unable to help, whereas biomedical understandings provide an alluringly simple framework and cure. Further, government and society have handed over to psychiatry the role of deciding whether people should be excluded from wider society due to perceived threat. This is often in the form of coercion and enforced sedation in the name of 'medical treatment' (see Rogers and Pilgrim, 2010, for further discussion). However, it is debatable whether clinical psychology would perform any better in this role of social arbitrator.

The rise of CBT and psychology: The saviour of context?

Given the severe limitations of an individualised biological notion of distress, we perhaps should applaud the interest shown in psychological ideas and support. However, any meaningful discussion of psychological thinking is currently strangulated by a preoccupation with cognitive behavioural therapy (CBT). Biogenetic explanations are based on diagnosis, the problem residing in the individual (therefore minimisation of context) and faulty neurones, whereas cognitive explanations are based on the continuation of diagnosis, the problem being within the individual (therefore minimisation of context), and faulty cognitions. Now that's a hard 'spot the difference' and perhaps why the Royal College of Psychiatrists is so keen to embrace CBT (RCPsych, 2008).

As clinical psychologists we have a responsibility to question an approach that is promoted as a universal panacea to psychological distress. There are a few key points worthy of consideration (see Epstein, 2006, for a more thorough examination). First, when different psychotherapeutic approaches are compared, the idea that any one (or more) therapeutic model would prove superior to others receives extremely limited support. Further, relationship and non-specific factors in therapeutic encounters appear to be the most important component of therapy (Bergin & Garfield, 1994; Hubble et al., 2005). Research that compares professionals and amateurs suggests that there are few real differences between them in effectiveness (Berman & Norton, 1985; Moloney, 2006). So if we do not need expert and technique-driven therapists, but perhaps people with empathy and interpersonal skills, why is there such a drive for expertise? Again to answer this, we need to consider in whose interest it is to control the access to 'expert' CBT knowledge and training. At this stage there are several mental health professions in competition for this powerbase, including cognitive behavioural therapists, clinical psychologists and psychiatrists (Midlands Psychology Group, 2007, 2008, has raised concerns over such issues). The confirmed loser in this battlefield is the service user whose context is obscured and cognitions challenged.

Clinical psychology rightfully needs to make sense of individual subjectivity. The mistake that much of psychology makes is not moving beyond the individual in its search for explanations (Smail, 1993). Subjectivity, behaviour and distress can only be properly understood by reference to the powerful socio-political forces that shape individuals

(Cromby, 2005; Smail, 1993). Whilst acknowledging critical perspectives in the profession, the ideology of business appears to have penetrated psychology so far that it has abandoned ideas of social justice and intellectual integrity, and instead pursues professional interest at any cost (Dineen, 1999; Rapley, 2003). These flaws appear to be reflected in much of clinical training and undergraduate psychology teaching, where social explanations and critical/questioning perspectives are not embedded (Cromby, Harper & Reavey, 2008; Prilleltensky & Nelson, 2002). Overall, the cult of corporate values and individualism within psychology means that its rise is unlikely to lead to fundamental change within mental health services.

Revealing

Given these powerful systems that obscure the social, material and historical reality of people's lives, how do clinical psychologists, who are mindful of the social and historical contexts of distress, help to positively influence this system? Due to the vested interests in maintaining the system status quo (Dineen, 1999; Prilleltensky, 1989; Sampson, 1993), including our own profession, it may feel difficult to mount a constructive challenge. Whilst there might be overwhelming powers we have little control over, we can look at what is within our own domain of influence. We have been investing our time in projects that we hope begin to reveal some of the social, material and historical contexts that are often obscured. Excellent examples of similar initiatives can be seen in Newnes, Holmes and Dunn (1999, 2001). We do not see the following developments as particularly new, nor do we consider that such projects will radically influence services. Nonetheless, it is our view that this development work should be within the domain of clinical psychology. This requires the profession to move outside the clinic, which it seems to have occupied with pride in recent years. These initiatives are not always seen as legitimate work given the drive for recorded contacts, interventions and psychology being seen as synonymous with therapy.

Given the dominance of an individualised understanding of distress (Johnstone, 2000; Rapley, 2003) and the obscuring of context, we have tried to publicise and highlight alternative understandings of suffering. One formal mechanism for this is the publication of *Clinical Psychology Bite-Size* within the Nottinghamshire Healthcare NHS Trust, which is received by all members of staff in adult mental health services. *Bite-Size* is a monthly two-page readable summary of psychological and social topics highlighting key research, theory and implications for practice. At the time of writing there are 32 *Bite-Size* articles. Topics have included making sense of paranoia and understanding voices and 'delusions' (Coles & Cromby, 2009; Coles, 2009; Collinson, 2008), which draw upon psychological research and literature around models of madness (Cromby & Harper, 2009; Newnes et al, 1999, 2001; Rapley, Moncrieff & Dillon, 2011; Read, Mosher & Bentall, 2004). *Bite-Size* has also covered topics on alternative ways of working, such as supportive conversations, deconstruction of CBT and alternatives to challenging beliefs (Diamond & Coles, 2010; Houghton, 2009; Coles, 2011). With such articles we have tried to remove the technical mystique that many psychological approaches come packaged with, and have attempted to make such ideas open and accessible to all staff. We see it as essential that psychologists working in psychiatric systems have a critical and questioning perspective regarding the values and practice that dominate mental health services and psychology, so literature by critical psychiatrists, psychologists and recipients of services is invaluable (e.g., Bracken & Thomas, 2005; Campbell et al., 2006; Diamond, 2008; Johnstone, 2000; Moncrieff, 2008; Sayce, 2000). We embed a critical perspective within *Bite-Size* publications, whilst also trying to engage a wide audience. Whilst we believe our profession can contribute to obscuring and individualising people's experiences, we also believe it has much to offer in terms of explanations of human despair, which should be shared with colleagues.

We provide substantive support and supervision to staff and teams; this involves individual supervision, and the majority of teams receive monthly group/team supervision. Recently we introduced a social, historical and psychological formulation protocol in supervision as a means of encouraging discussion beyond individual and psychiatric factors. Conducting these formulations with care coordinators allows us to ask questions and hold conversations that highlight the importance of a person's history and social circumstances and minimise the obscuring influence of the focus on symptoms, distorted cognitions and diagnosis. Such conversations can require interpersonal sensitivity to avoid staff feeling shamed for knowing little of a client's history (despite often working with them for many years). However, these formulations at times appear to have a short life in people's memories and it can often be disheartening but also predictable, given the dominant biomedical narrative, that many staff resort to individualising distress, particularly in meetings or completing paperwork that support a focus on 'individual pathology'.

One way of exposing some of the iatrogenic effects of the power imbalances and problematic practices within the psychiatric system is to provide a public space to openly debate such issues. To this end we have held a series of debates on topics such as CBT, risk, coercion, diagnosis and survivor knowledge (Keenan & Coles, 2012). We have tried to create a space where different ideas could be shared, discussed and critiqued. The debates were immensely popular, attracting a range of staff, survivors and service users as debaters and audience members. By having debaters provide polarised perspectives on a topic, a space was created for the audience to share, discuss and critique a diversity of ideas and opinions. This openness felt very different to the oppressive dominance of expert and individualistic ideas in day-to-day practice.

For a number of years our department encouraged and facilitated people with experiences of using services to be more vocal and active within and beyond their contact with services (Diamond, 1998, Diamond et al., 2003; Houghton, Shaw, Hayward & West, 2006). Historically, psychology has helped establish self-help groups on topics such as hearing voices and alternatives to medication (see Chapter 16 by Nottingham Mind Medication Group). The voice of people who use services and their expressed needs are often marginalised through professional discourse. In an attempt to redress this imbalance a self-assessment form, 'Meeting Your Needs', was developed in collaboration with several voluntary groups and is now incorporated as a standard part of the care programme approach. We believe that it is crucial to embed a service user-led and critical approach into our work within the psychiatric system.

We are part of a magical system that seeks to make the context and causes of distress disappear. Reality is obscured through the illusions of illness, diagnoses, 'cognitive distortions' and treatment, while psychiatry continues to conjure its white rabbit – the chemical cure. To avoid being assistants to this tawdry show it appears that the least we can do is to question how the tricks are done, perhaps heckle and to ask for a different type of act. Unfortunately, clinical psychology appears to have cheered another type of conjuror and has an eye on the magician's cape. Perhaps we should be encouraging people to demand their money back, or simply, walk out of the theatre?

References

Bergin, A., & Garfield, S. (1994). *Handbook of Psychotherapy and Behaviour Change.* New York: John Wiley.

Berman, J. S., & Norton, N. C. (1985). Does professional training make a therapist more effective? *Psychological Bulletin, 98,* 401–407.

Boyle, M. (1999). Diagnosis. In C. Newnes, C. Dunn & G. Holmes (Eds.), *This is Madness: A critical look at psychiatry and the future of mental health services* (pp. 75–90). Ross-on-Wye: PCCS Books.

Boyle, M. (2002). It's all done with smoke and mirrors. Or, how to create the illusion of a schizophrenic brain disease. *Clinical Psychology, 12,* 9–16.

Boyle, M. (2007). The problem with diagnosis. *The Psychologist, 20*(5), 290–292.

Bracken, P., & Thomas, P. (2005). *Postpsychiatry.* Oxford: Oxford University Press.

Campbell, P., Coldham, T., Coleman, R., Crepaz-Keay, D., Hart, L., Ingram, C., Linton-Abulu, A., Main, L., May, R., Read, J., Relton, P. & Wallcraft, J. (2006). Service user voices. *Openmind* (September/October), *141,* 8–13.

Coles, S. (2009). Understanding voices. *CPBS, 12,* 1–2.

Coles, S. (2011). An alternative to challenging unusual beliefs. *CPBS, 29,* 1–2.

Coles, S., & Cromby, J. (2009). Making sense of paranoia. *CPBS, 17,* 1–2.

Collinson, C. (2008). Understanding 'delusions'. *CPBS, 5,* 1–2.

Cromby, J. (2005). Theorising embodied subjectivity. *International Journal of Critical Psychology, 15,* 133–150.

Cromby, J., & Harper, D. (2009). Paranoia: A social account. *Theory and Psychology, 19*(3), 335–361.

Cromby, J., Harper, D., & Reavey, P. (2008). Mental health teaching to UK psychology undergraduates: Report of a survey. *Journal of Community and Applied Social Psychology, 18,* 83–90.

Department of Health. (2001). *Treatment Choice in Psychological Therapies and Counselling.* London: HMSO.

Department of Health. (2011). *Talking Therapies: A four year plan of action.* London: HMSO.

Diamond, B. (1998). Stepping outside and not knowing: Community psychology and enduring mental health problems. *Clinical Psychology Forum, 12,* 40–42.

Diamond, B. (2008). Opening up space for dissension: A questioning psychology. In A. Morgan (Ed.), *Being Human: Reflections on mental distress in society* (pp. 174–189). Ross-on-Wye: PCCS Books.

Diamond, B., & Coles, S. (2010). Contextualising distress III: *Therapeutic Conversations, 22,* 1–2.

Diamond, B., Parkin, G., Morris, K., Bettinis, J., & Bettesworth, C. (2003). User involvement: Substance or spin? *Journal of Mental Health, 12,* 613–626.

Dineen, T. (1999). *Manufacturing Victims: What the psychology industry is doing to people.* London: Constable.

Epstein, W. (2006). *Psychotherapy as Religion: The civil divine in America.* Reno, NV: University of Nevada Press.

Hagan, T., & Smail, D. (1997). Power-mapping – I: Background and basic methodology. *Journal of Community and Applied Social Psychology, 7,* 257–267.

Harper, D. (2001). Psychiatric and psychological concepts in understanding psychotic experience. *Clinical Psychology, 7,* 21–27.

Houghton, P. (2009). CBT for psychosis. *CPBS, 12,* 1–2.

Houghton, P., Shaw, B., Hayward, M., & West, S. (2006). Psychosis revisited: Taking a collaborative look at psychosis. *Mental Health Practice, 9*(6), 41–43.

Hubble, M. A., Duncan, B. L., & Miller, S. D. (2005). *The Heart and Soul of Change: What works in therapy.* Washington, DC: American Psychological Association.

Johnstone, L. (1993). Psychiatry: Are we allowed to disagree? *Clinical Psychology Forum, 100,* 31–34.

Johnstone, L. (2000). *Users and Abusers of Psychiatry* (2nd ed.). London: Routledge.

Joseph, J. (2003). *The Gene Illusion.* Ross-on-Wye: PCCS Books.

Keenan, S., & Coles, S. (2012). The art of debate. *Clinical Psychology Forum, 233,* 19–22.

Marshall, R. (1990). The genetics of schizophrenia: Axiom or hypothesis? In R. P. Bentall (Ed.), *Reconstructing Schizophrenia.* London: Routledge.

Meltzer, H., Singleton, N., Lee, A., Bebbington, P., Brugha, T., & Jenkins, R. (2002). *The Social and Economic Circumstances of Adults with Mental Disorders.* London: National Statistics Office.

Midlands Psychology Group. (2007). Questioning the science and politics of happiness. *The Psychologist, 20*(7), 422–425.

Midlands Psychology Group. (2008). Our big fat multi-million pound psychology experiment. *Clinical Psychology Forum, 181,* 34–37.

Miller, J., & McClelland, L. (2006). Social inequalities formulation. In L. Johnstone & R. Dallos (Eds.), *Formulation in Psychology and Psychotherapy.* London: Routledge.

Moloney, P. (2006). The trouble with psychotherapy. *Clinical Psychology Forum, 162,* 29–33.

Moncrieff, J. (2008). *The Myth of the Chemical Cure: A critique of psychiatric drug treatment.* Basingstoke: Palgrave Macmillan.

Newnes, C., Holmes, G., & Dunn, C. (1999). *This is Madness: A critical look at psychiatry and the future of mental health services.* Ross-on-Wye: PCCS Books.

Newnes, C., Holmes, G., & Dunn, C. (2001). *This is Madness Too: Critical perspectives on mental health services.* Ross-on-Wye: PCCS Books.

Pilgrim, D. (1991). Psychotherapy and social blinkers. *The Psychologist, 2*, 52–55.

Pilgrim, D. (2007). The survival of psychiatric diagnosis. *Social Science and Medicine, 65,* 536–544.

Prilleltensky, I. (1989). Psychology and the status quo. *American Psychologist, 44*(5), 795–802.

Prilleltensky, I., & Nelson, G. (2002). *Doing Psychology Critically: Making a difference in diverse settings.* Basisngstoke: Palgrave Macmillan.

Rapley, M. (2003). I want, therefore I am: A tribute to David Smail. *Clinical Psychology, 24,* 13–19.

Rapley, M., Moncrieff, J., & Dillon, J. (2011). *De-medicalizing Misery: Psychiatry, psychology and the human condition.* Basingstoke: Palgrave Macmillan.

Read, J., Mosher, L. R., & Bentall, R. P. (Eds.). (2004). *Models of Madness: Psychological, social and biological approaches to schizophrenia.* Hove: Brunner-Routledge.

Rogers, A., & Pilgrim, D. (2010). *A Sociology of Mental Health and Illness* (4th ed.). Maidenhead: Open University Press.

Royal College of Psychiatrists. (2008). *Psychological Therapies in Psychiatry and Primary Care.* London: RCPsych.

Sampson, E. E. (1993). Identity politics: Challenges to psychology's understanding. *American Psychologist, 48*(12), 1219–1230.

Smail, D. (1993). *The Origins of Unhappiness.* London: HarperCollins.

Smail, D. (2005). *Power, Interest and Psychology: Elements of a social materialist understanding of distress.* Ross-on-Wye: PCCS Books.

Sayce, L. (2000). *From Psychiatric Patient to Citizen: Overcoming discrimination and social exclusion.* Basingstoke: Macmillan.

Wilkinson, R., & Pickett, K. (2009). *The Spirit Level: Why equality is better for everyone.* London: Allen Lane.

Chapter 8

Manifesto for a Social Materialist Psychology of Distress

Midlands Psychology Group

This chapter explains the shared background and working practices of the authors; identifies the main assumptions of a social materialist psychology; and sets out a manifesto showing what it might mean to consider what are called mental health problems, i.e., distress, from a social materialist perspective. The chapter is aimed in part, but not exclusively, at people in the psy professions who seldom have any other vocabulary with which to talk about these issues, outside of psychiatry on the one hand, and talking therapy on the other. It marshals a wide range of theory and research on the kinds of misery that get treated by mental health professionals.

Introduction

We are a group of psychologists: clinical, counselling and academic. We have been meeting regularly since 2003. We call ourselves social materialist psychologists. This is not necessarily a formally worked-out philosophical stance. Most psychology is individual and idealist. It takes the individual as a given unit of analysis, and treats the social as a somewhat optional and often uniform context. Furthermore, in what is still at root a Cartesian move, it treats the material world as straightforwardly present, but simultaneously subordinate to the immaterial cognitions by which we reflect upon it.

It is by contrast to this that our psychology is social materialist. It is social because we affirm the primacy of the social, of collectivity, relationality and community, because we acknowledge that *individuals* are thoroughly social: ontogenetically, in their origins, and continuously and non-optionally during their existence. At the same time, it is materialist because

A version of this chapter was originally published as: Midlands Psychology Group. (2012). Draft manifesto for a social materialist psychology of distress. *Journal of Critical Psychology, Counselling and Psychotherapy, 12,* 93–107.

we acknowledge that the cognitions by which we reflect upon the world do not simply float free of its affordances, character and properties. Cognition is both social and material, rooted in the ring-fenced metacognitive resources we have acquired, the embodied capacities it recruits, and the resources and subjective possibilities our world supplies (Johnson, 2007; Tolman, 1994; Vygotsky, 1962).

By social materialist psychology, then, we do not mean to imply a mere inverse reflection of the mainstream, a negation, a futile rush to its polar opposite. Individuals exist, but their experiences are thoroughly social at the very same time as they are singular and personal. And cognitions occur, but their relation to the material world is neither determinate nor arbitrary. Our social materialist psychology is therefore aligned – in sentiment, if not content – with other contemporary initiatives that similarly refuse the naive separations of individual and social, experience and materiality: psychosocial studies, studies of subjectivity, process philosophy, the turns to language and to affect. In each of these perspectives (and more besides) we find resources, echoes and inspirations.

We write as we act: collectively. In this, we align ourselves with a tradition of psychologists (Curt, 1994), political theorists and activists (The Free Association, 2011), writers and artists (Home, 1991) who reject in practice the notion that ideas are simply the achievement of individuals. At a moment when collectivity, solidarity and mutual trust are so sorely needed, this simple act may take on significances beyond the pages within which it appears.

This manifesto is unfinished, a work in progress, a direction rather than a destination. We hope you find the ideas useful. Moreover it may inspire you to join with like-minded others, spending time sharing ideas and interests, as we continue to do.

1. Persons are primordially social and material beings

Before anything else, we are feeling bodies in a social world (Csordas, 1994; Merleau-Ponty, 2002; Schutz, 1970). Primordially, experience consists of a continuous flux of bodily feedback, or feeling. This feedback – which is the raw stuff of consciousness itself (Damasio, 1999) – reflects our embodied, material situation (hot, tired, hurting etc.). It situates us in a particular setting, and furnishes an ongoing sense of our bodily potentials: an embodiment. This feedback is also continuously social (influenced by the changing social relations of the lived moment) and socialised (somewhat habitual, shaped by the impress of prior experience). Bodily feedback, in the form of feelings, is the most elemental stuff of our being human.

However, the ineffability of the body means that the centrality of feeling often eludes reflection (Langer, 1967). Consequently, the most prominent component of thought itself is frequently what Vygotsky (1962) called inner speech. This running commentary on our own and others' actions has social origins: its cognitive aspects are secondary to the social, discursive relations that engendered it. It is also largely retrospective, serving to stabilise or represent what has just occurred. In doing so it can serve as a tool to guide our own (and others') actions, and in this way have some relatively limited influence on future circumstances.

Bodily, despite our somewhat fuzzy edges, we are discrete individuals. But this individuality is relationally and socially produced: ontogenetically, in the fusion of egg and sperm; developmentally, in the experience-dependent construction of important neural assemblies (Schore, 2001); and psychologically, through relations and interactions that inculcate the implicit habits and beliefs of selfhood. Because social relations shape our being, experience is not only specific to a particular trajectory of relational and familial social participation, it is also reflective of our epoch (Elias, 1978), class (Bourdieu, 1984), gender (Fine, 2010; Young, 1990) and – no doubt – other important social divisions.

This is not a denial of individuality. No one else will occupy precisely the same circumstances as you, with exactly the constellation of bodily capacities with which you are endowed: for this reason, we are each unique. However, this uniqueness is constituted from elements of the same flesh, the same social relations, the same material organisations of tools, objects, locations and institutions, the same cultural resources, artefacts and norms, the same discursive signs and symbols. Uniqueness and individuality are thoroughly social and material accomplishments.

2. Distress arises from the outside inwards

Distress is not the consequence of inner flaws or weaknesses. All mainstream approaches to 'therapy' locate the origin of psychological difficulty within the individual, usually as some kind of idiosyncrasy of past experience. A morally neutral 'normality' may thus be seen as having become 'neurotically' distorted via, for example, unconscious personal desires or errors of personal judgment (e.g., over-generalisation of negative experiences). Certainly this is the way we often experience our distress since such experience is *inevitably* interior. But experience and explanation are two very different things. Professional therapy tends to presume that both the *causes* and the *experience* of distress are interior, since this affords the therapist a legitimate ground of intervention: individuals can be worked on in ways that social and material circumstances cannot. Individuals thus quickly learn to see themselves as in some way *personally* defective when in fact their troubled experience arises from a defective environment (Smail, 2005).

Neither is distress the consequence of cognitive errors, or failures to process information correctly. Those therapeutic approaches that do not attribute distress to some kind of personal emotional defect (however acquired) often point instead to 'cognitive' failure. The possibility that individuals, through no fault of their own, have drawn the wrong conclusions from unfortunate eventualities may at least have the advantage of absolving them from the odour of blame or personal shortcoming that tends often to waft around more 'psychodynamic' approaches. Again, this kind of view allows the therapist an apparently legitimate field of operation in re-working the person's cognitive processes. It does so, however, at the expense of a truly convincing account of human learning. There is, surely, enough evidence of what a distressing place the world can be for us to avoid the necessity of concluding that the distress we experience is somehow mistaken (Smail, 2001a, 2005).

So-called 'individual differences' in susceptibility to distress are largely the consequences of prior socialisation. The fact that some of us seem to survive adverse experience unscathed while others are thrown into confusion or despair may be taken as pointing to 'interior', personal *qualities*: 'self-esteem', 'willpower', or most recently 'resilience'. However, it is far easier, and more credible, to point to the embodied advantages someone has acquired over time from the social/material environment than it is to postulate essentially mysterious and unanalysable personal qualities that originate from within. To mistake the gifts of providence for personal virtues is an all-too-common category mistake, and one that psychotherapies do little to rectify.

3. Distress is produced by social and material influences

Social and material influences are typically complex and multiple. None of them are either *necessary* causes or *sufficient* causes, but the more that they intersect the more likely clinical distress becomes. They include trauma, abuse and neglect; social inequality (organised in hierarchies of class, gender, ethnicity, sexuality and disability); and, somewhat more randomly, accidents, disability, severe illness and 'life events'.

For example, there is convincing evidence that we are more likely to experience clinical distress if we have experienced traumatic events, including abuse and neglect. Read, van Os, Morrison and Ross's (2005) meta-analysis suggests that at least 60–70 per cent of people experiencing visual or auditory hallucinations were subject to physical or sexual abuse in childhood. This body of evidence has received much less attention than the dominant psychiatric view that portrays distress as a consequence of biological or genetic influences.

Similarly, social inequalities that exclude or marginalise contribute significantly to the potential for distress. Poverty, impoverished housing and diet, threatening environments, limited resources, restricted choices, demeaning or poorly paid employment, discrimination, oppression and scapegoating are all causes of distress. People born in working-class areas to parents in manual labour are eight times more likely than controls to be given a diagnosis of schizophrenia as adults (Harrison, Gunnell, Glazebrook, Page & Kwiecinski, 2001). Being born to poorly educated parents doubles the risk of being given a diagnosis of depression; if neither parent is in skilled or professional employment the risk is tripled (Ritsher, Warner, Johnson & Dohrenwend, 2001). Non-white ethnic minorities in the UK are more likely to be given a diagnosis of schizophrenia, but only if they live in majority-white areas (Boydell et al., 2001). Women are roughly twice as likely as men to be given diagnoses of depression or anxiety disorder; in part, this is seemingly due to domestic violence (Garcia-Moreno, Jansen, Ellsberg, Heise & Watts, 2005). Clinical distress is consistently associated with markers of social inequality such as unemployment, low income and impoverished education, in countries including the UK, USA, Canada, Australia and the Netherlands (Melzer, Fryers & Jenkins, 2004). Wilkinson and Pickett (2009) have amassed extensive evidence showing that in societies where the gap between the richest and poorest is greater the prevalence of many health problems is higher.

We are more likely to experience distress the more our experiences are invalidated and the more isolated we become from one another. Equally, the further we are from supportive, nurturing relationships, the more that invalidation and isolation will engender distress. People stripped of ameliorative influences, such as a loving, supportive family and friends, comfortable, safe environments, and the trust, support and solidarity of others, are increasingly likely to experience clinical distress. In other words, the effects of trauma, social inequality and life events contingently interact with the less visible, less quantifiable effects of parenting, friendship, nurturing and caring. This is one reason why 'the same' event causes clinical distress in some, but not others.

4. Distress is enabled by biology but not primarily *caused* by it

Harré (2002) distinguishes between enabling and causing. All experience is *enabled* by the biological capacities which constitute our embodiment in the material world. For example, your experience of reading this paragraph is enabled by the musculature of your head, body and eyes, the light-sensitive cells of your retinas, the cortical pathways and neural assemblies that relay, collate and interpret the signals that these cells generate, and so on. But these biological capacities did not *cause* you to read it.

This distinction is useful in relation to distress, not least because it accords very well with the evidence. For a very small number of *organic* diagnoses (syphilis, respiratory or urinary tract infections in older adults, Korsakoff's syndrome, dementia) consistent biological causes of distress are known (although even these always interact with other influences). But for the overwhelming majority of *functional* diagnoses – schizophrenia, depression, generalised anxiety disorder, personality disorder and so on – there is no such consistent evidence. Over 100 years of extremely well-funded research using ever-more sophisticated technologies has so far failed to establish that *any* of these diagnoses are biological diseases. In the words of eminent psychiatrist Kenneth Kendler (2005, pp. 434–435):

> We have hunted for big, simple, neuropathological explanations for psychiatric disorders and have not found them. We have hunted for big, simple, neurochemical explanations for psychiatric disorders and have not found them. We have hunted for big, simple genetic explanations for psychiatric disorders, and have not found them.

But this does not mean that biology should be largely ignored, as is so often the case in social science and (predominantly cognitive) psychology. Embodied capacities lend shape and texture to distress, by enabling activities and by co-constituting perceptions, thoughts and feelings. This means we should strive to understand how *distress is produced by the adverse socialisation of embodied, biological capacities,* rather than by their impairment, disease or failure. This massively complex interdisciplinary undertaking will draw upon anthropology, social science, neuroscience, psychology and other disciplines. Despite some suggestive recent accounts (Schore, 2001) we have barely begun to conduct such research, nor to address the many methodological and conceptual difficulties it will encounter (Cromby, 2007; Newton, 2007; Rose, 1997).

5. Distress is influenced by biological variation to the extent that this variation provides non-specific capacities

Some biologically enabled capacities may facilitate people's transactions with the world and so help protect them from some forms of psychological distress or self-doubt. It may thus be an advantage to possess conventional physical beauty, sporting prowess, musical ability, unusual intellectual ability, and so on. More important, perhaps, (perceived) lack of such gifts may undermine a person's self-worth and render them more susceptible to distress.

An example: less conventionally attractive people encounter a more hostile social environment, have less chance of developing friendships and social skills, and experience fewer rewards (O'Grady, 1982). Meta-analyses by Langlois et al. (2000) suggest that conventional beauty – in children and adults – is associated with more favourable judgements and treatment by others. Farina et al. (1977) found that female psychiatric inpatients were judged less conventionally attractive than women selected from either a shopping centre or a university, and Napoleon, Chassin and Young (1980) showed that mental health service users were judged less attractive than high- or middle-income – but not low-income – controls.

Another example: sensitivity to others is a trait that might have a genetic component. Ordinarily this trait is adaptive, associated with maintaining good relationships, being a better employee, functioning well in groups, and so forth. But when someone with this trait is placed in a traumatic or abusive environment, the trait becomes maladaptive because it means that the effects of this toxic environment are felt more keenly. Tienari's (1991) adoption study found that, even amongst people with a family history of difficulties, the experiences associated with a psychotic-spectrum diagnosis emerged only in the context of unfavourable family dynamics.

This perspective is consonant with current molecular genetic research, which typically finds that effects are small, non-specific, produced by multiple DNA sequences, and always dependent upon environmental mediation (Joseph, 2006; Rose, 1997). Biological factors can influence susceptibility to distress, but this is not simply a matter of objective biological advantage which inevitably orders people along some or other dimension of human 'excellence'. The value placed upon biological capacities is always a *social* valuation, and their effects always depend upon social and material circumstances.

6. Distress does not fall into discrete categories or diagnoses

The quaint notion that distress can be neatly partitioned into robust categories reflects the mistaken belief that it is caused by organic diseases or impairments. If distress is understood instead as a kind of socially and materially inculcated experience, there is no reason to presume that we should be able to classify it in this way.

This may be why psychiatric diagnosis is notoriously both unreliable and invalid. Evidence of unreliability is provided by the lives of service users, who frequently receive different diagnoses during their contact with services. Further evidence comes from studies showing that, even in reliability trials where normal variation is artificially constrained (by video presentations, special training and broad categories), psychiatrists frequently disagree about the 'correct' diagnosis (e.g., Bentall, 2003, 2009; Pilgrim & Rogers, 2010; van Os et al., 1999). Evidence that diagnosis is invalid comes from studies of co-morbidity which show that patients who meet the criteria for one diagnosis most likely meet the criteria for at least one other (e.g., Boyle, 2002; Brady & Kendall, 1992; Dunner, 1998; Maier & Falkai, 1999; Sartorius, Ustun, Lecrubier & Wittchen, 1996; Timimi, 2011). Other evidence comes from studies of symptom profiles which show, for example, that the symptoms of people given a diagnosis of bipolar disorder do not cluster separately from those of people given a diagnosis of schizophrenia (Bentall, 2003). Because psychiatric diagnosis is neither reliable nor valid, *all* of its claimed benefits – in respect of aetiology, treatment, prognosis, service planning, inter-professional communication, reassurance to service users and their families – are compromised.

As a kind of experience, distress is on a continuum and continuously responsive to all other experiences. Its intrinsic variability is reflective of the great complexity of our social and material worlds, the many interacting, mediated contingencies that co-constitute our experience, and the primordially socialised embodiments each of us have acquired. Nevertheless, since we all occupy the same planet and belong to the same species, there are also similarities in our experiences of distress. These reflect shared embodied capacities: to feel sad when abandoned, to feel angry when insulted, to feel ashamed about sadness or frightened of anger; to get so overwhelmed by such mixtures of feeling that our very perceptions of the world get distorted (Cromby & Harper, 2009). They also reflect similar – but never 'the same' – experiences of power relations, social relations, material circumstances, and the contingent, mediated affordances they yield.

7. Distress is an acquired, embodied way of being in the world

Cognitive psychology studies processes such as memory, perception, reasoning, and judgement, and has influenced recent attempts within clinical psychology to explain and develop interventions for distress. These attempts are broadly based on the assumption that distress is caused by some problem or dysfunction with 'normal' cognitive processes: for example, within cognitive therapy, depressed mood is attributed to errors in reasoning such as 'over-generalisation'. Therapy attempts to help correct such errors, and so restore normal psychological functioning. However, this approach overemphasises individual psychology, and particularly consciousness; conflates (social and material) causes with (cognitive) effects; downplays bodily processes; and almost completely neglects those social and material causes of distress external to the person and their proximal situation. It also fails to address the ways in which cognitive psychology is itself an ideological construction, rather than a naturally scientific field investigating independently existing phenomena (Bowers, 1990; Sampson, 1981; Shallice, 1984).

Conversely, psychiatry tends to construe clinical distress as akin to a medical disease and focuses upon diagnosing and treating (usually with drugs) so-called 'mental illnesses': depression, schizophrenia etc. Although this acknowledges the body as the site of distress, it fails to adequately address the ways in which bodily manifestations of emotional distress are produced by, and consistently responsive to, social and material circumstances. Instead, psychiatry traces distress back to biological impairments and dysfunctions for which there is no credible, reliable and consistent evidence (Lynch, 2004).

Core to most psychological therapies is the development of 'insight'. For example, in cognitive therapy the therapist 'helps' the client become aware of cognitive processing errors, with the aim of helping to correct them. However, research in neuroscience and social psychology has shown that much of our experience, including emotional arousal, is not necessarily available to conscious introspection (Kahneman & Tversky, 1982; Schwitzgebel, 2011; Wilson & Dunne, 2004). Hence, when individuals from Western cultures are asked to talk about feelings of low mood they usually offer accounts that emphasise individual inadequacy and guilt, whereas those from non-Western cultures offer very different accounts (Fancher, 1996; Kleinman, 1986; Watters, 2010). Rather than providing reliable, accurate, direct accounts of experience, introspection is always mediated by cultural norms and linguistic resources that regulate what and how we can notice and report.

It is frequently difficult for us to make sense of, or explain to others, how we feel and why we feel the way we do. Complex feeling states are often triggered involuntarily in response to subtle environmental features, related to past events that have been forgotten, or that we do not connect with our current experience (Damasio, 1999; Kagan, 2007; LeDoux, 1999). We are often unaware of the many social factors that influence us: due to their complexity, or sometimes – in the case of advertising, tabloid media or politicians' speeches – the conscious manipulation of feelings by those in positions of power, with the intention of concealing such manipulation (Caldini, 1994; Freedland, 2012; Jones, 2011). Perhaps one of the useful aspects of therapy is the opportunity to try to make connections between events, past and present, and the feelings they evoke.

Both psychiatric and mainstream psychological explanations of distress are at best partial, at worst ideological, because they fail to capture the way in which experience is shaped over time by a social world that is frequently oppressive. The acquisition of what could be described as an affective 'default' position is sensibly interpreted by the person as reflecting the way the world is, has been, and will always be. This enduring, embodied aspect of distress means it is very difficult for us to change the way we experience ourselves and our world.

8. Social and material influence is always contingent and mediated

The ability to act is always contingent on the particular social, material and embodied resources available. In turn, the effects of these actions are not simply dependent on our intentions. They are also a function of the intentions and actions of others, and of the variable capacities and affordances of the (constantly changing) social and material world.

Bradley (2005) offers a startling example: stepping out and knocking a cyclist off his bike. In one circumstance, the man is largely unhurt and cycles away; in another, he is knocked into the path of an oncoming vehicle and killed. Intrinsically unpredictable combinations of interlocking factors (choices about where and when to travel; velocities, trajectories and reactions of cyclist, driver and walker; traffic flow and density; road and pavement layout) mean that three lives continue much as before in the first circumstance but are radically transformed in the second.

Contingency necessarily means that social and material influences are always mediated. They are in constant flow and exchange with each other and with the human characteristics and resources (habits, perceptions, affects, discourses, narratives) by which we understand and respond to them. Vitally, this does not mean that social and material influence is random: the contingencies and mediations by which it gets enacted are always already structured in relays of power. Nevertheless, power's influence therefore necessarily has an 'on average' character (cf. Bourdieu, 1977; Young, 1990). This means there are always potentials for movement, always immanent moments of becoming and change, even within what seem to be the most frozen and static regimes (Stephenson & Papadopoulos, 2007).

Adequate psychological accounts of causality therefore need to be multiple, complex and open-ended: they need to recognise the radical indeterminacy of social interaction (Shotter, 1993), the probabilistic character of social influence (Archer, 1995), and the influence of culture as a mutable system of normative guiding principles (Harré, 2002). But mainstream psychology is preoccupied with mechanistic notions of causality: consequently, it tends to read these indeterminacies, probabilities and norms in ways that consistently subordinate social and material circumstance to immaterial cognition. Social and material influence is therefore downplayed, in favour of individualistic conceptualisations against which these real influences typically appear only as mere context. When elaborated, this understanding provides further reasons why 'the same' events seemingly impact differently upon different people.

9. Distress cannot be removed by willpower

The notion of 'willpower' tacitly inhabits just about every theory of psychotherapy. Having been led, one way or another, to confront their personal failings, mistakes, or cognitive errors, it is assumed that patients can make the necessary correction by an act of will. If not, they are being uncooperative, 'resistant', etc. Never explicitly theorised, the notion of willpower lurks within such concepts as 'insight' and is typically assumed as an obvious, everyday human faculty that can be called on by all *in extremis*. Willpower constitutes a mysterious, interior moral force that cannot be measured or demonstrated – because, whatever its social utility, it doesn't exist (Smail, 2001a). To assume that it does, and to call upon patients to demonstrate it, can be positively cruel.

This does not mean that we are necessarily unable to choose a given course of action, nor that we are constrained to perform actions against our desires. 'Freedom', 'will' and 'power' are necessary and valid concepts. 'Willing' means choosing this or that; freedom means having the *power* to choose this or that. Whether or not we have the power to exercise our will depends upon the availability of the necessary social and material resources. Will and power are *two distinct capacities*: without resources, exercise of will is impossible.

So there is no immaterial force called willpower upon which we can call. The personal powers that make the exercise of will possible may be concurrently present in the world, or they may be acquired historically – embodied – from engagement with it. I will not be able to speak French (to 'will' a sentence in French) if I have not studied and practised the language sufficiently for it to become an embodied skill. Similarly, I will not be able to behave confidently in a given circumstance if I have not acquired and embodied the kind of experiences which engender the appropriate confidence. Most therapies, whether explicitly or not, invoke bootstrap-pulling as a vehicle of change, but bootstrap-pulling is no substitute for the necessary personal power (Smail, 2005).

10. Distress cannot be cured by medication or therapy

Distress is not an 'illness', so cannot be 'cured'. It is not bad genes, faulty cognitions or the Oedipus complex, but misfortune and the widespread abuse of power that mire so many in madness, addiction or despair. These are not symptoms of illness: they are states of being that encapsulate how most of us might respond to chronic adversity. The most widely cited evidence bases for psychiatric medication *and* talking therapy are overly optimistic catalogues of error and bias, featuring inadequate recruitment and blinding procedures, unreliable clinical outcome measures of limited real-life significance, and the selective publication of favourable results (Angell, 2004; Epstein, 2006; Kirsch, 2010). The more rigorous the study and the longer the post-treatment follow-up, the harder it is to demonstrate any superiority for the clinical treatment over dummy, placebo or alternative (Westen & Morrison, 2001). Neither drugs nor psychological therapies are magic bullets aimed at specific symptoms: whatever effects they have upon body and mind are quite general. The one reliable finding is that emotionally warm and attentive practitioners are more appreciated and get better results – an observation that applies equally to politicians, salespeople and prostitutes.

Indeed, the expectation that therapy or medication might 'cure' is itself harmful. Psychiatric drugs are marketed and prescribed relentlessly – cures for supposed chemical imbalances said to afflict up to a quarter of the population (Busfield, 2010). Likewise, the jargon and practices of over 400 schools of psychological therapy have invaded almost every corner of daily life: from the products of a lucrative 'self-help' industry to the running of schools, universities, business, clinics and prisons. The UK Government's *Improving Access to Psychological Therapies* (IAPT) programme promises to make psychological treatment 'available to all', as prophylactic for distress and happiness bromide: therapy on an industrial scale.

But the majority of psychoactive drugs cause mental and physical harm, especially with long-term use (Breggin, 1991; Moncrieff, 2006; Whitaker, 2010). The over-prescribing of so-called antipsychotics has unleashed an epidemic of psychosis throughout the world, as the effects of the dependency upon (and withdrawal from) medication have almost everywhere been mistaken for 'mental illness'. Whilst the talking therapies appear more benign, too often they are just a more insidious form of control, fostering the illusion that misery is an internal failure or breakdown, awaiting correction from an expert (Illousz, 2008; Parker, 2007). And – when medication or therapy frequently fails to generate the profound changes that were implicitly promised – those given these treatments then become those who simply *cannot be cured*.

11. Medication and therapy can make a difference, but not by curing

Sometimes, medication can usefully anaesthetise the distressed to their woes, yielding brief bubbles of respite or clarity. During these short, chemically induced holidays from their misery, those with the resources may initiate life changes that alleviate their problems and establish positive future trajectories. But whether this occurs is a function, not simply of the medication, but of the resources and circumstances within which it is ingested: consequently, medication can also make things worse (Moncrieff, 2008).

Therapy can also help, though again not by 'curing'. Understood generically, therapy provides comfort (you are not alone with your woes), clarification (there are sound reasons why you feel the way you do) and support (I will help you deal with your predicament) (Smail, 2001b). In an atomised, fragmented, time-poor society, where solidarity and collectivity are derided, time limited, and relationships consistently infected with a toxic instrumentalism, these are valuable, compassionate functions.

At its best, psychological therapy can help the sufferer to understand their distress, not as a (more or less wilful) failure of insight, motivation or learning, but as the inevitable result of living in a noxious world. Moreover, both medication and therapy can help people make better use of the powers and resources already available to them. Both may draw attention to unrecognised resources (e.g., solidarity with others); make it feel permissible to use available powers and resources; change the ways that people use available powers and resources; or explicitly support people to cease viewing themselves as 'the problem'.

With the exception of iatrogenic poisoning and disciplinary self-regulation, neither therapy nor medication has any other significant influence.

12. Successful psychological therapy is not primarily a matter of technique

When therapy succeeds it seems to be primarily a matter of two kinds of influence: on the one hand relationality (ordinary human compassion and understanding); on the other, coincidence with social and material circumstances and resources.

In the therapy literature it is well established that the clients who do best are generally young, attractive, verbal, intelligent and successful – YAVIS (Pilgrim, 1997). By contrast, the people whose needs are described as 'complex' and requiring long-term treatment are usually the poorest (Davies, 1997; Hagan & Donnison, 1999). Where people have (or can obtain) more resources then they will have more scope to act upon whatever insights they might have gained.

It is also well established in this literature that so-called 'non-specific factors' are a consistent predictor of good outcomes: in other words, that the therapist and client are able to establish a good relationship (Mair, 1992; Norcross, 2010). Indeed, unlike professional therapists, service users frequently declare the most ordinary aspects of therapy the most helpful: listening, understanding, respectfulness.

Despite this, therapy is mostly presented as a matter of technique. Cognitive behavioural therapy, psychoanalysis, and almost all other schools of therapy appear as specialist technologies of subjectivity, skilled interpersonal practices founded on specific assumptions, locked in place by particular theories and evidence bases. In a thoroughly commodified society it is perhaps understandable that some practitioners will want to have branded, marketable products, just as in a professionalised culture some will want to identify themselves as bearers of highly specialised knowledge and skills. Like everyone else, therapists must earn a living, so it is only to be expected that interest should influence how they present themselves and their work. Nevertheless, doing so distracts attention from the actual causes of distress by bolstering the belief that it is a mysterious state amenable only to professional help; it disables friends and family, who may feel that they could not possibly understand; and it negates the contribution of community, solidarity and trust. The presentation of therapy as specialised technique cheapens and oversells psychology itself; leads to resources being wasted comparing the marginal differences between this brand and that; and deflects effort and attention from the very real opportunities for psychological research and insight that are supplied by the highly privileged situation of the therapeutic encounter.

References

Angell, M. (2004). *The Truth about Drug Companies: How they deceive us and what to do about it.* New York: Random House.

Archer, M. (1995). *Realist Social Theory: The morphogenetic approach.* Cambridge: Cambridge University Press.

Bentall, R. P. (2003). *Madness Explained: Psychosis and human nature.* London: Allen Lane.

Bentall, R. P. (2009). *Doctoring the Mind: Why psychiatric treatments fail.* London: Penguin.

Bourdieu, P. (1977). *Outline of a Theory of Practice* (R. Nice, Trans.). Cambridge: Cambridge University Press.

Bourdieu, P. (1984). *Distinction.* London: Routledge.

Bowers, J. (1990). All hail the great abstraction: Star Wars and the politics of cognitive psychology. In I. Parker & J. Shotter (Eds.), *Deconstructing Social Psychology* (pp. 127–140). London: Routledge.

Boydell, J., van Os, J., McKenzie, K., Allardyce, J., Goel, R., McCreadie, G., et al. (2001). Incidence of schizophrenia in ethnic minorities in London: Ecological study into interactions with environment. *British Medical Journal, 323,* 1336–1338.

Boyle, M. (2002). *Schizophrenia: A scientific delusion?* (2nd ed.). London: Routledge.

Bradley, B. (2005). *Psychology and Experience.* Cambridge: Cambridge University Press.

Brady, E., & Kendall, P. (1992). Comorbidity of anxiety and depression in children and adolescents. *Psychological Bulletin, 111*(2), 244–255.

Breggin, P. (1991). *Toxic Psychiatry.* New York: St. Martin's Press.

Busfield, J. (2010). 'A pill for every ill.' Explaining the expansion in medicine use. *Social Science and Medicine, 70,* 934–941.

Caldini, R. (1994). *Influence: The psychology of persuasion.* New York: Morrow.

Cromby, J. (2007). Integrating social science with neuroscience: Potentials and problems. *Biosocieties, 2*(2), 149–170.

Cromby, J., & Harper, D. (2009). Paranoia: A social account. *Theory and Psychology, 19*(3), 335–361.

Csordas, T. (Ed.). (1994). *Embodiment and Experience: The existential ground of culture and self.* Cambridge: Cambridge University Press.

Curt, B. (1994). *Textuality and Tectonics: Troubling social and psychological science.* Buckingham: Open University Press.

Damasio, A. R. (1999). *The Feeling of What Happens: Body, emotion and the making of consciousness.* London: William Heinemann.

Davies, D. (1997). *Counselling in Psychological Services.* Buckingham: Open University Press.

Dunner, D. L. (1998). The issue of co-morbidity in the treatment of panic. *International Clinical Psychopharmacology, 13*(Apr, Suppl. 4), s19–24.

Elias, N. (1978). *The History of Manners: The civilising process* (Vol. 1) (E. Jephcott, Trans.). Oxford: Basil Blackwell.

Epstein, W. (2006). *The Civil Divine: Psychotherapy as religion in America.* Reno, NV: University of Nevada Press.

Fancher, R. (1996). *Cultures of Healing: Correcting the image of American mental health care.* San Francisco: W. H. Freeman & Co.

Farina, A., Fischer, E., Sherman, S., Smith, W., Groh, T., & Mermin, P. (1977). Physical attractiveness and mental illness. *Journal of Abnormal Psychology, 86,* 510–517.

Fine, C. (2010). *Delusions of Gender.* London: Icon Books.

The Free Association. (2011). *Moments of Excess: Movements, protest and everyday life.* Oakland, CA: PM Press.

Freedland, J. (2012). Bash the poor and wave the flag – how this Tory trick works. *The Guardian,* 28/1/2012. Retrieved 2 February 2012 from http://gu.com/p/354a2

Garcia-Moreno, C., Jansen, H. A. F. M., Ellsberg, M., Heise, L., & Watts, C. (2005). *The WHO Multi-country Study on Women's Health and Domestic Violence against Women.* Geneva: World Health Organisation.

Hagan, T., & Donnison, D. (1999). Social power: Some implications for the theory and practice of cognitive behaviour therapy. *Journal of Community and Applied Social Psychology, 9,* 119–135.

Harré, R. (2002). *Cognitive Science: A philosophical introduction.* London: Sage Publications.

Harrison, G., Gunnell, D., Glazebrook, C., Page, K., & Kwiecinski, R. (2001). Association between schizophrenia and social inequality at birth: Case-control study. *British Journal of Psychiatry, 179,* 346–350.

Home, S. (1991). *The Assault on Culture: Utopian currents from Lettrism to class war.* Edinburgh: AK Press.

Illousz, E. (2008). *Saving the Modern Soul: Therapy, emotions and the culture of self-help.* Berkeley, CA: University of California Press.

Johnson, M. (2007). *The Meaning of the Body: Aesthetics of human understanding.* Chicago: University of Chicago Press.

Jones, O. (2011). *Chavs: The demonisation of the working class.* London: Verso.

Joseph, J. (2006). *The Missing Gene: Psychiatry, heredity and the fruitless search for genes.* New York: Algora.

Kagan, J. (2007). *What is Emotion?* New Haven, CT: Yale University Press.

Kahneman, D., & Tversky, A. (Eds.). (1982). *Judgement under Uncertainty: Heuristics and biases.* Cambridge: Cambridge University Press.

Kendler, K. (2005). Towards a philosophical structure for psychiatry. *American Journal of Psychiatry, 162,* 433–440.

Kirsch, I. (2010). *The Emperor's New Drugs: Exploding the antidepressant myth.* New York: Basic Books.

Kleinman, A. (1986). Social origins of distress and disease: Depression, neurasthenia, and pain in modern China. *Current Anthropology, 24*(5), 499–509.

Langer, S. (1967). *Mind: An essay on human feeling* (Vol. 1). Baltimore, MD: Johns Hopkins University Press.

Langlois, J., Kalakanis, L., Rubenstein, A., Larson, A., Hallam, M., & Smoot, M. (2000). Maxims or myths of beauty? A meta-analytic and theoretic review. *Psychological Bulletin, 126*(3), 390–423.

LeDoux, J. (1999). *The Emotional Brain.* London: Phoenix.

Lynch, T. (2004). *Beyond Prozac: Healing mental distress.* Ross-on-Wye: PCCS Books.

Maier, W., & Falkai, P. (1999). The epidemiology of comorbidity between depression, anxiety disorders and somatic diseases. *International Clinical Psychopharmacology, 14*(Suppl. 2), s1–6.

Mair, K. (1992). The myth of therapist expertise. In W. Dryden & C. Feltham (Eds.), *Psychotherapy and Its Discontents.* Buckingham: Open University Press.

Melzer, D., Fryers, T., & Jenkins, R. (2004). *Social Inequalities and the Distribution of the Common Mental Disorders.* Hove: Psychology Press.

Merleau-Ponty, M. (2002). *Phenomenology of Perception* (C. Smith, Trans.). London: Routledge.

Moncrieff, J. (2006). Why is it so difficult to stop psychiatric drug treatment? It may be nothing to do with the original problem. *Medical Hypotheses, 67*(3), 517–523.

Moncrieff, J. (2008). *The Myth of the Chemical Cure: A critique of psychiatric drug treatment.* London: Palgrave.

Napoleon, T., Chassin, L., & Young, R. (1980). A replication and extension of 'physical attractiveness and mental illness'. *Journal of Abnormal Psychology, 89,* 250–253.

Newton, T. (2007). *Nature and Sociology.* London: Routledge.

Norcross, J. (2010). The therapeutic relationship. In B. Duncan, S. Miller, B. Wampold & M. Hubble (Eds.), *The Heart and Soul of Change: Delivering what works in therapy.* Washington, DC: APA.

O'Grady, K. (1982). Sex, physical attractiveness and perceived risk for mental illness. *Journal of Personality and Social Psychology, 43*(5), 1064–1071.

Parker, I. (2007). *Revolution in Psychology.* London: Pluto Press.

Pilgrim, D. (1997). *Psychotherapy and Society.* London: Sage.

Pilgrim, D., & Rogers, A. (2010). *A Sociology of Mental Health and Illness.* Maidenhead: Open University Press/McGraw Hill Education.

Read, J., van Os, J., Morrison, A. P., & Ross, C. A. (2005). Childhood trauma, psychosis and schizophrenia: A literature review with theoretical and clinical implications. *Acta Psychiatrica Scandinavica, 112,* 330–350.

Ritsher, J. E. B., Warner, V., Johnson, J. G., & Dohrenwend, B. P. (2001). Intergenerational longitudinal study of social class and depression: A test of social causation and social selection models. *British Journal of Psychiatry, 178*(Suppl. 40), s84–90.

Rose, S. (1997). *Lifelines: Life beyond the gene.* Oxford: Oxford University Press.

Sampson, E. E. (1981). Cognitive psychology as ideology. *American Psychologist, 36*(7), 730–743.

Sartorius, N., Ustun, T. B., Lecrubier, Y., & Wittchen, H. U. (1996). Depression co-morbid with anxiety: Results from the WHO study on psychological disorders in primary health care. *British Journal of Psychiatry, 168*(Suppl. 30, Jun), s38–43.

Schore, A. (2001). The effects of early relational trauma on right brain development, affect regulation, and infant mental health. *Infant Mental Health Journal, 22*(1), 201–269.

Schutz, A. (1970). *On Phenomenology and Social Relations.* Chicago: University of Chicago Press.

Schwitzgebel, E. (2011). *Perplexities of Consciousness.* Cambridge, MA: MIT Press.

Shallice, T. (1984). Psychology and social control. *Cognition, 17,* 29–48.

Shotter, J. (1993). *Conversational Realities: Constructing life through language.* London: Sage.

Smail, D. J. (2001a). *The Nature of Unhappiness.* London: Robinson.

Smail, D. J. (2001b). *Why Therapy Doesn't Work.* London: Robinson.

Smail, D. J. (2005). *Power, Interest and Psychology: Elements of a social materialist understanding of distress.* Ross-on-Wye: PCCS Books.

Stephenson, N., & Papadopoulos, D. (2007). *Analysing Everyday Experience: Social research and political change.* London: Palgrave Macmillan.

Tienari, P. (1991). Interaction between genetic vulnerability and family environment: The Finnish adoptive family study of schizophrenia. *Acta Psychiatrica Scandinavica, 84*(5), 460–465.

Timimi, S. (2011). *The Myth of Autism: Medicalising men's and boys' social and emotional competence.* London: Palgrave.

Tolman, C. (1994). *Psychology, Society, Subjectivity: An introduction to German critical psychology.* London: Routledge.

Van Os, J., Gilvarry, C., Bale, R., van Horn, E., Tattan, T., White, I., et al. (1999). A comparison of the utility of dimensional and categorical representations of psychosis. UK700 Group. *Psychological Medicine, 29*(3), 595–606.

Vygotsky, L. S. (1962). *Thought and Language* (E. Hanfmann & G. Vakar, Trans.). Cambridge, MA: MIT Press.

Watters, E. (2010). *Crazy Like Us: The globalisation of the American psyche.* New York: Free Press.

Westen, D., & Morrison, K. (2001). A multi-dimensional meta-analysis of treatments for depression, panic and generalised anxiety disorder: An empirical examination of the status of empirically supported therapies. *Journal of Consulting and Clinical Psychology, 69*(6), 875–899.

Whitaker, R. (2010). *Anatomy of an Epidemic*. New York: Random House.

Wilkinson, R., & Pickett, K. (2009). *The Spirit Level: Why equality is better for everyone*. London: Penguin.

Wilson, T., & Dunne, E. (2004). Self-Knowledge: Its limits, value and potential for improvement. *Annual Review of Psychology, 493–518*.

Young, I. M. (1990). *Throwing like a Girl and Other Essays in Feminist Philosophy and Social Theory*. Bloomington, IN: Indiana University Press.

Chapter 9

Soteria: Contexts, practice and philosophy

Philip Thomas

In the second half of the twentieth century a scientific revolution transformed medical care. Developments in molecular biology and genetics delivered new insights into many diseases and more effective treatments. This revolution, which began in the laboratory, has since moved into the clinic, where evidence-based medicine (EBM) has introduced scientific principles into day-to-day clinical decision making. Not wanting to be left behind, anxious to prove that it was as rigorously scientific as the rest of medicine, psychiatry fell under the spell of this revolution. But EBM has had unintended consequences in mental health care; it has drawn attention to the poor quality of the evidence that currently informs treatment decisions.

Concern about the quality of drug trial evidence used to justify the use of neuroleptic drugs in 'schizophrenia'[1] is nothing new (Thornley & Adams, 1998); recent work raises serious questions about their effectiveness in the short-term (Bola, 2006; Bola, Kao & Haluk, 2012) and long-term management of the condition (Harrow, Jobe & Faull, 2012). There are concerns, too, about their safety. Long-term neuroleptic use is associated with higher rates of mortality from cardiovascular disease, diabetes, and reduced life expectancy (Hennessy et al., 2002; Ray, Chung, Murray, Hall & Stein, 2009; Casey, Rodriguez, Northcott, Vickar & Shihabuddin, 2011;

---

1 A note on the use of the word 'schizophrenia' is necessary here. My preferred expression for the range of experiences that are included under this rubric (and for that matter, other psychiatric diagnoses) is 'madness'. The word 'mad' is an ancient one. According to the Shorter Oxford English Dictionary it originated in Old High German between a thousand to fifteen hundred years ago. It is thus unsullied by contemporary meaning. However, it seems to me that refusing to use the word 'schizophrenia' for whatever reasons is to deny an historical reality. No matter how much we may object to it, pretending that it does not exist will not change the fact that it has existed. For this reason I use the word in single quotation marks where other writers have used it in their work. Otherwise, I use the word madness.

This chapter has benefited from the wisdom of Judy Schreiber and Pat Bracken. I am grateful to them both for their constructive comments on an earlier version.

Wildgust, Hodgson & Beary, 2010). Their long-term use is associated with cortical atrophy (reduced brain volume) and the negative symptoms thought to be an integral feature of the 'disease process' associated with poor outcome (Moncrieff & Leo, 2010; Ho, Andreasen, Ziebell, Pierson & Magnotta, 2011). The diagnosis of 'schizophrenia' has no validity; a recent literature review failed to find any evidence that people given a diagnosis of 'schizophrenia' differed in any way biologically or psychologically from people who did not have it (Anckarsäter, 2010). Even academic psychiatrists question the value of the category, pointing out that 150 years of scientific research into the condition has yielded no significant insights that are of benefit to patients (Kingdon, 2007).

Despite this, psychiatry lumbers along, stuck in a biological groove, unable to stutter its way out, incapable of articulating more meaningful ways of engaging with distress. Some forms of madness may have a physical basis, but at present this is grounded not in science but scientism, an ideology driven by the pharmaceutical industry's drive for greater profit. Most people who use mental health services want more than medication, yet the only alternative available for most is cognitive behavioural therapy, if they can gain access to it. They want something different, but what exactly?

In this chapter I propose that one way forward is through the work of the late Loren Mosher, who set up the first Soteria House in California. Soteria (a Greek word meaning 'deliverance' or 'salvation') was the product of an approach that regarded madness as potentially meaningful and understandable. The individual's search for meaning is an essential component of recovery (Leamy, Bird, Le Boutillier, Williams & Slade, 2011), and Soteria relied not on drugs or therapy, but the quality of relationships between staff and residents to guide this quest. It was a product of the 1960s, a time when psychoanalysis, social milieu therapy and therapeutic communities influenced thought as to how people experiencing madness should be helped. The influence of these ideas may have waned, but Soteria is as relevant today as it was 40 years ago. Indeed, its focus on the quality of the relationships between residents and staff could and should extend to acute admission units, secure units, early intervention services, assertive outreach teams and community development projects. It reminds us that the human spirit's capacity for compassion and care defies containment within institutions, theories, and therapies.

Here, I will describe the influences that shaped Soteria, including the view of psychosis that informed Loren Mosher's work. This has implications for the use of medication in psychosis. But the main focus is interpersonal phenomenology, Loren Mosher's adaptation of existential philosophy, which is at the heart of Soteria. I will briefly describe this, and then argue that this way of engaging with madness is profoundly different from the contemporary technological paradigm. I make no apologies for dwelling at length on the philosophy that lies behind Loren Mosher's work. The influence of existentialism in psychiatry has waned since the 1960s (Spandler & Thomas, 2012) and most readers will be unfamiliar with it. Finally, I will end by considering some of the barriers to its wider implementation.

The influences that shaped Soteria

Soteria was the product of the life and work of the American psychiatrist, Loren Mosher. He was born in California in 1933, and graduated from Harvard Medical School with honours in 1961.[2] After training in psychiatry at Harvard he worked at the National Institute for Mental Health's (NIMH) Intramural Research Program, before spending a year at the Tavistock Clinic. On returning to America he was appointed the first Chief of NIMH's Center for Studies of Schizophrenia, a post he held from 1968 to 1980. During this period he was the founding editor of *Schizophrenia Bulletin*. The first Soteria House opened in San Jose, California in late 1971, and closed through lack of funding in 1983. Another house, Emanon, opened in California to replicate the work of Soteria, but this too closed through lack of funding (Mosher & Burti, 1994).

Like most young doctors, Mosher struggled early in his career to come to terms with the existential problems raised by his first encounters with the reality of death. He describes his powerlessness to do anything to help his dying patients, other than trying to understand their experiences of it, something his medical education had ill-prepared him for (Mosher, 1999). So he turned to existential phenomenology in an attempt to grapple with the dilemmas posed by his awareness of mortality. He discovered Rollo May et al.'s *Existence* (May, Angel & Ellenberger, 1958) and this led him to the work of a number of existential/phenomenological writers, including Allers (1961), Boss (1963), Husserl (1967) and Sartre (1958). In an era of

---

2 Much of the following account of Loren Mosher's career is taken from his biography available at http://www.moshersoteria.com/bio-of-loren-mosher-soteria/ accessed 7 February 2012, and in Mosher, Hendrix and Fort, 2004.

theory-driven rationalism he was attracted by their open-minded, non-categorising approach to the problems of suffering. When he was at the Tavistock (1966–1967), he spent time with R. D. Laing at Kingsley Hall. Laing (1960, 1967) was, of course, the pre-eminent authority on existentialism and madness, and it was here that Mosher began to think about how a community-based social milieu could facilitate the reintegration of psychologically disintegrated individuals, while minimising the harm of institutional care and psychiatric drugs.

Although Laing's influence is apparent in Mosher's work, it is important to state that Mosher was not an 'anti-psychiatrist' (a term that, in any case, Laing rejected). He was sceptical of models of 'schizophrenia' because he believed they stood in the way of a phenomenological view of psychosis (Aderhold, Stastny & Lehmann, 2007). He regarded madness as a way of coping with traumatic events that caused the person to retreat from reality. He saw the experiences of madness – terror, irrationality and mystical experiences – as extremes of ordinary human responses.

In his early career he worked with Sullivanian analysts at Harvard. Harry Stack Sullivan pioneered psychoanalytic work with people suffering from schizophrenia (Sullivan, 1931). He was also one of the first to recognise the value of employing people with no specialist mental health background in working with psychotic people. Freda Fromm-Reichmann (1948) was another important influence; she pioneered psychoanalysis in 'schizophrenia', famously depicted in the novel *I Never Promised You a Rose Garden* (Green, 1964). The influence of the object relations school of psychoanalysis is also apparent in Mosher's work, especially that of Ronald Fairbairn, the Edinburgh psychoanalyst who was primarily interested in the relationships *between* people, not the drives *within* them. Most significantly, his work is grounded in a phenomenological tradition that had been translated into practice by R. D. Laing, David Cooper and Meddard Boss. Indeed, Mosher set up Soteria to create a therapeutic environment capable of testing the critiques of Laing and Franco Basaglia.

From the outset, Soteria was inspired by the philosophical tradition of Kingsley Hall, where the Philadelphia Association opened a community to help people experiencing psychosis. A belief common to Kingsley Hall and Soteria was the '… innovative conception of the psychotic experience – usually viewed as irrational and mystifying – as one which, if treated in an open, non-judgmental way, could be valid and comprehensible' (Mosher, Hendrix & Fort, 2004, p. 4). Unlike Kingsley Hall, which eventually closed in response to pressure from local residents, staff in Soteria worked hard not to antagonise the local community. The project was set up and funded as a research project to investigate whether Soteria was as effective in promoting recovery from first-episode 'schizophrenia' as the drug-based treatment offered by a local psychiatric unit. It was evaluated through randomised controlled trials (e.g., Bola & Mosher, 2003), and a recent systematic review has found that Soteria was at least as effective as traditional hospital-based treatment, but with much lower levels of neuroleptic drug use (Calton, Ferriter, Husband & Spandler, 2008).

The House

The original Soteria House was situated in a multicultural working-class district of San Jose, California. It had 12 rooms, accommodating up to six residents, two full-time staff members, volunteers and helpers. It was furnished to provide a comfortable 'domestic' ambience. The intention was to have a roughly equal mix of residents in crisis, and other residents who were sufficiently advanced on the path to recovery to act as helpers. Staff were non-professional (with the exception of part-time input from a house psychiatrist), and were selected for their ability to contribute to a safe, supportive, warm and relaxed environment. They were also selected on the basis of having an open mind about the nature of madness. Everyone, staff and residents, shared domestic duties.

When the house was first set up there were three rules. Violence to self and others was prohibited. Visitors were allowed only with the prior permission of the residents. No street drugs were permitted in the house, and although alcohol was permitted, it was occasionally banned if someone in the house was abusing it. There was no rule prohibiting sexual relationships between residents, but an 'incest taboo' prohibiting sexual relations between staff and residents was introduced shortly after the house opened. This followed the admission of a young female resident who was vulnerable, disorganised, and sexually disinhibited with staff. Although members of staff were generally encouraged to follow and engage with residents' behaviours, everyone agreed that this was a clear exception.

Soteria and psychosis

Mosher et al. (2004) set out a view of madness that helps us to understand how a therapeutic milieu aimed at helping people to recover should function. In this view, an acute episode of 'schizophrenia' is an altered state of consciousness in response to a crisis. This is associated with a sense of loss of self, brought about by fragmentation of the personality:

> As modalities of experience blend with one another, inner being becomes difficult to distinguish from outer, ambivalence reigns, and the disturbed person's terror is reinforced by others in his/her environment, who feel their own sanity challenged by the events taking place. Mystical experiences are common in this state beyond reason. (Mosher et al., 2004, p. 11)

Mystical experiences were regarded as metaphorically comprehensible, a task made easier by the early 1970's Californian *zeitgeist*. Indeed they make an analogy between the role of staff working with people in psychosis, and that of a 'trip guide', someone who accompanies a person experimenting with LSD, but who doesn't necessarily take the drug themselves.

From this emerges the possibility of growth and reintegration. Staff were encouraged to engage with residents' feelings, beliefs and experiences, and to see in them the potential for psychological growth and reconstitution. This feature of Mosher's view of madness carries the imprint of Erikson's developmental view of human growth and the importance of crises in progressing from one stage of development to the next. This was facilitated by a strong view that the experiences of psychosis were simply extreme expressions of what are fundamentally human experiences.[3] This view was further reinforced by staff values that respected individuality, tolerance, equality, and which resisted any pressure that people should conform. If we see the experiences of psychosis as symptoms of a disease, there is the risk that we negate the person. If their experiences are assumed to be meaningless, we place them beyond the ability of others to engage with them. This relegates the person to the status of a non-person. Instead:

---

3 An implication of this is that the experiences of psychosis lie on a continuum, that there is no point of discontinuity between non-psychotic and psychotic experience. There are strong empirical arguments in support of this view (van Os, 2003; Bentall, 2003). In addition, this view reinforces the ethical position of seeing someone who is mad as human. This is important because of a disturbing tendency in some recent academic writing that interprets loss of narrative in madness as evidence of loss of the person (see Thomas, 2008).

> Soteria saw the individual experiencing a 'schizophrenic' reaction as someone to *be with* – tolerated, interacted with, indeed appreciated. (Mosher et al., 2004, p. 12)

The emergence of a psychosis also affects the social environment in which that individual is embedded, so it was important to work with families and friends in ways that fostered recovery outside.

Medication

Mosher famously resigned from the American Psychiatric Association (APA), claiming that its acronym more accurately reflected its metamorphosis into the American Psychopharmacological Association (Mosher, 1998), but it is wrong to assume that he was completely opposed to the use of medication in madness. He objected to the disingenuity of a system whose theories benefited the pharmaceutical industry, whilst claiming a spurious scientific validity. But he was a pragmatist and he recognised that some people benefited from medication, so he used neuroleptics and benzodiazepines sparingly and judiciously. The overriding consideration in his use of medication, however, was his view that the medium and long-term use of neuroleptic drugs could impede recovery.

The basis for this view was his conviction that 20 years of research (from the late 1950s on) had yielded no evidence that neuroleptics cured 'schizophrenia', whereas it was well established that they caused extremely distressing, sometimes irreversible, toxic effects. For the first six weeks in Soteria all residents were as far as possible drug-free in order to give interpersonal phenomenology a chance to work. During this period medication was used only to reduce otherwise uncontrollable violence or self-destructive impulses, or to damp down unremitting psychological distress that had not responded to interpersonal phenomenology. It was also used if residents specifically requested it. During the first five years of operation, fewer than 10 per cent of residents received continuous medication. They also occasionally used benzodiazepines for the short-term management of severe anxiety and sleep disturbances. There is evidence that these drugs are as effective as neuroleptics in the short-term management of 'schizophrenia' (Wolkowitz & Pickar, 1991).

Being with[4]

Being with was the main way of engaging and working with people experiencing psychosis in Soteria. It was the closest thing to an intervention, although it would be utterly incorrect to describe it as such for reasons that will become clear. It originated in Mosher's interpretation of phenomenology, but in practice it developed out of the vigil used by Rappaport and Silverman (Rappaport, Hopkins, Hall, Belleza & Silverman, 1978), and used in Soteria as a means for interceding in the psychotic process. Rappaport and Silverman's vigil involved pairs of staff (usually one female, one male) spending consecutive shifts of between four to eight hours with the person in crisis, in a comfortable room set aside for the process. The staff had no other demands on their time, so they could spend uninterrupted periods with the person. If the individual wanted to walk about outside they were free to do so accompanied by staff. It was, literally, a case of being with the person continually. Experience indicated that this proved to be a very effective way of engaging with people in acute psychosis.

Being with, '… the basic mode of the Soteria process' (Mosher et al., 2004, p. 169), grew out of the vigil, and took place in three stages. First, staff established and maintained continuous contact with the psychotic person (bonding). The second stage focused on developing ordinary social interactions between the resident and other residents and staff. The third stage encouraged the resident to initiate and engage in activities more generally within and outside the house. This might include involvement in domestic and leisure activities.

Mosher et al. (2004) provide a detailed description of being with through the vigil of a young man, Chuck. This took place over a period of six weeks, during which time members of staff stayed with him for extended periods. During these periods of intense focus, staff set their own needs for sustenance and sleep to one side. This would be impossible to achieve in a conventionally organised acute admission unit, where staff are constantly changing in the endless cycle of shifts. Reliance on agency and bank staff would confound any opportunity to establish relationships based in being with.

---

4 In order to be clear about the use of terms, 'being with' used without a hyphen and italics signifies Loren Mosher's use of the expression. In contrast, '*being-with*' signifies its use by the philosopher Martin Heidegger.

From the descriptions of how staff related to residents in Soteria it is clear that being with involved much more than simply sitting with someone for eight-hour shifts. After all, this happens today on many acute psychiatric inpatient units under the name of 'close observation'. Being with in Soteria demanded a quite specific form of engagement between staff and residents. Some of this was achieved through close physical proximity, and the judicious use of touch and physical contact. It also involved a non-judgemental approach to the experience of another person. This meant that staff had to be open to the world as the resident found it. This openness involved an acceptance of the reality of the other person's experiences, without having to do anything about it, like trying to convince them they were wrong to have the experiences they had. Only from this position, which is a form of concern, is it possible to start the process of entering into the other person's world.

There is a major difficulty in trying to convey anything about the existential or phenomenological aspects of human life. Words are inadequate. Being with is a human process, and as such is greater than the sum of the individual components of human subjectivity, thought and language, feeling and emotion, perception, posture, touch and expression. It reflects a struggle to reach into and grasp the world of another human being. There is a profound philosophical difference between a phenomenological approach to human experience and that of scientific modes of thought. One way of grasping this difference is through a thought experiment, discussed below.

Phenomenology and existentialism

A phenomenological perspective on human life deals primarily with our relationship with the world we encounter before us. The expression used by the philosopher Heidegger (1962) to describe this, *being-in-the-world*, conveys the inseparable nature of our relationship with the world. As an extension of this more general view, *being-with* deals with our relationship to the human beings we encounter in the world. There is a strong element of choice in the way we engage with the world, and the others we encounter in it. In an attempt to make this clear, I will use a simple thought experiment that you can try yourself.

I would like you to think carefully about an image that means a great deal to you. It might be a photograph of someone special, a painting, or some other image that moves you. In front of me is an image captured by Don McCullin, the photographer, called *Shell-shocked Marine, Hue, Vietnam, 1968* (McCullin, 2003).[5] Right now, I remember vividly the first time I encountered it. I was waiting for a tram in Piccadilly Station, Manchester, two or three years ago. The image was on the other side of the platform, advertising an exhibition of Don McCullin's photographs at the Imperial War Museum North. The following weekend I had to see it. I stood in front of it and was drawn to the soldier's eyes. Even today they strike me as intense and glazed at the same time. How can that possibly be the case? It doesn't make sense to have eyes that are glazed *and* intense, but that's how they seem to me. He stares through me, but I don't know what he is staring at. Then it struck me; that's not true. The truth is I'd rather not think about what he's staring at. I dread to think about the horrors this man has witnessed, flickering in the space a thousand yards behind my head. At the same time the fixity and terror of his gaze is at odds with his appearance. He seems to have no neck. As he cowers in fear his head seems to be set directly on his shoulders, and is also somehow too big for his body. This gives him a faintly mechanical appearance, like a child's puppet frozen in time. Perhaps that is how he sees himself, were it possible for him to have seen himself in the state he was in. Then I wonder if this is how he felt, a petrified toy soldier, an automaton without any will, under someone else's control. His fingers curl around the barrel of his rifle as though they were carved from the same piece of wood. He is inseparable from his gun; they are one and the same. All these reflections, conflicting, paradoxical, puzzled, flashed through me the first time I saw the image. Finally, I think about the man who took the photograph, of Don McCullin and the camera he used to capture the image. It wasn't any camera, but a Nikon, a particular model, a Nikon F. And Don McCullin's Nikon F was uniquely tied to his life in a terrifying way. In Vietnam a sniper's bullet hit the camera, saving his life.

Now I look at the image again, two or three years after my first encounter with it. At first the marine still arouses the same responses, but this time I am aware of something else. As I look at it I ask myself a question, how is it possible for this image to be present in front of me? Again I think of Don McCullin's battered camera, and as I try to answer

---

5 This image is available online at http://www.guardian.co.uk/artanddesign/gallery/2010/feb/ 07/don-mccullin-war-photographs#/?picture=358984551&index=1 accessed 12 March 2012.

this question I think of the lens and its optical elements, the diaphragm that set the aperture to regulate the depth of field, the shutter screen and the intricate mechanisms for controlling its speed, and thus the amount of light that reaches the film. That light impinged on the invisible silver salts in the emulsion, where photons caused physico-chemical changes that resulted in the release of visible silver particles. Then I move to the darkroom where more light and lenses, this time in an enlarger, were followed by more chemical processes as the first image developed. More recently someone has scanned the image and converted the light reflected off its surface into binary information to store and manipulate it in a computer so it can be printed out in the book that sits on my desk.

When I try to answer the question, how did this image come before me? I find myself making a deliberate effort to break it down into discrete stages or processes involving optics, chemistry, quantum physics and the manipulation of digital data. Each has its own set of rules and laws, none of which I understand. But in trying to answer the question it is not necessary for me to understand them; all I need is a general awareness that they exist. But as I try to answer the question, something changes in my relationship with the image. It is not possible for me to answer the question of how this image came before me, *and* be engaged with it at the same time. I have to disengage from the image so that it is no longer present to me in the way that it was when I first encountered it in Piccadilly Station, a powerful icon of war and suffering. On that first occasion the image had a powerful emotional impact on me. It stood out as something that I could not avoid grappling with, the soldier, the suffering he was involved with, his suffering, and the courage of the man who took the photograph. In this mode of being I am drawn into the image. It preoccupies me and fills my awareness to the exclusion of everything else, evoking a range of responses, some contradictory, but never ending. Each time I engage with it in this way I become aware of new responses, and in that sense the image is endless and never fixed, impossible to be determined. Indeed, we may see the question 'how?' and the scientific explanations that arise from this, as simply one aspect of my continuing responses to the presence of the image before me. However, as soon as I ask the question 'how?', I stand back from the image and disengage from it. And as soon as that happens it ceases to be something special to me. It wouldn't have mattered if the image were the soldier at Hue or an image of a bowl of porridge. The answer to the question, how did this image come to be before me? would have been the same.

To grasp the difference between Soteria's interpersonal phenomenology and the technological paradigm in psychiatry, we replace the soldier's image with a person in distress.

The purpose of the thought experiment is to draw attention in a simple manner to an aspect of phenomenology[6] necessary to understand Loren Mosher's being with: that of Heidegger's *being-in-the-world*. The work of the philosophers Heidegger (1962) and Merleau-Ponty (1962) is critical of the view that scientific theories are capable of generating a complete account of our experience of the world. This does not mean that scientific accounts of experience are wrong, or that they have no role in accounting for madness or distress, simply that it is important that we are aware of the limitations of these accounts. Why is this?

Merleau-Ponty (1962) argues that scientific modes of thought arise from the fact of our *being-in-the-world*, which stands for our immediate experience of the world as it already presents itself to us, as we are already immersed and engaged in it. Before we ever begin to think about the world in scientific terms, we are already in that world, grappling with it, interpreting it, struggling to make sense of it. This is broadly how I experienced the soldier's image when I first encountered it. The human activities of scientific thought and inquiry are themselves products of this struggle to meaning.[7] The difficulty is that scientific modes of thought have become so influential over the last four centuries that we assume they provide a view of the world as it really is. This puts the cart before the horse. Existential philosophy holds that scientific accounts of human experience do not stand outside that experience; they are created by it.[8]

Pat Bracken has written about the implications of this in relation to understanding the suffering of those who have experienced trauma (Bracken, 2002). He points out that Heidegger writes about different types

6 Although well beyond the scope of this chapter, it is important to note in passing that there are different strands of thought in phenomenology. The phenomenological tradition in which interpersonal phenomenology is based is that influenced by the philosophers Martin Heidegger and Maurice Merleau-Ponty. This must not be confused with the phenomenological tradition that has dominated psychiatric thought, that of Karl Jaspers (1963). Pat Bracken and I (2005) have argued that Jaspers regarded his approach as primarily scientific in nature.

7 Echoing Sartre's famous dictum, we are condemned to freedom, Merleau-Ponty said we are condemned to meaning.

8 Some have argued that Merleau-Ponty was anti-science; I maintain that a close reading of his work reveals that this was not the case. He simply wanted to place science in a more appropriate relationship to human experience. My position is not that I am opposed to scientific approaches to suffering, but it is important that we are aware of their limitations, that what they seek to exclude is important and valuable in clinical work. See Thomas, Bracken and Timimi (2012).

of care and caring. One variety involves taking over the world of the other person and dominating them. For example, we can 'intervene' in people's lives, and do things to them or for them. This is what happens when psychiatrists force people to have medication against their wishes. Under less extreme circumstances, such as when someone suffers from a chronic sadness and suffering, it may be difficult for the person to retain control. This is a well-recognised problem in psychotherapy, where the person may be dominated by his or her therapist, or be dependent on them. In contrast there is a form of care that can liberate, or what Heidegger calls authentic care. This does not involve rushing in and taking over for the other person, but being at hand for them, respectful, receptive and ready to stand with them in facing the world. This is exactly what Mosher's being with entails.

Barriers to Soteria

Given the evidence that Soteria is at least as effective as conventional psychiatric inpatient care, why has it not been adopted more widely? There are houses in Berne (Ciompi & Hoffman, 2004), Zwiefalten, Munich, and Budapest, and there was a house in Stockholm until it was merged into a crisis programme. The influence of Soteria can also be seen in Open Dialogue (Seikkula et al., 2003) and the Needs-Adapted approach (Alanen, Lehtinen, Rakkolainen, Aaltonen, 1991) both in Finland, and the Swedish 'Parachute' Project (Cullberg, Levander, Holmqvist, Mattsson & Wieselgren, 2002). All three are community-based support systems for people experiencing acute psychosis; and all three have been formally evaluated and shown to be effective in the short term with good long-term outcomes. The Soteria Network UK[9] works to promote the development of drug-free and minimal medication approaches based in Loren Mosher's ideas. But the question remains, why has Soteria had such a limited influence? There are four possible explanations.

First, Soteria demedicalised psychosis. It rejected the notion that 'schizophrenia' is a medical condition, but it did so when the influence of psychotherapeutic and social interventions for psychosis was waning. The publication in 1980 of the holy text of scientific psychiatry, *DSM-III*, marked the beginning of a barren period for non-scientific ways of engaging with madness. The rise of EBM, and the insistence that interventions had to have their efficacy established through controlled trials, has made it

---

9 See http://www.soterianetwork.org.uk/ Retrieved 9 May 2012.

even more difficult to argue the case for Soteria. There is a fundamental paradigmatic conflict between the randomisation necessary for EBM, and the emphasis on personal choice that is central to Soteria. Mosher et al. (2004) give an excellent account of this tension.

Second, there are political factors. Mosher et al. (2004) describe the political pressures that Soteria encountered in the 1970s and 1980s. Some of these persist today, such as the insistence that Soteria conforms to scientific requirements of evaluation. There is also the political resistance of a psychiatric profession dominated by the interests of the pharmaceutical industry. But today there is also the perceived dangerousness of people identified as suffering from 'schizophrenia', and the role of medication in managing this risk. Technological psychiatry has created the myth that 'schizophrenia' is a disease amenable to treatment with drugs. Against the context of the risk culture in which we live, this is a powerful factor maintaining the dominance of technological psychiatry (Moncrieff, 1997). The proposition that psychosis does not require treatment with drugs is likely to encounter the question of risk.

The third barrier is the waning influence of psychodynamic and social ways of understanding and responding to madness, although this in turn relates to the rise of scientific psychiatry. Soteria was explicitly set up to work in a way that did not conform to positivist psychiatry. In addition, since the 1960s and the work of Laing, the influence of existentialism (an important branch of twentieth-century continental philosophy) has waned in British psychiatry.

The fourth barrier is the challenge to professional authority posed by Soteria, which explicitly preferred to employ staff with no specific mental health knowledge or training. Indeed, former residents who had been through Soteria were frequently employed as staff members. Thus the widespread adoption of Soteria would represent a significant threat to the professional power of psychiatrists, mental health nurses, psychologists and other professional groups.

Conclusions

The failure of technological psychiatry to improve the outcome for people who experience psychosis, the serious harm associated with the long-term use of neuroleptic medication, and at a fundamental level, the failure of science to explain madness, have resulted in a crisis in contemporary psychiatry. This, I have argued, means that the core values and philosophy of Soteria are more relevant today than they were back in the 1970s. Mental health care desperately needs a new direction, and in these days of post-institutional care, Soteria offers a way forward.

References

Aderhold, V., Stastny, P., & Lehmann, P. (2007). Soteria: An alternative mental health reform movement. In P. Stastny & P. Lehmann (Eds.), *Alternatives Beyond Psychiatry*. Berlin: Peter Lehmann Publishing.

Alanen, Y. O., Lehtinen, K., Rakkolainen, V., & Aaltonen, J. (1991). Need-adapted treatment of new schizophrenic patients: Experiences and results of the Turku Project. *Acta Psychiatrica Scandinavica, 83,* 363–372.

Allers, R. (1961). *Existentialism and Psychiatry.* Springfield, IL: Charles C. Thomas.

Anckarsäter, H. (2010). Beyond categorical diagnostics in psychiatry: Scientific and medicolegal implications. *International Journal of Law and Psychiatry, 33,* 59–65.

Bentall, R. P. (2003). *Madness Explained: Psychosis and human nature.* London: Allen Lane.

Bola, J. R. (2006). Medication-free research in early episode schizophrenia: Evidence of long-term harm? *Schizophrenia Bulletin, 32*(2), 288–296.

Bola, J. R., Kao, D., & Haluk, S. (2012). Antipsychotic medication for early-episode schizophrenia. *Schizophrenia Bulletin, 38*(1), 23–25.

Bola, J. R., & Mosher, L. R. (2003). Treatment of acute psychosis without neuroleptics: Two-year outcomes from the Soteria Project. *Journal of Nervous and Mental Disease, 191,* 219–229.

Boss, M. (1963). *Psychoanalysis and Daseinsanalysis.* New York: Basic Books.

Bracken, P. (2002). *Trauma: Culture, meaning and philosophy.* London: Whurr Publishers. (See especially pp. 124–127.)

Bracken, P., & Thomas, P. (2005*). Postpsychiatry: Mental health in a postmodern world.* Oxford: Oxford University Press.

Calton, T., Ferriter, M., Husband, N., & Spandler, H. (2008). A systematic review of the Soteria paradigm for the treatment of people diagnosed with schizophrenia. *Schizophrenia Bulletin, 34,* 181–192.

Casey, D., Rodriguez, M., Northcott, C., Vickar, G., & Shihabuddin, L. (2011). Schizophrenia: Medical illness, mortality, and aging. *International Journal of Psychiatry in Medicine, 41,* 245–251.

Ciompi, L., & Hoffman, H. (2004). Soteria Berne: An innovative milieu therapeutic approach to acute schizophrenia based on the concept of affect-logic. *World Psychiatry, 3,* 140–146.

Cullberg J., Levander S., Holmqvist R., Mattsson M., & Wieselgren I.-M. (2002). One-year outcome in first episode psychosis patients in the Swedish Parachute project. *Acta Psychiatrica Scandinavica, 106,* 276–285.

Fromm-Reichmann, F. (1948). Notes on the development of treatment of schizophrenics by psychoanalytic psychotherapy. *Psychiatry, 11,* 263–273.

Green, H. (1964). *I Never Promised You a Rose Garden.* London: Gollancz.

Harrow, M., Jobe, T., & Faull, R. (2012). Do all schizophrenia patients need antipsychotic treatment continuously throughout their life time? A 20-year longitudinal study. *Psychological Medicine, 42*(10), 2145–2155. DOI: 10.1017/S0033291712000220

Heidegger, M. (1962). *Being and Time* (J. Macquarrie & E. Robinson, Trans.). Oxford: Basil Blackwell. (See especially Division 1.4, p. 26)

Hennessy, S., Bilker, W. B., Knauss, J. S., Margolis, D. J., Kimmel, S.E., Reynolds R. F., et al. (2002). Cardiac arrest and ventricular arrhythmia in patients taking antipsychotic drugs: Cohort study using administrative data. *British Medical Journal, 325,* 1070.

Ho, B.-C., Andreasen, N., Ziebell, S., Pierson, R., & Magnotta, V. (2011). Long-term antipsychotic treatment and brain volumes: A longitudinal study of first-episode schizophrenia. *Archives of General Psychiatry, 68,* 128–137.

Husserl, E. (1967). *The Paris Lectures.* The Hague: Martinus Nijhoff.

Jaspers, K. (1963). *General Psychopathology* (J. Hoenig & M. Hamilton, Trans.). Manchester: Manchester University Press.

Kingdon, D. (2007). Research into putative biological mechanisms of mental disorders has been of no value to clinical psychiatry. *British Journal of Psychiatry, 191,* 285–290.

Laing, R. D. (1960). *The Divided Self: An existential study in sanity and madness.* London: Tavistock Publications.

Laing. R. D. (1967). *The Politics of Experience.* New York: Ballantine.

Leamy, M., Bird, V., Le Boutillier, C., Williams, J., & Slade, M. (2011). Conceptual framework for personal recovery in mental health: Systematic review and narrative synthesis. *British Journal of Psychiatry, 199,* 445–452.

May, R., Angel, E., & Ellenerger, H. (Eds.). (1958). *Existence: A new dimension in psychiatry and psychology.* New York: Basic Books.

McCullin, D. (2003). *Don McCullin.* London: Jonathan Cape.

Merleau-Ponty, M. (1962). *Phenomenology of Perception* (C. Smith, Trans.). London: Routledge & Kegan Paul.

Moncrieff, J. (1997). Psychiatric imperialism: The medicalisation of modern living. *Soundings, 6*(Summer).

Moncrieff, J., & Leo, J. (2010). A systematic review of the effects of antipsychotic drugs on brain volume. *Psychological Medicine, 40,* 1409–1422.

Mosher, L. R. (1998). Letter of resignation from the American Pychiatric Association. Retrieved 7 February 2012 from http://www.moshersoteria.com /articles/resignation-from-apa/

Mosher, L. R. (1999). Soteria and other alternatives to acute psychiatric hospitalization: A personal and professional review. *Journal of Nervous and Mental Disease, 187,* 142–149.

Mosher, L. R., & Burti, L. (1994). *Community Mental Health: A practical guide.* (pp. 127–142). New York & London: W. W. Norton & Company.

Mosher, L. R., Hendrix, V., & Fort, D. (2004). *Soteria: Through madness to deliverance.* Bloomington, IN: XLibris.

Rappaport, M., Hopkins, H., Hall, K., Belleza, T., & Silverman, J. (1978). Are there schizophrenics for whom drugs may be unnecessary or contraindicated? *International Pharmacopsychiatry, 13,* 100–111.

Ray, W. A., Chung, C. P., Murray, K., Hall, K., & Stein, C. (2009). Atypical antipsychotic drugs and the risk of sudden cardiac death. *New England Journal of Medicine, 360,* 225–235.

Sartre, J.-P. (1958). *Being and Nothingness.* London: Methuen.

Seikkula, J., Alakare, B., Aaltonen, J., Holma, J., Rasinkangas, A., & Lehtinen, V. (2003). Open dialogue approach: Treatment principles and preliminary results of a two-year follow-up on first episode schizophrenia. *Ethical Human Sciences and Services, 5,* 163–182.

Spandler, H., & Thomas, P. (2012). *A Survey of Existentialism in Mental Health Practice in the UK.* Manuscript in preparation, 2012.

Sullivan, H. (1931). The modified psychoanalytic treatment of schizophrenia. *American Journal of Psychiatry, 11,* 519–540.

Thomas, P. (2008). Towards a critical perspective on 'narrative loss' in schizophrenia. In A. Morgan (Ed.), *Being Human: Reflections on mental distress in society* (pp. 24–39). Ross-on-Wye: PCCS Books.

Thomas, P., Bracken, P., & Timimi, S. (2012). The anomalies of evidence-based medicine in psychiatry: Time to rethink the basis of mental health practice. *Mental Health Review Journal, 17*(3), 152–162.

Thornley, B., & Adams, C. (1998). Content and quality of 2000 controlled trials in schizophrenia over 50 years. *British Medical Journal, 317,* 1181–1184.

Van Os, J. (2003). Is there a continuum of psychotic experience in the general population? *Epidemiologia e Psychiatria Sociale, 12*(4), 242–252.

Wildgust, H., Hodgson, R., & Beary, M. (2010). The paradox of premature mortality in schizophrenia: New research questions. *Journal of Psychopharmacology, 24*(Suppl. 4), s9–15.

Wolkowitz, O., & Pickar, D. (1991). Benzodiazepines in the treatment of schizophrenia: A review and reappraisal. *American Journal of Psychiatry, 148,* 714–726.

Part Two

Exploring the Liberation
of Madness

Recovery, Discovery and Revolution: The work of Intervoice and the Hearing Voices Movement

Eleanor Longden, Dirk Corstens & Jacqui Dillon

According to Kuhn's (1962) famous treatise on the cause and correlates of scientific revolution, intellectual shift occurs when spiralling anomalies and contradictions begin to undermine the basic hypotheses upon which the 'old rules' were founded. Furthermore, as in the case of political dissent, this rebellion is enacted in a context of increasing social crisis, professional anxiety, and personal discontent, wherein the failures and incongruence of the original paradigm fuels a search for more appropriate, compatible models. The ultimate outcome is conceptual revolution, and a shift from 'ordinary to extraordinary' research, theory, and practice.

Correspondingly, this chapter describes how the pessimism and pathology of traditional biomedical approaches to hearing voices was the means of energising a revolutionary new paradigm for understanding the experience. We will explore how these social, political, clinical, and philosophical assumptions became collectively embedded within what has come to be known as the Hearing Voices Movement, before discussing the role of Intervoice: The International Network for Training, Education and Research into Hearing Voices (www.intervoiceonline.org) in coordinating these activities at a local, national, and international level. In doing so, we will draw on social movement theory to demonstrate how the Hearing Voices Movement fits within a broader framework of collective protest and social reform. Finally, we will discuss how the ethos of the Hearing Voices Movement, most notably the premise of accepting and making sense of voices, can be applied in clinical practice to create frameworks for supporting clients in holistic, humanistic ways.

Redefining hearing voices

The philosophy, practice, and politics of the Hearing Voices Movement originate in the work of Dutch social psychiatrist Marius Romme and his co-researcher Sandra Escher. Romme and Escher's (1993, 2000) ground-breaking approach, which was devised in partnership with voice hearers themselves, is based on the principles that (1) hearing voices is a normal human experience, that (2) can be understood in the context of life events and interpersonal narratives, and which (3) is often precipitated and maintained by events that overwhelm and disempower the individual. Correspondingly, they have advocated a process of accepting voices, making sense of them, and acknowledging the subjective reality of the voice hearer.

Although destined to become an international concern, Romme and Escher's research was initially disseminated in the Netherlands in the late 1980s. Amongst other achievements, this led to the establishment of Stichting Weerklank (Foundation Resonance), a supportive network of voice hearers and allies organised outside of the psychiatric system. The approach was swiftly adopted in the UK, with the Hearing Voices Network (HVN) launched in Manchester in 1988. A traditional home of radical politics and progressive social change, Manchester has been described as 'the international gateway' for the Hearing Voices Movement (James, 2001, p. 47), and since its inception HVN has earned a reputation as a critical and progressive organisation that wields increasing influence over psychiatry (Dillon & Longden, 2011; Hornstein, 2012; Johnstone, 2011).

Today there are Hearing Voices networks in 21 countries, including Australia, Denmark, Germany, Italy, New Zealand, and most recently, the USA. In turn, these national networks are coordinated, promoted, and supported via Intervoice. These initiatives are rooted in what is now collectively known as the Hearing Voices Movement, and together have elaborated a way of understanding voice hearing that is a complete contradiction of the illness model espoused by biological psychiatry (see Box 1). Although initially perceived as contentious and marginal, these ideas have become increasingly mainstream, with many of the movement's basic assumptions gathering rapid academic and clinical support in the last 10 years. This includes, for example, the association between voices and trauma (e.g., Read, van Os, Morrison, & Ross, 2005); the suggestion that voice content is psychologically significant and meaningful (e.g., Beavan & Read, 2010); that structural voice characteristics are reliably similar between psychotic patients, non-psychotic patients and non-clinical groups (e.g., Longden, Madill & Waterman, 2012); and that links between voice hearing and mental health problems may primarily be determined by an individual's interpretation of and/or emotional response to their voices (e.g., Romme, Escher, Dillon, Corstens & Morris, 2009).

Box 1. Aims and Assumptions of Intervoice and the Hearing Voices Movement

Normalising voices

Psychiatry has traditionally portrayed voice hearing as a bizarre and unusual experience that is indicative of serious psychopathology. In contrast, the Hearing Voices Movement argues that voice hearing is a normal human variation – a sign of difference and diversity – that is by no means the sole province of the mentally distressed. This contention is supported by recent research (e.g., Beavan, Read, & Cartwright, 2011), which indicates voice-hearing prevalence in the general population may be as high as 13 per cent. To put this in perspective, these figures suggest that in a Western nation, one is more likely to be a non-patient voice hearer than to be left-handed (10 per cent of the population), to be a vegetarian (6 per cent of the population), to have a PhD (3 per cent of the population), or to experience a stammer (1 per cent of the population).

Correspondingly, Intervoice challenges negative, stereotypical views of voice hearing that reinforce its association with chaotic emotions and disturbed, disordered behaviour. While conventional illness models endeavour to 'change' the voice hearer, Intervoice can therefore be seen as trying to combat shame and stigma by challenging society's and psychiatry's prejudicial views. Indeed, Romme (2000) argues that voice hearer 'emancipation' is comparable to the civil rights movements of the 1960s, in which psychiatry was forced to revise its punitive, persecutory attitudes towards homosexuality.

Personal meaning

Although not disputing that voices can terrorise and demoralise the hearer, the fact that many people hear voices whilst living happy, high-functioning lives suggests that voice presence, in itself, may not be the true problem. Conversely Intervoice suggests that what distresses individuals is their inability to cope with voice hearing and/or with the painful, unresolved life events that evoked it. Rather than working within diagnosis and illness frameworks, Intervoice therefore advocates an exploration of emotions, life events, and personal interpretations. Voices are seen as 'messengers' that represent important information about life problems (Romme, 2000), and which can therefore be utilised as a means of solving social and emotional conflict. This is a startling contrast to traditional views of voices as a meaningless, aberrant symptom of illness.

While Intervoice espouses psychosocial understandings of voice hearing, it is not directive about the 'true' cause of voices. Instead, it encourages individuals to seek solutions within their own preferred frame of reference (e.g., spiritual, parapsychological, medical, cognitive). In this way, it provides a tolerant, non-judgemental space in which voice hearers are respected and validated; supported to understand their experiences and develop their own ways of coping; and to ultimately use this knowledge to grow, strengthen, and develop in their own way.

Individual agency and expertise

Intervoice strongly critiques the traditional view of dominant, expert clinician, and passive, recipient patient. Instead, it argues that every voice hearer has unique expertise and insight about her own experiences, circumstances and needs. This includes formulating the meaning of one's voices, but also extends to crediting the role of agency and self-determination in the recovery process. While not denying the value some voice hearers find in interventions like medication – and whilst also acknowledging the significant social and material adversities that can hinder recovery – Intervoice believes individuals should be supported to find opportunities to reclaim ownership of their own healing through activities like peer support, self-management, and self-directed coping. By helping voice hearers to empower themselves and reclaim mastery of their experiences, Intervoice believes they can ultimately take ownership of their own recovery.

Intervoice

Intervoice was first established in 1997 as an organisational structure that could provide administrative and coordinative support to the numerous initiatives taking place as part of the Hearing Voices Movement. In 2007 it was incorporated as a not-for-profit company under UK law (International Hearing Voices Projects Ltd.) with Marius Romme as its president and, since 2009, the psychiatrist Dirk Corstens as chairperson.

The Intervoice board includes individuals from Australia, Denmark, the Netherlands, the UK, and the USA, and is comprised of a combination of voice hearers and mental health workers.

Intervoice locates itself within the broader framework of a civil rights movement, perceiving that its members are being denied various social benefits (e.g., safety, respect, opportunities) simply because of their identity as voice hearers. As such, it aims to 'emancipate voice hearers and people who support them' by enhancing awareness of voice hearers' civil rights, and developing best practice in working with distressed individuals in ways that serve recovery (Intervoice, 2012). This goal is enacted within a respectful alliance between experts by experience (voice hearers) and experts by profession (mental health workers, academics, activists). This process of partnership informs much of Intervoice's decision making, in that a variety of perspectives bridge 'the personal and professional' by breaking down the divide between worker and psychiatric survivor (Intervoice, 2012).

Closely related to this mission is Intervoice's second primary goal: disseminating hopeful, positive information about voice hearing and ensuring that its innovative approach becomes increasingly familiar with voices hearers, mental health professionals, and the general public. Current strategies include the Intervoice website, social media, multilingual publications, peer support initiatives, self-help groups, media coverage, training events and the annual World Hearing Voices Congress. Intervoice also has its own Research Committee, comprised of voice hearers as well as internationally renowned academics, which is designed to promote Intervoice's emancipatory ethos via scientific channels.

The emergence of a social and civil rights movement

Social movements represent a significant, sustained form of communal protest, solidarity, and action, in which groups of ordinary individuals work together to challenge established systems. Some of the most outstanding social movements have been the means of enacting permanent political and cultural transformations (e.g., women's suffrage, gay liberation, the civil rights movements, environmental activism). The Hearing Voices Movement can be seen as a reformative, group-focused, global movement that works to transform a minority experience from a position of shame and persecution to one of collective empowerment.

Social movement theory (e.g., Engel, 2001; McAdam, 1997) provides a comprehensive framework for understanding the inception and development of social movements. Amongst other observations, the model suggests that these are shaped and maintained by two interrelated processes: perceived *threat*, and sufficient *opportunity* to challenge and rectify it. In the following section, we will use social movement theory to explore the formation and maintenance of the Hearing Voices Movement. In this respect, while the latter's emergence can be understood as the creative initiative of three individuals (Marius Romme, Sandra Escher, and the voice hearer Patsy Hage: see James, 2001) it is important to realise that this endeavour occurred within a context of fundamental structural shifts in both society and the psychiatric system: in effect, an ideal confluence of perceived threat and opportunity. Correspondingly, the Hearing Voices Movement can be understood as part of a broader systemic process that followed the same developmental lines as other social movements.

Movement development
The inception of any social movement depends on three broad factors: changing opportunity structures (*why* the movement developed), engaging existing resources (*how* it developed), and recruiting relevant stakeholders (*when* it developed).

Why: Changing opportunity structure
Taken together, shifts within traditional psychiatric structures, a growing dissatisfaction towards the treatment of psychiatric patients, and the emergence of novel theoretical and research-based approaches created opportunities to develop attitudes around voice hearing that were based on empowerment, inclusion, and de-medicalisation.

The moral and political reaction to ineffective, inhumane psychiatric treatments led to the dismantling of traditional, large-scale institutions in many Western societies. Thousands of ex-patients were discharged into urban areas, where they in turn fell victim to extremes of isolation, exclusion, and marginalisation. Services capable of promoting genuine social integration were rarely on the political agenda, prompting a growing dissatisfaction from families, mental health charities, and society itself at the plight of many service users.

This period, in which psychiatric patients were becoming increasingly visible within society, coincided with a growth in epidemiological research investigating the prevalence of 'psychotic-like phenomena' in the general population. This work (see Longden et al., 2012) repeatedly supported the contention that hearing voices, far from being a rare, extraordinary experience, was surprisingly common amongst those in good psychological health. Correspondingly the innovative and intellectual work of Julian Jaynes (1976) – a perfect example of creative theorising during a period of transition – articulated the argument that voice hearing may have played a pivotal role in the evolution of human consciousness. In turn, Jaynes' work influenced the creative social action of the early protagonists of the Hearing Voices Movement, with Marius Romme and Patsy Hage appearing on Dutch television to try and identify non-patient voice hearers and learn how they coped with their voices.

The fate of American veterans after the Vietnam War led to a new awareness of the psychological impact of trauma, prompting the development of the diagnostic category of post-traumatic stress disorder. In turn, trauma and adversity played a formative role in Romme and Escher's explanatory model of voice hearing.

How: Pre-existing organisations

The emergence of the service user/survivor movement in the 1980s and 1990s heralded a new level of protest against prevailing medical ideologies and the dehumanising regimes of traditional psychiatric services. Simultaneously, coalitions of families and carer groups became a political force that highlighted the neglect and maltreatment endured by many patients. However, although the user movement became increasingly articulate and politically engaged, it exerted only nominal impact on psychiatric practice and developed relatively small initiatives within society. The user movement generally embraced the ideas that emerged from the anti-psychiatry movement, especially the political emphasis on the 'mad society' and the 'identified patient', yet the psychotherapeutic approach harboured by rebel protagonists like Laing and Szasz found little resonance in traditional psychiatric practice.

At the same time, psychotherapeutic centres like Chestnut Lodge in the USA offered a promise of more humane, holistic treatment for individuals with complex mental health needs. The Soteria Project became a well-researched, hopeful initiative that worked within the confines of classical psychiatric diagnoses but offered respectful treatment based on solidarity and pragmatic reasoning. The recovery movement also gathered momentum, propagating a powerful focus on the individual as author and arbitrator of her own healing. Social psychiatry developed in countries like the Netherlands, with community mental health centres becoming increasingly prevalent in other parts of Europe. Psychologists, especially in England, became interested in psychosis and the feasibility of treating it in a psychological way (British Psychological Society, 2000). In turn, this provided ammunition against the clinical concept of schizophrenia (e.g., Boyle, 2002), although it was ultimately unsuccessful in diminishing the powerful medical model of biological psychiatry.

During this transition, where numerous organisations and initiatives competed to offer alternatives to orthodox concepts of mental distress, the experience of voice hearing – a paradigmatic psychotic 'symptom' – emerged as the basis for a powerful collective identity. In turn, this was strongly reinforced by the organisation of annual conferences in which, for the first time in history, voice hearers and their allies were able to gather together to articulate their needs, hopes, and aspirations.

When: An emerging collective identity

Collective identity refers to an individual's sense of shared status: 'a cognitive, moral, and emotional connection with a broader community, category, practice, or institution' (Polletta & Jasper, 2001, p. 85). For the Hearing Voices Movement, this process involved dismantling narratives based on disease, impairment and chronicity by substituting the concept of 'the schizophrenic' with that of the 'voice hearer.'

Indeed, while individuals 'often join [Intervoice] with a "diagnosis" as their identity ... the process of membership often leads to significant change in people's perception of themselves as contributors and as whole people' (Intervoice, 2012). This is particularly important in terms of acknowledging and valuing an experience that has traditionally been derided or labelled as deviant and abnormal. As Elisabeth Svanholmer states 'creating a "fellowship" around voice hearing gives the experience, the recognition, the weight of reality, the value, that it truly has to every voice hearer' (quoted in Romme et al., 2009, p. 82).

As part of this imperative, the Hearing Voices Movement supports voice hearers to hone and celebrate their sense of themselves as experience-based experts. Experiential knowledge is accorded equivalent value to scientific or training-derived knowledge, with individuals supported to disseminate their expertise through publications, training, and conference presentations. Correspondingly, this input is remunerated equally, with voice hearers receiving the same fees as professional speakers like doctors and researchers. Other initiatives to reclaim voice hearing as a valuable, non-stigmatised identity include development projects that educate the public about the acceptability and significance of voice hearing (e.g., speaking in schools, civic buildings, and community centres), and promoting respectful, enlightening portrayals in the media.

Movement maintenance

The mobilisation of social movements incorporates similar dynamics to their formation. Specifically, maintenance depends on the input of component organisations; however, while the movement itself generally operates outside of a 'ruling' system, institution, or ideology, these groups and networks often interact and navigate within them in order to raise awareness and institute reform.

Interest groups

Interest groups (sometimes called 'pressure groups') are collectives of individuals, organised outside of official governing parties, who advocate a specific cause and promote its interests in terms of public and political policy. Intervoice itself is an interest group, although it also works in partnership with other organisations in order to publicise its message, advance its cause, and share strengths and resources with like-minded colleagues. Interest groups currently affiliated with Intervoice include local Hearing Voices groups, national Hearing Voices networks, non-governmental organisations, and professional bodies that espouse critical psychiatric practice.

Political institutions and traditional psychiatric services

It is necessary for social movements to interact and collaborate with dominant institutions if they are to influence philosophies and practice, and effectively promote destigmatisation, emancipation, and empowerment. An example of such cooperation in the Hearing Voices Movement is a unique service created in the Danish city of Aarhus. The municipality finances and supports a community support worker and several voice hearers, who oversee the formation of city-wide self-help groups and provide national training initiatives. The values of the Hearing Voices Movement are therefore disseminated in a way that is adapted to the specific situation of that country (for example, self-help groups are guided by professionals), thereby carefully and cumulatively influencing psychiatric practice. Similarly, Voices Vic (based in Melboune, Australia) is a well-resourced network of voice hearers, carers, and professionals that supports the development of peer-support initiatives, educates the wider community about voice hearing, and organises regular training events and an annual conference. In the UK, HVN considers itself a psychiatric service which offers recovery-oriented initiatives and strategies to transform the lives of voice hearers. HVN members work in traditional psychiatric services (e.g., acute wards, forensic institutions) to support the development of self-help groups and challenge pessimistic, paternalistic medical beliefs by demonstrating individual progress and empowerment.

Intervoice board members similarly deliver training, lectures and consultation in various countries to promote change in psychiatric services and improve the treatment of voice hearers. Whereas the emphasis in the early years of the Hearing Voices Movement was critiquing traumatic, stigmatising aspects of traditional treatments, there is a growing appreciation that change in psychiatric services will happen more effectively through a process of cooperation with these services and recruiting allies within them.

Academic studies into voice hearing have increased substantially since the development of the Hearing Voices Movement 20 years ago. Simultaneously, research that supports the Movement's values and aims is indispensable in order to enhance and reinforce these developments. Intervoice deliberately created a research branch in order to strengthen its impact on public and scientific debate. Its next ambition is to challenge the academic focus on 'objectivity' in research by propagating the value of more subjective approaches which emphasise the 'evidence' provided by personal stories of recovery (e.g., Romme et al., 2009).

Fuel

As with other social movements (see Edwards & McCarthy, 2004), the Hearing Voices Movement is mobilised and energised through the deployment of various resources. These sources of 'fuel' include moral/ cultural factors (solidarity and emotional and intellectual support); organisational factors (social networks, professional bodies); material assets (donations and other financial capital); and human input, including volunteers and paid workers. Current resource mobilisation includes: joining traditional systems (e.g., peer-support workers, introducing hearing voices groups on acute wards, using research to enact evidence-based change, intervention and innovation); media coverage; training; the Internet, including social media (e.g., Intervoice has its own website and Facebook page, as do many national Hearing Voices networks); social action, debate and demonstration; and national and international conferences.

Current challenges

Intervoice envisages a society that understands voice hearing as an expression of personally and culturally significant information and respects it as a normal human variation; in effect, a society that supports the needs of individuals who hear voices and values them as full citizens. There are numerous obstacles in meeting these goals. The challenge for Intervoice is to use its ideological urge to 'change the world' as fuel, but in daily practice to operate strategically and realistically. Prioritising these challenges is paramount in order to forge connections with relevant political forces, to thrive, and to enact change. In no particular order, some of the current challenges facing Intervoice include:

- combating negative media portrayals of voice hearing and promoting social inclusion and citizenship
- challenging the dominance of reductionist biological paradigms and promoting the Hearing Voices Movement approach as a legitimate alternative
- disputing de-humanising clinical language (e.g., 'schizophrenics', 'hallucinators', 'mental disease')
- promoting user-informed research that offers clear benefits for voice hearers
- developing positive, productive relationships with other psychiatric services
- using early intervention strategies to benefit young people and prevent chronic stigma and distress
- delivering systematic training on an international scale
- promoting services that are primarily user led
- engaging with cultural, social, and ethnic minorities
- reaching out to non-industrialised countries.

In addition to its social, systemic, and political concerns, the Hearing Voices Movement also outlines a clear rationale for individual change and empowerment. In the final section, we will briefly outline how these tenets can be applied in clinical practice to support distressed voice hearers in holistic, recovery-orientated ways.

Clinical applications

Various authors have advanced Pierre Janet's (1889/1973) 'phase-oriented' model of recovery (most notably Herman, 1992; although see also Courtois, 2010; Dillon, 2011; May & Longden, 2010; Putnam, 1989). According to this theory, distressed individuals must attain: (1) a sense of *safety* before (2) *integration and resolution* can take place, whereby trauma is processed and associated losses mourned for. Finally, a process of (3) *reconnection* occurs, in which the skills of the previous stages are incorporated into daily life. Although these phases are sequential they are not prescriptive, nor strictly linear, and many individuals will iterate between them as they navigate through their healing process (Dillon, 2011).

Correspondingly, Romme and Escher's (1993) three-stages model, derived from interviews with numerous patient and non-patient voice hearers, describes a progressive shift from intense fear and disorientation (the startling phase) to a time of exploration and meaning making (the organisational phase) before finally achieving acceptance and growth (the stabilisation phase). In this section we have combined Romme and Escher's findings with Janet's three-phase model to propose interventions that workers may usefully employ throughout a voice hearer's recovery journey.

Establishing safety (the 'startling phase')

A defining feature of psychological trauma is powerlessness and loss of control (Herman, 1992). Establishing a sense of security, stability, and self-command therefore takes priority over commencing other tasks, including therapeutic work (Putnam, 1989). When delineating the 'startling phase' (i.e., voice hearing onset) Romme and Escher likewise acknowledge how even positive voices can initially be experienced as shocking and intrusive. A central task is therefore achieving some level of safety and calmness, not only in terms of the voices, but in regard to personal and interpersonal security, self-care strategies, and the regulation of distressing emotions.

The associations between voice hearing and exposure to victimisation, oppression, and other experiences of injustice, means many voice hearers can derive benefit from the kind of safety strategies endorsed in trauma-based therapies (Longden et al., 2012; Moskowitz & Corstens, 2007; Romme, 2009). Examples include relaxation skills, meditation, yoga, breathing exercises, and guided imagery. Grounding techniques, mindfulness, and the use of comforting associational cues or self-hypnosis can likewise be used to reorient oneself during episodes of intense panic or dissociation (Dolan, 2000). Conversely, vigorous physical activity can help alleviate tension and anxiety. May and Longden (2010) suggest that finding non-violent ways to express anger can be beneficial for those whose voices represent unprocessed rage and/or who encourage aggressive behaviour. For voice hearers suffering feelings of guilt or shame, compassionate mind techniques (Gilbert & Procter, 2006), self-soothing, positive visualisations, mantras and/or affirmations can provide an alternative to habitual disparaging beliefs about the self. Advance planning is also of value; for example, Dillon (2011) advocates devising a list of '20 things to do when desperate' for use during crisis.

Supportive relationships are of considerable value at this stage, particularly ones in which voices can be discussed without fear of censure or prejudice. This is something which self-help groups are particularly well placed to provide, in that their emphasis on solidarity and shared experience fosters 'a safe-haven where people feel accepted and comfortable' (Downs, 2005, p. 5). The benefit of hearing voices groups has been well documented (see Dillon & Longden, 2011), and can generally be characterised as: social (e.g., reducing isolation and alienation; improving opportunities and aptitude for socialising; providing respect and validation); psychological (e.g., building confidence, self-esteem and self-determination; prompting reflexivity); and 'clinical' (e.g., providing frameworks for understanding one's experiences; generating hope and inspiration; sharing and augmenting coping strategies). Most national Hearing Voices networks retain databases of available groups, although only those maintaining a user-led philosophy tend to be endorsed.

Voice hearing's taboo status may fill individuals with a sense of shame that they are 'going mad', or that others will reject or ridicule them. Psychoeducation is therefore helpful in terms of fostering hope and overcoming confusion and fear: for example, the provision of recovery stories, coping/self-help materials, and normalisation literature (e.g., famous people who have heard voices, the prevalence of voice hearing in non-clinical groups). It may also be beneficial to represent voice hearing as a meaningful response to overwhelming events; in effect, an ingenious, creative survival strategy that provides insights into previous threats and challenges that the individual has faced (Knols & Corstens, 2011). This input should ideally be framed within empathic, yet empowering language, in which the person is supported to redefine their sense of themselves as someone who is capable of making positive changes and reformulating the identity of 'sufferer' (i.e., a passive victim of pathology and/or circumstance) to that of survivor, thriver, and victor (Coleman, 2011). Intervoice's website contains multilingual information on a range of available resources, including first-person accounts, advice and testimony, as well as more scholarly and clinical materials.

A further purpose of psychoeducation is supporting individuals to begin attending more closely to their voices. A good example of this is a 'Voice Diary' (e.g., Smith, Coleman, & Good, 2003), which provides a framework for identifying patterns and triggers (e.g., particular people, emotions, and/or social circumstances that provoke the voices). Anticipating voices in this way can provide important insights into their role in the person's life (see next section) but in the short term can augment their sense of confidence and control by helping avoid known triggers and/or preparing coping strategies in advance. Furthermore, a written record may provide a valuable tool for reflecting more fully on one's thoughts and feelings about the voices.

Integration and resolution (the 'organisational phase')
In this stage, the person embarks on processing painful memories (and associated emotions) within the context of a safe, healing environment and in the presence of an ally – possibly a therapist – who acts as a supportive witness (Courtois, 2010). Previously acquired skills are utilised throughout in order to bolster safety, security, and self-regulation. This is a time of mourning, but also a time of exploration and transformation (Herman, 1992).

Romme and Escher (1993) likewise describe this phase as when individuals begin 'organising' their experiences through experiential making-sense processes. A central theme is exploring the symbolic meaning of one's voices in terms of painful emotions and interpersonal conflict, and finding new ways to control and express these experiences (Corstens,

Escher, & Romme, 2008). For example, interviews with 50 recovered voice hearers (Romme et al., 2009) identified integrative processes such as acknowledging and accommodating voices as part of one's self, acceptance and exploration of one's experiences, taking ownership of voices, accepting oneself by accepting one's emotions, and negotiating boundaries and relationships with voices, as healing and instructive in terms of reducing distress and regaining control.

In order to successfully 'organise' experience, individuals may benefit from making time to selectively listen to their voices rather than evade all contact with them (Corstens et al., 2008). Techniques like 'time-sharing' (e.g., Smith et al., 2003) break down avoidance by helping individuals schedule time-limited listening, possibly supplemented by interacting with the voices in a respectful, yet assertive way, asking them questions, and recording the responses. As well as enhancing one's sense of choice and control, this strategy is consistent with research that suggests constant suppression of voices may heighten their activity, much in the same way as ignoring intrusive thoughts increases the likelihood of occurrence (Valmaggia & Morris, 2010). Thus while constant attempts at distraction can be exhausting and restricting, accepting and acknowledging voice presence can facilitate growth and self-determination, for example, by deflecting emotional energy and behavioural resources away from efforts to evade and contain voice activity and towards more rewarding social and psychological goals (Shawyer et al., 2007).

Psychological therapy is likely to be of benefit at this stage, particularly that which attempts to incorporate voices within the person's contextual and intersubjective circumstances. For example, in order to elucidate associations between voices and adverse life events, Romme and Escher (2000) advocate devising 'a construct', a method of psychological formulation for exploring the links between voice content/characteristics, and experiences of trauma and loss in the person's life. Subsequent information can be utilised within an individual psychotherapeutic recovery plan through addressing two central queries: who or what the voices may represent, and what interpersonal problems they embody (see also Corstens et al., 2008; Longden, Corstens, Escher, & Romme, 2011). Similarly, the concept of 'talking with voices' (Corstens, Longden, & May, 2011) uses dialoguing approaches to directly engage with the voice(s) in order to instigate a process of integration and reconciliation, enhance awareness of voice characteristics, and explore relevant factors in voice emergence and 'purpose.'

Reconnection (the 'stabilisation phase')

According to Herman (1992), a central task of the final stage of recovery is achieving a sense of empowerment and reconnection. Correspondingly, Romme and Escher (1993) suggest that this is the point at which voice hearers attain some kind of positive acceptance, harmony and equilibrium. In the long term, individuals can ideally learn to take pride in their experiences, exhibit compassion and respect towards themselves (and their voices) and engage in a process of personal and interpersonal growth.

Many people in this phase of recovery opt for some kind of 'survivor mission', in which experiences of injustice are addressed in a restorative way (Herman, 1992). This commonly involves seeking collective, social, or political dimensions to one's suffering, and using it as a basis to protect others and/or raise public awareness. For example, individuals may choose to disseminate respectful, informative accounts of voice hearing through training professionals or participating in community education initiatives, media projects, or voice hearing networks (May & Longden, 2010); or find ways to assist others through direct support and/or by challenging and exposing wider societal injustice (Dillon, 2011). In addition to developing new skills, these activities can prove affirming and empowering by providing a sense of recognition, solidarity, and connectedness. Intervoice supports this process by organising annual conferences that emphasise both individual stories and the collective identity of 'proud voice hearer.'

In order to reconnect to (or newly discover) feelings of power and confidence, individuals may benefit from setting themselves controlled, achievable challenges. Assertiveness classes might help a submissive, victimised voice hearer reassert feelings of dignity and self-determination. Alternatively, physical pursuits like self-defence courses or extreme sports can be a way for a previously terrorised individual to achieve 'psychological mastery and physiological reconditioning' (Herman, 1992, p. 198). Other congruent initiatives include reconnecting with previous social responsibilities, and/or instituting new ones. This may incorporate a search for meaningful and valued activities, roles, and relationships, or examining one's dreams, hopes, ambitions, and aspirations: to become more adventurous in the world (Herman, 1992). This pertains to the concept that 'living well is the best revenge' (Dolan, 2000) and that rediscovering the capacity for joy, taking satisfaction from one's life, and striving for a bright future regardless of one's painful past are fundamental rights for every voice hearer.

Conclusions

Redefining voice hearing as a normal human variation, conducting experiential-based research, and organising conferences for voice hearers and their allies paved the way for the emergence of the Hearing Voices Movement and its organisational body, Intervoice. The former now constitutes numerous local, national and international projects that disseminate hopeful messages and offer support for people struggling to reclaim ownership of their voices and their lives. We have used social movement theory to illustrate how the formation and development of these initiatives were grounded in changing opportunity structures and pre-existing resources. Movement maintenance is supported by national and international networks that serve as alternative psychiatric services, supporting individuals in their recovery journeys and connecting interest groups to allies in various political bodies and formal psychiatric organisations. In the future, Intervoice will need to act strategically so to continue to develop the movement. Finally, clinical applications of the Hearing Voices Movement ethos offer a strong model to guide holistic, recovery-based practice.

The paradigm shift from voice hearing as a 'symptom' to an understanding of voices as a meaningful experience that can direct personal change and recovery has appealed to many voice hearers, workers and family members, ultimately creating a new language and practice of hope. Together, the Hearing Voices Movement and Intervoice offer a collective identity; a locus for dignity, respect and citizenship; and a positive practice to empower voice hearers: in essence, a form of social and psychiatric revolution.

References

Beavan, V., & Read, J. (2010). Hearing voices and listening to what they say: The importance of voice content in understanding and working with distressing voices. *Journal of Nervous and Mental Disease, 198*(3), 201–205.

Beavan, V., Read, J., & Cartwright, C. (2011). The prevalence of voice hearers in the general population: A literature review. *Journal of Mental Health, 20*(3), 281–292.

Boyle, M. (2002). *Schizophrenia: A scientific delusion* (2nd ed.). London: Routledge.

British Psychological Society. (2000). *Recent Advances in Understanding Mental Illness and Psychotic Experiences.* London: BPS.

Coleman, R. (2011). *Recovery: An alien concept?* Fife: P&P Press.

Corstens, D., Escher, S., & Romme, M. (2008). Accepting and working with voices: The Maastricht approach. In A. Moskowitz, I. Schäfer & M. J. Dorahy (Eds.), *Psychosis, Trauma and Dissociation: Emerging perspectives on severe psychopathology* (pp. 319–332). Oxford: Wiley-Blackwell.

Corstens, D., Longden, E., & May, R. (2012). Talking with voices: Exploring what is expressed by the voices people hear. *Psychosis: Psychological, social and integrative approaches, 4*(2), 95–104. DOI: 10.1080/17522439.2011. 571705

Courtois, C. A. (2010). *Understanding Complex Trauma, Complex Reactions, and Treatment Approaches.* Retrieved 18 January 2012 from, http:// giftfromwithin.org/html/cptsd-understanding-treatment.html

Dillon, J. (2011). The personal *is* the political. In M. Rapley, J. Moncrieff & J. Dillon (Eds.), *De-Medicalizing Misery: Psychiatry, psychology and the human condition* (pp. 141–157). Basingstoke: Palgrave Macmillan.

Dillon, J., & Longden, E. (2011). Hearing voices groups: Creating safe spaces to share taboo experiences. In M. Romme & S. Escher (Eds.), *Psychosis as a Personal Crisis: An experience-based approach* (pp. 129–139). London: Routledge.

Dolan, Y. (2000). *Beyond Survival: Living well is the best revenge.* London: BT Press.

Downs, J. (2005). *Starting and Supporting Hearing Voices Groups.* Manchester: HVN.

Edwards, B., & McCarthy, J. D. (2004). Resources and social movement mobilization. In D. A. Snow, S. A. Soule, & H. Kriesi (Eds.), *The Blackwell Companion to Social Movements* (pp. 116–152). Oxford: Blackwell.

Engel, S. M. (2001). *The Unfinished Revolution: Social movement theory and the gay and lesbian movement.* Cambridge: Cambridge University Press.

Gilbert, P., & Procter, S. (2006). Compassionate mind training for people with high shame and self-criticism: Overview and pilot study of a group therapy approach. *Clinical Psychology and Psychotherapy, 13,* 353–379.

Herman, J. L. (1992) *Trauma and Recovery.* New York: Basic Books.

Hornstein, G. A. (2012). *Agnes's Jacket: A psychologist's search for the meaning of madness.* Ross-on-Wye: PCCS Books.

Intervoice. (2012). *About Us.* Retrieved 24 February 2012 from, http:// www.intervoiceonline.org/about-intervoice

James, A. (2001). *Raising Our Voices: An account of the Hearing Voices Movement.* Gloucester: Handsell.

Janet, P. (1973). *L'Automatisme Psychologique.* Paris: Société Pierre Janet. (Original work published 1889)

Jaynes, J. (1976). *The Origin of Consciousness in the Breakdown of the Bicameral Mind.* Boston: Houghton Mifflin.

Johnstone, L. (2011). Voice hearers are people with problems, not patients with illnesses. In M. Romme & S. Escher (Eds.), *Psychosis as a Personal Crisis: An experience-based approach* (pp. 27–36). London: Routledge.

Knols, M., & Corstens, D. (2011). Tuning in: A story by a patient and a therapist about making sense of voices. *Mental Health Today, Nov/Dec,* 28–32.

Kuhn, T. S. (1962). *The Structure of Scientific Revolutions.* Chicago: University of Chicago Press.

Longden, E., Corstens, D., Escher, S., & Romme, M. (2011). Voice hearing in biographical context: A model for formulating the relationship between voices and life history. *Psychosis: Psychological, social and integrative approaches, 4*(3), 224–234. DOI: 10.1080/17522439.2011.596566

Longden, E., Madill, A., & Waterman, M. G. (2012). Dissociation, trauma, and the role of lived experience: Toward a new conceptualization of voice hearing. *Psychological Bulletin, 138*(1), 28–76.

May, R., & Longden, E. (2010). Self-help approaches to hearing voices. In F. Larøi & A. Aleman (Eds.), *Hallucinations: A guide to treatment and management.* Oxford: Oxford University Press.

McAdam, D. (1997). The classical model of social movements examined. In S. M. Buechler & F. K. Cylke (Eds.), *Social Movements: Perspectives and issues* (pp. 135–148). Mountain View, CA: Mayfield Publishing Co.

Moskowitz, A., & Corstens, D. (2007). Auditory hallucinations: Psychotic symptom or dissociative experience? *The Journal of Psychological Trauma, 6*(2/3), 35–63.

Polletta, F., & Jasper, J. (2001). Collective identity and social movements. *Annual Review of Sociology, 27,* 283–305.

Putnam, F. (1989) *Diagnosis and Treatment of Multiple Personality Disorder.* New York: Guilford Press.

Read, J., van Os, J., Morrison, A. P., & Ross, C. A. (2005). Childhood trauma, psychosis and schizophrenia: A literature review with theoretical and practical implications. *Acta Psychiatrica Scandinavica, 112,* 330–350.

Romme, M. (2000). *Redefining Hearing Voices.* Based on a speech given at the launch of The Hearing Voices Network, Manchester, UK, Summer 2000. Retrieved 24 February 2012 from, http://www.psychminded.co.uk/critical/marius.htm

Romme, M. (2009). Psychotherapy with hearing voices. In M. Romme, S. Escher, J. Dillon, D. Corstens & M. Morris (Eds.), *Living with Voices: 50 stories of recovery* (pp. 86–94). Ross-on-Wye: PCCS Books.

Romme, M., & Escher, S. (1993). *Accepting Voices.* London: Mind.

Romme, M., & Escher, S. (2000). *Making Sense of Voices.* London: Mind.

Romme, M., Escher, S., Dillon, J., Corstens, D., & Morris, M. (Eds.). (2009). *Living with Voices: 50 stories of recovery.* Ross-on-Wye: PCCS Books.

Shawyer, F., Ratcliff, K., Mackinnon, A., Farhall, J., Hayes, S. C., & Copolov, D. (2007). The Voices Acceptance and Action Scale (VAAS): Pilot data. *Journal of Clinical Psychology, 63*(6), 593–606.

Smith, M., Coleman, R., & Good, J. (2003). *Psychiatric First Aid in Psychosis: A handbook for nurses, carers and people distressed by psychotic experiences.* Fife: P&P Press.

Valmaggia, L. R., & Morris, E. (2010). Attention training technique and acceptance and commitment therapy for distressing auditory hallucinations. In F. Larøi & A. Aleman (Eds.), *Hallucinations: A guide to treatment and management.* Oxford: Oxford University Press.

Chapter 11

Experiential Knowledge and the Reconception of Madness

Peter Beresford

Introduction

These are times of ambiguity and major change in relation to madness and mental distress. On the one hand, for decades now, policy and practice in the UK (and indeed in many other countries) have been overlaid with the rhetoric of empowerment, inclusion and participation. On the other hand, currently in the UK (and similar trends can be identified elsewhere), there are powerful political forces working to stigmatise and exclude mental health service users/survivors. These are often presented in the name of 'welfare reform' and social inclusion, framed in terms of getting people into paid work, rather than receiving state benefits. Thus many individual service users are currently feeling under unprecedented personal attack, in some cases this is resulting in people having suicidal thoughts, while as a group, they are receiving more invitations than ever before to 'give their views' and get involved (Campbell, 1999; Beresford & Andrews, 2012).

Influenced by this confusing context, this chapter is primarily concerned with addressing four key questions:

- Is it possible to theorise or write about madness now without referring to the direct views of people included as mad or 'mentally ill'?

- Can service users' understandings of madness justifiably be ignored?

- Does it matter if they are?

- What are the possible advantages and disadvantages of including them?

Two things sparked off my writing this chapter in its present form. The first was accidental; the second is deeply rooted in my life's experience.

First was coming across a recent text about madness by a distinguished academic author on a bookshop's shelves. The second was the growing realisation that my own understanding, or perhaps lack of understanding, of 'madness' when it happened to me was both a cause of many of the difficulties I encountered and also the reason for many of the things I have subsequently done, which have helped me make sense of it.

First, though, as is so often the case in discussions about 'mental health' issues, there needs to be some consideration of terminology. 'Psychosis' and 'neurosis' have become key categories in medicalised understandings of madness. In this discussion, I prefer to use the terms 'madness' and 'mental distress', but it should be said that these are not offered as equivalents or synonyms for psychosis and neurosis, since I take a critical view of these medicalised concepts and terms. Equally, it needs to be acknowledged that there is no general consensus or agreement even among mental health service users about language in this field. All the terms that have come into use: 'service user', 'consumer', 'patient', 'survivor', may be liked by some, but are disliked by others. While terms like 'emotional' or 'mental distress' have found considerable favour, madness remains a heavily contested concept even among mental health service users/psychiatric system survivors. This is true internationally. In a study which I was involved in, mental health service users expressed some very strong views about 'madness':

> I stick to my guns and I don't like the word madness. I think it ought to be done away with.
>
> It's a negative.
>
> It's labelling and stigmatizing.
> (Beresford, Nettle & Perring, 2009, p. 22)

At the same time there are other survivors who value the word and seek to reclaim it, as has been reflected in the emergence of developments like Mad Pride, MAD Art and mad culture. In this chapter the words 'madness' and 'distress' will be preferred, although it is difficult to avoid talking about 'mental health' because it has gained such common currency in policy and services. While being distanced from concepts of 'illness' and 'disorder', the notion of mental health nonetheless still originates from them.

Ignoring experience

In his book, *Madness: A Very Short Introduction*, one of a series of high-profile introductory texts published by Oxford University Press, Andrew Scull, the noted international academic, acknowledges from the start that 'madness is no longer an acceptable word to use in polite company' (Scull, 2011, p. 1). Yet it is his term of choice and he readily shifts from using it as a descriptor to an objective reality – 'something that frightens and fascinates us all' (p. 1). While it is a short text, it is up to date and all-embracing, examining the social, historical, cultural and ideological context and relations of madness. Its time span ranges from the Old Testament to the present. Its sweep includes anti-psychiatry and antipsychotics, Baudelaire and Bedlam, syphilis and Szasz. But nowhere do we hear directly what service users have to say. There is no mention of their ideas or explanations. In a chapter entitled 'Madness and Meaning' there is no mention of meanings that mad people or service users may give to their emotions or experience. There is not one reference to the work or writings of service users or their organisations, with one exception – mad men as artists. Thus we do hear about Van Gogh. Richard Dadd's paintings get a mention. Perhaps most importantly we are offered something of the story of one mental health service user's experience, Sylvia Plath – but as the author of *The Bell Jar* (1963), rather than as a service user. Scull offers *his* reflections of what she was a 'victim' of, which led to her suicide, rather than her account and analysis of her life and situation (Scull, 2011, p. 95). This is the closest we get to mental health service users, their understandings, viewpoints and critiques.

However, as Peter Campbell, the mental health service user activist, made clear in his 1996 chapter, 'The History of the User Movement in the United Kingdom', the emergence of a mental health service user/survivor movement can readily be traced back to the mid-1980s and a strong claim can be made for the existence of service user organisations like the Mental Patients Union from the early 1970s. There have been organisations and movements internationally for nearly as long. The modern survivor movement can be traced back far further; Campbell refers back as far as the early seventeenth century for documented instances of collective protest by mad people (Campbell, 1996, pp. 218–219). While the development of such collective action has made it possible for mental health service users to gain a greater reach and profile for their accounts and perspectives, reporting their views and experience has not been conditional on this. While often hidden and marginalised, personal accounts and stories have been produced and available for many years.

Now in the twenty-first century, there are local, national, European and global organisations of mental health service users/survivors. They have formed international movements, with their own cultures, arts, literatures and bodies of work. Survivor research, including research based in some of the most prestigious academic institutions, like the world-famous Institute of Psychiatry at King's College London with its Service User Research Enterprise (SURE), have generated user-led projects with findings that are disseminated internationally.

Despite this, Andrew Scull has found no place for service users' own accounts, ideas or perspectives in his book on madness. It might be argued that his is a small text and that there was insufficient space for this to be included. But given the breadth of his focus and the space he has, for example, devoted to other critiques of psychiatry, like anti-psychiatry and Goffman's anti-institutionalisation (Goffman, 1961), this seems a difficult argument to sustain. Scull's editorial decision certainly offers an answer to the first question raised here:

Is it possible to theorise or write about madness now without referring to the direct views of people included as mad or 'mentally ill'?

That answer would seem to be yes. It is possible and it does happen. Scull's book is not an isolated example. Much of the 'mental health' literature, particularly the medically and laboratory-based research literature, is similarly based on 'expert' or 'academic' analysis and interpretations, rather than fully including material from service users. Historically, service users, in the main, have only featured as a data source, with analysis and findings offered by non-service-user researchers and reflecting their professional and research standpoints. This is true even of apparently progressive sources. Thus, progressive writer and psychotherapist Suzy Orbach (2012) wrote critically of the government's 'wellbeing' agenda, drawing a connection between collective distress and the consumerist capitalist society in which we live. But again there is no reference to the perceptions of people experiencing such distress; no mention of what they might have to say on the subject. The frequently negative and stigmatising tabloid media presentation of mental health service users, which is seen to play a large part in their scapegoating and 'othering' – that is, being treated as alien and separate – also notably tends to avoid the inclusion of first-hand voices (Philo et al., 1996).

Can service users' understandings of madness justifiably be ignored?

Thus, we can see that it is still possible in the second decade of the twenty-first century to ignore the understandings and ideas of mental health service users/survivors. However, this leads to our second question, can this be justified? If we turn to mainstream UK public policy, the answer would seem to be not. It would be difficult to sum this up better than Peter Campbell did in 2009:

> [Mental health] services now set out to 'put the user at the centre'. Information and opportunities for individuals to influence their care and treatment have increased. Collectively, service users are extensively involved, indeed are required to be involved, in the monitoring of existing services and the planning of new ones. It is now hardly possible to embark on major mental health debates without at some point seeking out the views of those with direct, personal experience of madness and mental health services. (Campbell, 2009, p. 46)

Mental health service user involvement is now routinely required in policy, professional practice, education, research and evaluation. This has made it possible for their perspectives and insights to be included routinely, where once they were almost entirely ignored. Pressure for this has followed from the consumerist agendas of UK governments from Mrs Thatcher's onwards. Certainly after New Labour came into power in 1997, 'legislation, policy pronouncements, Department of Health guidance and initiatives by the major mental health professions ... made it clear it was no longer acceptable not to involve service users' (Campbell, 2009, p. 49). As Campbell highlights, it has also been linked with the increasing pressure exerted by UK service user organisations and movements. Individually and collectively, service users have increasingly demanded to be involved (Campbell, 1996). To different degrees and with varying success and effectiveness, this development has been apparent internationally. Thus market-inspired political ideology and pressures from service users for involvement, empowerment and the democratisation of policy and provision have combined to make service users' involvement and inclusion the default position. These two often-opposed forces, of market ideology and service user pressure, have worked in complex interaction to help make this happen. They have taken us beyond traditional assumptions which can be traced to the eighteenth-century enlightenment with its concern with 'reason' and 'order', which in turn gave rise to the age of science and with it, psychiatry.

Science came to be seen as the best way to engage with madness (Bracken & Thomas, 2009, pp. 78–79). As commentators from Porter (1987) to Foucault (1971) have highlighted, this logic led to segregating, in large institutions, people seen as 'unreasonable' and upsetting 'order', ranging from the mad and criminal to people who were seen as intellectual or moral 'imbeciles'. Thus mad people were seen as having little or nothing to contribute to understanding because they were irrational and lacking reason, pathological and defective, with spoiled identities. Now in an age of *post*-modernity, where different and competing viewpoints are acknowledged and may be taken into account, such assumptions have come under increasing challenge.

Does excluding service users' views matter?

This brings us to third question raised in this chapter. Does it matter if mental health service users, their viewpoints and views, are ignored and excluded? Significantly, the general consensus seems to be that it does – even though we know that their viewpoints and views still frequently are ignored. Many arguments, including moral, ethical, ideological, political and policy arguments, have been raised against their exclusion. From a consumerist standpoint, taking no account of what mental health service users want and think ignores the basic tenets of market research and makes for inefficiency. It leaves products, which are now taken to include public services, and their providers, uninformed by customer preferences. This, in market terms, increases the risk of making provision that is unwanted, inappropriate and doesn't work (Simmons, Powell & Greener, 2009).

For service users, such exclusion is morally and ethically unsustainable, because it can represent a denial of their human and civil rights. They are being prevented from influencing policy and provision that impact particularly on their lives and may have major and detrimental effects on them. More to the point, they are being prevented from speaking for and about themselves (Campbell, 2009). Speaking for yourself, or self-advocacy, has emerged as the cornerstone principle of the modern disabled people's and service users' movements (Campbell & Oliver, 1996; Beresford & Campbell, 2004). As mental health service users/survivors have themselves highlighted, this tends to result in them being presented in distorted, patronising and pathologising ways (May, 2004; Trivedi, 2009). This is what seems to happen when any oppressed or excluded group's understandings are ignored or rejected, whether on the basis of sexuality, gender, race, age, culture, class, belief or disability. They can expect to be presented as inferior, deviant or defective. The evidence also highlights that the negative effects for mental health service users/survivors are compounded if they are different in other ways, for example, in relation to gender, sexuality or race – all of which historically have resulted in inferior treatment in the psychiatric system (see, for example, Chambers, 2009).

However, the devaluing and denial of people's viewpoints as a result of their being oppressed or seen as different, as has been the case with mental health service users, has an additional destructive effect. If someone has had such experience, they can then expect routinely to face further discrimination and be further marginalised by being seen as having less credibility and being a less reliable source of knowledge. This further invalidates people who are already heavily disadvantaged (Beresford, 2003). It means that their interpretation of themselves and their situation will always tend to be seen as inferior to those of others without their experience – a double discrimination.

What are the effects of including mental health service users/ survivors?

So far, we have seen a major contradiction emerge in relation to madness and distress. The perspectives of people with direct experience are now meant to be included in debates and developments. There is widespread consensus that they should be, and strong arguments offered in support of this. Nonetheless, their viewpoints are still often excluded or marginalised. This leads us to our final question. What are the effects of this likely to be? What possible advantages and disadvantages are there from including mental health service users/survivors and their perspectives and understandings? There is increasing interest in what has come to be called the 'impact' of user involvement. This has extended to including and involving service users in all areas, from policy and practice to research and evaluation. The term 'impact' is used to mean what difference do they make; what effects does their involvement have? (Staley, 2009; Robinson, Newton & Dason, 2012).

The negative potential of involvement

These effects may be both positive and negative. Involving mental health service users/survivors and their perspectives may have both advantages and disadvantages. Let's start with possible disadvantages. While there is strong pressure for their involvement, as indicated earlier, service users have frequently highlighted that such involvement is often not meaningful or productive, but rather can be tokenistic, bureaucratised and ineffective (Campbell, 1999). Sophie Staniszewska and others highlight that negative experiences seem to be 'related to the predominantly top-down nature' of many participatory initiatives, seeking to fit people into 'existing systems and practices', rather than involving them on their own terms (Staniszewska, Mockford, Gibson, Herron-Marx & Putz, 2012, p. 141). Instead of providing an opportunity for service users to effect change, or to develop their critiques and discourses, involvement may only work to incorporate them in dominant psychiatric discourses. An important current example of this is the way that many service users have been enlisted to support the 'recovery' model in mental health; a model generated by professionals in the United States, which reinforces an essentially medicalised individual model of mental illness and is tied into integrating mental health service users into the labour market, regardless of the many barriers they face and its discriminatory and damaging effects upon them (Beresford, 2012, pp. 159–160).

Thus the potential of our involvement depends on our circumstances as well as the nature of the involvement itself. The more disempowered we are, the more it is likely to be circumscribed. At the beginning of this chapter I referred to my own initial encounter with madness and distress. As I said, I found it very difficult to make sense of it, to know what was happening, or how to deal with it. I was anxious, frightened and unprepared. The experience was utterly confusing and disorientating. I did none of the things I or anybody else might usually do when we face a problem. I had no one I knew to ask for guidance and advice. I didn't think to turn to what available information there might be, as in other circumstances I might have – I just didn't think to. The experts, who in due course I did turn to, took me down the usual road of medicalised understanding, formal diagnosis and drug-based 'treatment', which just added to my problems. It was only later that a skilled and supportive psychologist put me on the road to regaining control. Many of us in this situation are only familiar with the dominant interpretations of our experience. We only 'know' what we have heard and been told. Often what we do is internalise these understandings. We are likely only to be able to see what is happening to ourselves in terms of psychiatric explanation and diagnosis. That's why some mental health service users are so pleased to receive a diagnosis, because it legitimates their experience to them. But it is actually more likely to distance them from their own analysis and undermine the chances of them arriving at their own understanding of what is happening.

We accept public stereotypes, fears and misconceptions because, like everyone else, we have been exposed to them. We believe what psychiatry tells us because that is the only model we have to refer to. This does not put us in a strong position to contribute our understandings to making sense of madness and distress. The effects are the opposite and serve to alienate us from our experience. If we are fortunate, what may happen is that we will travel a long road to come to make our own sense of our emotions, experience and feelings. However, just involving mental health service users/survivors who have not had a chance to work through what is happening to them may not really open up discussion to their insights and understandings, because they are mediated and subverted by dominant discourses.

The positives of involvement

What can particularly help mental health service users/survivors to challenge existing psychiatric interpretations and develop their own viewpoints and ideas is getting together and working with others with shared experience. Disability and service user activists (just like those in other liberatory and new social movements) have repeatedly highlighted the value of becoming involved in collective action, not only to create political and social change, but also to undergo the personal change that is key to achieving this (Campbell & Oliver, 1996). Empowerment is thus seen as a personal and political process best achieved through such collectivity.

These processes make it possible to liberate and develop the unique contribution that people with experience of madness and distress have to offer – their experiential knowledge. This key quality distinguishes mental health service user knowledge from all other forms of knowledge within the field of madness and mental health. Thus:

> Experiential knowledge is truth learned from personal experience with a phenomenon rather than truth acquired by discursive reasoning, observation or reflection on information provided by others. (Borkman, 1976, p. 446)

Service users 'know' from their direct experience of the issues concerned. Their knowledge alone is primarily based on direct *experience* of madness and distress and associated policy and provision *from the receiving end*. Service users' knowledge grows out of their personal and collective experience of policy, practice and services. Their views are not based solely on an intellectual, occupational or political concern. Traditionally mental health policy and practice have been dominated by 'expert' knowledge, whether framed as scientific, professional, academic, research or psychiatric knowledge. This has been based on the knowledge claims of others about the experience of mad people and mental health service users. Others, therefore, have played the key role in interpreting service users' experience, while the latter's own interpretations have been excluded or devalued.

As with all identity-based groupings and movements, like the black civil rights, women's and lesbian, gay, bisexual and transgender (LGBT) movements, service users' knowledge or knowledges[1] are experientially based. Thus the introduction of service users' knowledges into the discussion, analysis and development of 'mental health' policy and thinking brings into the arena a crucially different relationship between experience and knowledge and between direct experience and 'mental health' discourses. The importance of this cannot be overstated. As we will see, it is likely to have fundamental implications for the understanding of 'mental health'. Phil Cotterell and Carolyn Morris highlight two important elements of experiential knowledge: first, that 'it arises from personal participation in the phenomenon and incorporates a reflective stance on this experience' and second, that the individual holds belief and trust in this knowledge 'based on their experience of the phenomenon in question' (Cotterell & Morris, 2012, p. 58).

---

1 The word 'knowledges' is used deliberately to indicate that there is no one service user knowledge, instead there are different knowledges, which reflect different experiences, survivor identities etc.

The knowledge of mental health service users/survivors is both individual and collective. It has developed formally and informally, growing through the contact that service users have with each other, within and beyond the service system; in self-advocacy and service user groups and organisations, at meetings and in campaigns. There is a massive body of unrecorded and hidden service user knowledge, which remains alive in the memories of service users. Such knowledge has increasingly begun to be recorded in the form of service users' accounts, testimonies, critiques and discussions (Read & Reynolds, 1996; Beresford, Stalker & Wilson, 1997; Campbell & Oliver, 1996). Such accounts are to be found in service users' newsletters, journals and other publications and now increasingly in professional publications and mainstream print and broadcast media. In addition, service users are now producing and contributing to their own histories (Campbell, 1996; Campbell & Oliver, 1996; James, 2001; Wallcraft, with Read & Sweeney, 2003). Service users' experiential knowledge base is also becoming more diverse, both individual and collective, including the wide range of mental health service users'/survivors' experience and backgrounds, like, for example, those with experience of forensic services, and people from black and minority ethnic and LGBT communities.

Mental health service users' knowledges are also being advanced by their increasing involvement in research and their development of their own 'survivor research'. Such research is concerned with changed, more equal and participatory research relationships, research committed to the empowerment of service users and broader social change to support their human and civil rights (Sweeney, Beresford, Faulkner, Nettle, & Rose, 2009; Wallcraft, Schrank, & Amering, 2009; Russo, 2012). It is developing an evidence base which supports the inclusion of service user perspectives. It is also beginning to influence research priorities, agendas, focus, ethics and outcomes, as well as research methods and methodology. It has highlighted the importance of social factors in and the social relations of madness, reflecting service users' own concerns, rather than the individualising emphasis of psychiatry, with its longstanding preoccupations with medicalised diagnosis and drug therapy.

Just as survivor research has challenged the traditional values and concerns of research, so service users' perspectives and knowledge more generally are reshaping the conceptualisation of madness, distress and mental health. They have been the inspiration for radical new critiques and understandings. In 2009, a Joseph Rowntree Foundation-funded project reported that most service users believed that a medical model based on deficit and pathology still dominated public and professional understandings of mental health issues shaping attitudes and policy. They largely saw such a medical model as damaging and unhelpful, instead seeing social approaches to mental health issues as much more helpful. They felt that broader issues needed to be taken more into account to counter the individualisation of mental health issues (Beresford, Nettle & Perring, 2009). Survivors' different and ground-breaking ways of thinking have also been reflected in their reconception of some of the major manifestations of madness and distress that they experience. This has led to the Hearing Voices Movement and to creative harm-minimisation approaches to self-harm and eating distress, which instead of treating them as individual pathologies, puts them in their context as responses to broader oppression, discrimination and disempowerment.

Survivor knowledge also has the potential to transform understanding of helpful responses to madness and distress. Survivors are now also challenging the histories that others have written about them, based on their own first-hand knowledge (Survivors History Group, 2012). As well as highlighting the importance of recognising and addressing the broader relations of madness and distress, whether these concern relationships, abuse, loss, employment and occupation, spirituality or material wellbeing, this helps engender an appreciation of the holistic nature of the person and their situation. Elsewhere I have written about the kind of principles that seem to be emerging, based on survivor experience, to underpin a liberatory approach and response to madness and distress. These include:

- prioritising self-advocacy
- being rights-based
- building on the philosophy of independent living
- self-management and self-support
- commitment to anti-oppressive practice
- supporting race equality and cultural diversity
- minimising compulsion
- breaking the bad/mad link

- prioritising participation

- equalising power relations. (Beresford, 2010, p. 64)

Service users emphasise the value of peer support, self-management, holistic and complementary approaches, self-run schemes for personal support, outreach and community development and user-controlled services and organisations. They blur traditional distinctions between 'helper' and 'helped', seeing shared experience and experiential knowledge as having key contributions to make in supporting people. Thus much work has gone into developing 'user trainers' and training as well as user involvement in professional education, to support the learning of professionals and other workers, as well as into efforts to highlight the value of direct experience as a relevant and much valued qualification for working with and supporting mental health service users/survivors (Beresford, 2010).

Key next steps

There aren't, as yet, survivor-controlled conceptualisations of madness and distress, or what the survivor researcher Jasna Russo has called 'a first-person-defined model of madness' (personal communication, March 2012). But in time we can expect to see these emerging. We can expect survivors to generate their own constellation of models and theories about madness which extend beyond analysis to include critiques of the maddening effects of society and new survivor-led approaches to offering help and support. However survivor knowledge, from which this follows, is far from secure, as we have seen. It is liable to be ignored, excluded, marginalised, misrepresented and subverted. It must be safeguarded for the future in all its diversity and richness. Key to this is supporting the development of a wide range of survivor-led organisations. All the evidence suggests that this is likely to be the most helpful way of fostering and enhancing mental health service users'/survivors' experiential knowledge. These organisations make possible alliance and equal relationships between service users and the service system, rather than co-option and assimilation. They enable confidence building at a personal level and collective capacity building. In England, there have been commitments from government to develop a national network of such local 'user-led organisations' as part of an 'independent living strategy'. However, this network is far from being achieved and both local and national survivor organisations remain insecure and underfunded. Supporting such organisations must be the priority for the future if user knowledge is to have the flowering it warrants and be ensured the presence that is increasingly emerging as essential for making sense of madness.

References

Beresford, P. (2003). *It's Our Lives: A short theory of knowledge, distance and experience*. London: Citizen Press in association with Shaping Our Lives.

Beresford, P. (2010). *A Straight Talking Guide to Being a Mental Health Service User*. Ross-on-Wye: PCCS Books.

Beresford, P. (2012). Psychiatric system survivors: An emerging movement. In N. Watson, A. Roulstone, & C. Thomas (Eds.), *Routledge Handbook of Disability Studies* (pp. 151–164). London/New York: Routledge.

Beresford, P., & Andrews, A. (2012). *Caring for Our Future: What service users say* (Programme Paper, March 2012). York: Joseph Rowntree Foundation. Retrieved 2 December 2012 from, http://www.jrf.org.uk/publications/caring-our-future-what-service-users-say

Beresford, P., & Campbell, P. (2004). Participation and protest: Mental health service users/survivors. In M. J. Todd & G. Taylor (Eds.), *Democracy and Participation: Popular protest and new social movements*. London: Merlin Press.

Beresford, P., Nettle, M., & Perring, R. (2009). *Towards a Social Model of Madness and Distress? Exploring what service users say*. 22 November. York: Joseph Rowntree Foundation. Available for download at http://www.jrf.org.uk/publications/social-model-madness-distress

Beresford, P., Stalker, K., & Wilson, A. (1997). *Speaking for Ourselves: A bibliography*. London: Open Services Project in association with the Social Work Research Centre, University of Stirling.

Borkmann, T. (1976). Experiential knowledge: A new concept for the analysis of self-help groups. *Social Services Review, 50,* 445–456.

Bracken, P., & Thomas, P. (2009). Postpsychiatry: A new direction for mental health. In J. Reynolds, R. Muston, T. Heller, J. Leach, M. McCormick, J. Wallcraft & M. Walsh (Eds.), *Mental Health Still Matters*. Basingstoke: Palgrave.

Campbell, J., & Oliver, M. (1996). *Disability Politics: Understanding our past, changing our future*. London: Routledge.

Campbell, P. (1996). The history of the user movement in the United Kingdom. In T. Heller, J. Reynolds, R. Gomm, R. Muston & S. Pattison (Eds.), *Mental Health Matters*. Basingstoke: Macmillan.

Campbell, P. (1999). The service user/survivor movement. In C. Newnes, G. Holmes & C. Dunn (Eds.), *This Is Madness* (pp. 195–209). Ross-on-Wye: PCCS Books.

Campbell, P. (2009). The service user/survivor movement. In J. Reynolds, R. Muston, T. Heller, J. Leach, M. McCormick, J. Wallcraft & M. Walsh (Eds.), *Mental Health Still Matters.* Basingstoke: Palgrave.

Chambers, P. (2009). What black women want from the mental health system. In J. Reynolds, R. Muston, T. Heller, J. Leach, M. McCormick, J. Wallcraft & M. Walsh (Eds.), *Mental Health Still Matters.* Basingstoke: Palgrave.

Cotterell, P., & Morris, C. (2012). The capacity, impact and challenge of service users' experiential knowledge. In M. Barnes & P. Cotterell (Eds.), *Critical Perspectives on User Involvement* (pp. 57–69). Bristol: Policy Press.

Foucault, M. (1971). *Madness and Civilisation: A history of insanity in the age of reason.* London: Tavistock.

Goffman, E. (1961). *Asylums.* Garden City, NY: Anchor Books.

James, A. (2001). *Raising Our Voices: An account of the Hearing Voices Movement.* Gloucester: Handsell Publications.

May, R. (2004). Making sense of psychotic experiences and working towards recovery. In J. Gleeson & P. McGorry (Eds.), *Psychological Interventions in Early Psychosis* (pp. 245–260). New York: John Wiley.

Orbach, S. (2012). The sad truth. *Royal Society of Arts Journal, Spring,* 16–19.

Philo, G., Secker, J., Platt, S., Henderson, L., McLaughlin, G., & Burnside, J. (1996). Media images of mental distress. In T. Heller, J. Reynolds, R. Gomm, R. Muston, & S. Pattison, (Eds.), *Mental Health Matters.* Basingstoke: Macmillan.

Plath, S. (1963). *The Bell Jar* (under the name of Victoria Lucas). New York: Heinemann.

Porter, R. A. (1987). *A Social History of Madness: Stories of the insane.* London: Weidenfeld & Nicolson.

Read, J., & Reynolds, J. (Eds.). (1996). *Speaking Our Minds: An anthology.* Basingstoke: Macmillan.

Robinson, L., Newton, J., & Dason, P. (2012). Professionals and the public: Power or partnership in health research? *Journal of Evaluation in Clinical Care, 18*(2), 276–282.

Russo, J. (2012). Survivor-controlled research: A new foundation for thinking about psychiatry and mental health. *Forum: Qualitative Social Research, 13*(1), Art. 8 Retrieved 2 December 2012 from, http://www.qualitative-research.net/index.php/fqs/article/view/1790

Scull, A. (2011). *Madness: A very short introduction.* Oxford: Oxford University Press.

Simmons, R., Powell, M., & Greener, I. (Eds.). (2009). *The Consumer in Public Services: Choice, values and difference.* Bristol: Policy Press.

Staley, K. (2009). *Exploring Impact: Public involvement in NHS, public health and social care research.* Eastleigh: NIHR Involve.

Staniszewska, S., Mockford, C., Gibson, A., Herron-Marx, S., & Putz, R. (2012). Moving forward: Understanding the negative experiences and impacts of patient and public involvement in health service planning, development and evaluation. In M. Barnes & P. Cotterell (Eds.), *Critical Perspectives on User Involvement* (pp. 129–141). Bristol: Policy Press.

Sweeney, A., Beresford, P., Faulkner, A., Nettle, M., & Rose, D. (Eds.). (2009). *This Is Survivor Research*. Ross-on-Wye: PCSS Books.

Survivors History Group. (2012). Survivors History Group takes a critical look at historians. In M. Barnes & P. Cotterell (Eds.), *Critical Perspectives on User Involvement* (pp. 7–18). Bristol: Policy Press.

Trivedi, P. (2009). Are we who we say we are – or who they think we are? In J. Reynolds, R. Muston, T. Heller, J. Leach, M. McCormick, J. Wallcraft & M. Walsh (Eds.), *Mental Health Still Matters*. Basingstoke: Palgrave.

Wallcraft, J. (with Read, J. & Sweeney, A.). (2003). *On Our Own Terms: Users and survivors of mental health services working together for support and change.* London: The Sainsbury Centre for Mental Health.

Wallcraft, J., Schrank, B., & Amering, M. (Eds.). (2009). *Handbook of Service User Involvement in Mental Health Research*. Chichester: World Psychiatric Association, Wiley-Blackwell.

Chapter 12

Service User-led Research on Psychosis: Marginalisation and the struggle for progression

Jan Wallcraft

This chapter explores the exclusion of people defined as psychotic from research about psychosis[1] and looks at how this is now changing, with new opportunities for service user involvement and leadership of research as well as barriers to progress. The first section considers how the marginalisation and diminished citizenship granted to people labelled psychotic has limited their credibility as legitimate creators of knowledge about mental health. This is despite such diminished social status being challenged by the UN Convention on the Rights of Persons with Disabilities (CRPD). The second section highlights how the dominant approach to research in mental health of positivism further excludes the active involvement of services users in the creation of knowledge. The dominant professional knowledge of psychiatric diagnosis has justified its status through the use of positivist methods and has again marginalised the perspective of those labelled. The final sections look at service user attempts to gain some control and legitimacy in mental health research, in terms of: playing a role in mainstream research; attempting to redefine what constitutes knowledge; and utilising the ideas from the Hearing Voices Movement. It is argued that personal experience must be considered one form of legitimate knowledge.

Psychosis – Whose evidence?

In researching the area called psychosis, it is important to consider which group of people are currently given legitimacy to create the knowledge base – as this knowledge will shape how we make sense of the diversity of

---

1 The term 'psychosis' is used throughout this chapter, though less medically oriented forms of terminology have been coined which some people with these experiences prefer, e.g., 'non-ordinary experiences', or 'hearing voices' if this is the primary experience.

experiences labelled as psychosis. If people who have been labelled psychotic are denied an opportunity to help define and describe psychosis and to state what kinds of help they need, how can we be sure psychosis research is reliable, valid and useful?

The opinions and perspectives of those labelled psychotic have often been seen as globally lacking credibility and have been marginalised. People diagnosed with psychoses have effectively been deprived of citizenship under mental health laws which allowed psychiatrists to confine and treat them against their will. In addition, such people have received treatment that results in long-term damage (Breggin, 1991; Lehmann, 2005) and suffer from pervasive social stigma (Mehta, Kassam, Leese, Butler & Thornicroft, 2009), which increases marginalisation. Not surprisingly, once diagnosed as 'psychotic', people rarely took part in democratic processes and movements for citizen involvement. This began to change in the late twentieth century, largely due to popular social movements. The service user movement, emerging in the 1970s and 1980s (Chamberlin, 1978; Campbell, 2009), led to patients' councils and mental health advocacy projects which supported people diagnosed with psychoses to speak out (Peck & Parker, 1998).

The emergence of the UN Convention on the Rights of Persons with Disabilities (CRPD) (UN, 2008) is a challenge to this marginalisation. The struggle to restore human rights to people with psychiatric diagnoses culminated in the successful lobbying by former patients at the United Nations to ensure the CRPD fully included the rights of people with psychiatric disabilities (UN, 2008). According to a key lobbyist (Minkowitz, 2011), a lawyer as well as a survivor of psychiatry:

> CRPD Article 14, coming out of historic demands of users and survivors of psychiatry for an end to this regime of detention, requires States Parties to ensure that 'the existence of a disability shall in no case justify a deprivation of liberty.' No mental health law, no matter how narrowly framed, can ever meet the requirements of Article 14, so long as it contains any provision whatsoever that allows involuntary confinement of people with psychosocial disabilities for purposes of treatment or preventive detention, or for any other reason linked in legislation to the existence of the disability. (Minkowitz, 2011, pp. 2–3)

The implication of this UN document on national mental health laws has not yet been fully taken on board, even though the UK Government has ratified the CRPD. However, the attempted restoration of people deemed psychotic as having basic human rights and citizenship granted to all others, helps press the case for credibility and legitimacy of service users in reforming the mental health research base (Sweeney, Beresford, Faulkner, Nettle & Rose, 2009; Wallcraft, Amering & Schrank, 2009). There is no case for this process to be solely the prerogative of psychiatrists.

Why does traditional mental health research disregard personal experience?

To understand why mental health research has failed to reflect personal experience it is helpful to look at the philosophical theories of knowledge (epistemologies) on which the research is based. The three main approaches found in mental health research will be briefly summarised here.

Positivist psychiatric research

The positivist approach can be understood as applying conventional scientific methods to studying mental health. Tew et al. (2006) argue that positivist researchers treat research subjects as 'passive objects that are done to by the technologies and practices of expert professionals' (p. 3). They state that in positivist research, questions of meaning are determined by the researchers, not the people researched.

Government concerns with ensuring NHS-funded treatments are evidence based have reinforced positivist research in psychiatry. The National Institute for Health and Clinical Excellence (NICE) adopts the general hierarchy of evidence as follows (Greenhalgh, 1997):

1. Systematic reviews and meta-analyses
2. Randomised controlled trials with definitive results
3. Randomised controlled trials with non-definitive results
4. Cohort studies
5. Case-control studies
6. Cross sectional surveys
7. Case reports

Systematic reviews and randomised controlled trials (RCTs) take priority. Such methods are beyond the resources of service users to undertake. Rose

(2009) argues that the voice of service users is excluded from systematic research reviews, due to the type of outcome measures used. Researchers seek one primary outcome, leaving out other possible effects of treatment. There is no opportunity for personal testimony. RCTs therefore are likely to continue to reinforce medical assumptions about psychosis rather than to challenge them. Beresford and Rose (2009) question whether RCTs are appropriate in the field of mental health, in which interventions are often far more complex than in physical medicine, and outcomes less straightforward and consensual. Thomas and Bracken (2004) make a similar point about positivism in general, saying:

> Positivism is simply unable to deal with the complexity of social and cultural environments. In reality, these worlds are rich in meaning and resist linear causal models ... This means that understanding and interpretation should be central to our approach to psychosis. (Thomas & Bracken, 2004, p. 363)

Phenomenological research

Phenomenology considers that each phenomenon is unique and no two situations are identical. Researchers using this perspective seek the fullest possible understanding of experience. They take into account the fact that researchers have an impact on the situations and the people whom they observe, and that there may be different interpretations of reality.

Phenomenological research is typically based on narratives or stories. People are encouraged to tell their stories in their own words. Roberts (2000) says that narrative approaches address people's individuality, which is otherwise lost in statistical averaging. Similarly Pennebaker and Seagal (1999) argue that narrative research can benefit people's mental health through enabling them to 'put their emotional upheavals into words' (p. 1244).

Davidson, Stayner, Lambert, Smith and Sledge (1997) carried out phenomenological research where long-term patients with 'serious mental illness' were invited to talk about what would help them stay out of hospital. The results of the research were helpful in designing support to help people live independently. They argue that positivist approaches fail to explain why people in this group are repeatedly readmitted to hospital, because they leave out patients' own views.

Critical theory research

Critical theorists try to understand social phenomena in their social context. They assume that social reality is historically constituted and that people continually produce and reproduce social realities. They take the view that although people can and do try to change their individual circumstances, their ability to do this is limited by social, cultural and political forces. Critical research is a way to challenge this, and tends to be politically committed, rather than objective or focused on the individual experience.

Foucault (1965, 1972) used the concept of 'psychopathology' (mental illness) to demonstrate his method of discourse analysis, arguing that mental illness does not exist as a real object, outside the particular historical context in which the concept was developed. He dates the emergence of the concept of mental illness to the early nineteenth century, when science and technology began to replace religion as the main influence on society, law and government. Foucault (1965) argued that the authority of doctors based on their status as wise men was replaced at that time by authority based on positivist science and knowledge. Foucault's approach allows the possibility of deconstructing concepts such as 'psychosis' which have become apparent 'common sense' to the extent we may not realise that these concepts were originally constructed to suit the interests and beliefs of particular groups.

Another important form of critical theory research is 'action research'. Action researchers assume the need for social change. Researchers initiate changes and evaluate their impact, for example, through setting up community projects. Researchers in the disability and mental health fields have developed participatory and emancipatory forms of action research. Participatory research encourages involvement of communities in the research about them. Emancipatory research aims to help people to gain skills and take more control over their lives (Mahone et al., 2011; Oliver, 1997).

Current psychosis research

Although the positivist approach is predominant in psychosis research, there are examples of other types of research receiving public funding. In England, the state-funded Mental Health Research Network (MHRN) supports and co-ordinates public mental health research. Its database of research includes studies run by mental health trusts and universities along with some pharma industry studies. A scan of the database at the time of writing revealed 55 separate studies relating to the diagnosis of schizophrenia. There were 32 controlled trials, mostly randomised, 13 other treatment observation studies, and 10 qualitative studies. One of the qualitative studies specifies that it takes a phenomenological approach to decision-making capacity. However, it can be seen from the predominance of controlled trials on the MHRN database that the positivist perspective still holds sway, even in the public sector. In the private sector, pharma industry-funded research is likely to be entirely positivist in nature.

In summary, although there are at least three very different approaches to researching psychosis, most research funding is spent on positivist research, which has the highest status. It also marginalises service user experience and it is the phenomenological and critical theory approaches which offer the greatest opportunities for service user involvement and leadership.

Positivist psychiatric research and the creation of spurious diagnoses

Biomedical research in psychosis is based on positivist assumptions that it is possible to identify and categorise mental diseases. The process of creating diagnoses is based on international consensus building about symptoms and categories among psychiatric professionals. This is needed, since there is no laboratory test for a psychosis. The consensus does not hold up, however, if a wider range of expert views are taken into account, including those of psychologists, social workers, families and last but not least, patients and service users. Patients have challenged psychiatrists since the creation of the original madhouses, as this quote illustrates:

> Regarding his committal to Bethlem [in the seventeenth century], the Restoration playwright Nathaniel Lee reputedly said, 'They called me mad, and I called them mad, and damn them, they outvoted me.' (Porter, 1991, p. 1)

Lee was a lone voice, but in recent years, the collective challenges of patients have had an impact at an international level. Professional organisations of psychiatrists, led by the World Psychiatric Association (WPA), work continually at updating diagnoses. The influence of service users on the revision of *ICD* (the *International Classification of Diseases,* a diagnostic system widely used in Europe) was noted in a recent issue of the WPA journal:

> The user community in mental health has been increasingly aligned
> with the disability rights movement, adopting the motto of 'Nothing
> about us without us!', rejecting what they see as medical paternalism,
> and demanding to be consulted about the decisions that affect their
> lives. The ICD revision process must encompass substantive and
> serious opportunities for participation of user groups, not just
> symbolic and ritualistic gesture. (IAGR-ICD-10, 2011, p. 88)

The above quote shows that international bodies are now beginning to recognise the need to include service users in the consensus building on diagnostic criteria. However, it is also clear that service users have had to fight hard for this recognition. The same writers recognise that the process of classifying groups of psychiatric symptoms may unhelpfully result in the creation of disease categories which serve the needs of psychiatric research rather than the needs of patients. Examples from history of the creation of spurious diagnoses to suit the times include 'drapetomania' (Kanani, 2011), a diagnosis which was given to slaves who ran away from their masters in the United States. Another example is the diagnosing and treatment of deviancy in homosexuals which only ended in 1974 (Palfy, 2011).

The creation of 'psychosis' (and the range of 'psychotic' diagnoses including 'schizophrenia') is arguably equally spurious. Read (2004) argues that psychiatrists, determined to establish their profession in the nineteenth century, urgently looked for physical causes of mental illness. He describes how Kraepelin (a leading psychiatrist) was funded by the Rockefeller Foundation to categorise madness so that it could be treated. The Rockefeller Foundation owned the petroleum industry, from which, at a later date, medicines were produced. Kraepelin grouped together 'mad' behaviours for which no physical cause had been discovered. He named this category 'dementia praecox', or 'early dementia', on the assumption that people with these problems only got worse, not better (Read, 2004). Bleuler later altered the concept and renamed it 'the group of Schizophrenias'. He dropped the certainty of degeneration, and admitted there was still no physical evidence of causes, nor any way to predict outcomes.

Boyle (2002) argues that 100 years later the diagnosis of schizophrenia has still not been successfully validated, and therefore has no scientific basis. More recently it has been argued that the diagnosis of schizophrenia is racially discriminatory (Fernando, 1988, 1989). A study confirming high rates of 'schizophrenia' in people from black and minority ethnic

(BME) groups (Fearon & Morgan, 2006) was strongly criticised by academics and BME voluntary sector organisations for raising racist fears of an epidemic of psychosis among black people:

> We know from a number of reports that rather than being a reflection of the true incidence of mental illness, it is the result of medicalising cultural differences, social problems and institutional racism. (O'Hara, 2010, *The Guardian*, 3rd February)

The controversy over the diagnosis of schizophrenia continues, yet a large amount of money is still given to genetic and biochemical research based on the assumption that it is a brain disease. Johnstone (1989) and Moncrieff (2003) draw attention to the extent of the influence of drug companies on psychiatric research:

> The industry is now heavily involved in the organisation of research into psychiatric drugs and the dissemination of research findings. This raises questions about the scientific objectivity of this research and the extent to which the industry is able to shape the research agenda. (Moncrieff, 2003)

In summary, critics of the positivist scientific basis for psychosis research, i.e., diagnosis, argue that it has a shaky and unproven foundation. It has also been used to exclude the perspective of those labelled. However, there is now some acceptance that service users have a right to a say in the revision of diagnoses.

Service users creating the knowledge base

Involvement in mental health research

Service users have been marginalised in mental health research, being the objects of research rather than the creators of the research; however, there are tentative signs of progression. UK governments are now emphasising patient-led services and involvement in every aspect of health. A government white paper (DH, 2010) on partnership for patient-centred care, quotes research that shows involvement improves healthcare outcomes, patient satisfaction, adherence to treatment, and may also reduce costs. These policy changes have encouraged national bodies such as MHRN (2012) to support service user involvement in mental health research. MHRN-supported studies have to show how they will involve service users. Progress is slow, however, as shown in a recent evaluation of service user involvement in MHRN (Staley, 2012). Only 20 per cent of studies involve service users as co-researchers, while in the majority of studies involvement is still limited in scope. Service users still do not have much opportunity to develop research questions and specify the methodology and outcomes sought.

In theory, there are opportunities for service users to be involved in mainstream psychosis research but it is still hard for them to make a real impact. For instance, the National Institute for Health and Clinical Excellence (NICE) involved service users in revising its guidance on the treatment of 'schizophrenia' (NICE, 2009). The panel of twenty-six people included five psychiatrists, three psychologists, and fifteen other professionals, with only two service users and one carer. In such circumstances, service users have a limited voice and restricted power to challenge underlying assumptions (see Campbell, 2009). While national policies state that service users should be involved in everything to do with mental health, they have limited power and are not yet able to have a strong impact on psychosis research.

Service user-led research

Despite being on the margins of academic and professional research, service users and survivors have been carrying out their own research projects since the late 1970s (Wallcraft et al., 2009; Sweeney et al., 2009). Some have worked as researchers for statutory and non-governmental organisations (NGOs), writing up the results of service user events. Others have carried out research looking at alternatives to hospital and drugs, often using participatory and emancipatory research methods (Beresford & Wallcraft, 1997; Lehmann, 2005; Read, 2009; Beresford & Rose, 2009). Another form of user-led research is the collection of narratives, where people tell their own stories of coping with psychosis (e.g., Susko, 1991; Read & Reynolds, 1996; Leibrich, 1999; Curtis, Dellar, Leslie, Watson & Monstersmith, 2000; Gray, 2006). One service user relates her experience of being treated with paroxetine, a controversial drug. She found that clinical researchers had ignored the service user voice, but that users were coming together to be heard:

> It was not until a critical mass of people who were experiencing disabling and dangerous withdrawal symptoms and side effects came together to share knowledge and take action that the pharmaceutical

company was forced to acknowledge the problem. To me, the whole situation exposed the perilous shortcomings of biomedical research that dismisses or suppresses the direct experiences of the people taking the medication. It also showed the power of the collective to bring about change. (Coldham, Russo et al., 2009, pp. 182–183)

Recently, the Institute of Psychiatry (IoP) enabled service users to take on research leadership roles. Rose (2009) and Fleischmann (2009) describe the work of the Service User Research Enterprise (SURE) at the IoP. They carried out two user-led reviews including 'grey' (unpublished) literature and personal testimony. Fleischmann (2009) concludes that 'the challenge for user/survivors and academic reviews is to ensure that systematic reviewing is demystified and that a truly participative model is developed' (p. 96).

Research by service users has been described as 'challenging the underlying assumptions and world-views on which traditional mental health research is based, in small, incremental ways, and in radical, fundamental ways' (Wallcraft & Nettle, 2009, p. 1). Lindow (2001) has argued that it is essential that research is completed from a service user perspective to find out what works, given the limitations of current medical and social services. Such research would help to devise outcomes that were defined by services users rather than services.

Overall, service users are developing a range of skills in research through their own efforts and through involvement in mainstream organisations. Much of their work challenges the biomedical discourse and positivist scientific methodology.

Service users taking a lead in hearing voices and unusual beliefs research

Many service users with the types of experience classed as 'psychotic' are involved in the user/survivor movement. In the late 1980s a specialist group, the Hearing Voices Network (HVN) emerged (Johnstone, 1989; James, 2001; Coleman & Smith, 2002). HVN was inspired by the work of Romme, a psychiatrist in the Netherlands (Romme & Escher, 1993). James (2001) recounts how HVN began to develop in Manchester in 1988 when service users were enabled to talk about their experiences of hearing voices without this being medicalised or seen as problematic:

For the first time in the UK ... schizophrenics were redefining themselves as voice-hearers, and so making the first collective attempt to de-pathologise their experience … their voices were being validated as real and meaningful experiences rather than an 'auditory hallucination'. (James, 2001, p. 48)

This movement provided a basis for survivor-led research in psychosis through establishing a new way of looking at the experience of voice hearing, outside the positivist assumption that voice hearing is a symptom of 'schizophrenia'. HVN has contributed greatly to the work of critiquing the biomedical approach to schizophrenia and allowing the possibility of new perspectives to emerge. Since the development of HVN, many people have begun to speak and write about how they cope with voices and other non-ordinary experiences and manage their lives with less psychiatric treatment or even without any at all (e.g., Coleman, 1999). Govers (2011) gives an account of how she overcame 'schizophrenia', with the help of psychotherapists and doctors who were willing to listen and encourage her to tell her life story and to write it down. Klafki writes:

> The main reason I have not needed a hospital or psychiatric drugs since 1997 is surely due to the fact that I have become involved in the hearing voices movement … People who hear voices do not want to be excluded from society or solely be treated with psychiatric drugs any more. Instead they want to learn the reasons for their voices so that they can live in peace with them. (Klafki, 2007, pp. 130–131)

A recent collection of narratives (Cordle, Fradgley, Carson, Holloway & Richards, 2011) is focused on stories of recovering from psychosis. Contributors speak of their spiritual and creative side which is neglected or denied by doctors, and the value of hearing voices groups. One person said: 'Hearing voices is a common human experience which needs to be normalised, not pathologised … we need to get rid of the whole diagnostic procedure and treat people as people' (p. 163).

Knight (2006) worked with a local unusual beliefs self-help group linked to HVN. She evaluated the group by carrying out a focus group with some of the members. She found that people gain support and acceptance from each other, and can talk about new ways of coping with their experiences. People's beliefs are not referred to as 'illness', but are accepted and respected, allowing members to speak freely. The group subsequently made links with the local clinical psychology training scheme and has collaborated on the development of new research into the meanings people give to their experience of unusual beliefs.

In summary, people who hear voices and have other non-ordinary experiences have carried out pioneering work through the HVN locally and nationally, and their work, including individual and collective narrative accounts and evaluation of HVN support groups, provides a major challenge to biomedical assumptions of voice hearing as a symptom of psychotic illness.

Conclusion

Although service users are not yet in a powerful position in relation to the research agenda, they are contributing to a new research approach based on personal testimony, narrative accounts of experience and collective empowerment. People who have been diagnosed 'psychotic' are creating the nucleus of a new evidence base which could be built on and used in the education and re-education of all mental health professionals, including psychiatrists. The literature emerging from service user groups including HVN networks challenges entrenched predominant thinking about psychosis based on the outdated and poorly validated work of the psychiatrists of the nineteenth and twentieth centuries.

Widespread narrative research, led by service users, would be of value to the participants who would gain from telling their stories, to the service user researchers who would gain confidence through doing the work, and to mental health professionals who could continually update and refresh their knowledge through hearing a wide range of life stories, viewpoints and approaches to recovery and wellness.

Research funders and academic researchers need to do more than invite service users to sit on panels to discuss research where the assumptions have already been established. It is time to recognise the opportunities that service users have demonstrated for addressing the life-limiting effects of the diagnosis and treatment of psychosis and the stigma that is inextricably linked with the biomedical approach. Change will require a collaborative approach and a respect for personal experience, which has been absent from the previous 150 years of the development of biomedical psychiatry.

References

Beresford, P., & Rose, D. (2009). Background. In A. Sweeney, P. Beresford, A. Faulkner, M. Nettle, & D. Rose (Eds.), *This is Survivor Research* (pp. 11–21). Ross-on-Wye: PCCS Books.

Beresford, P., & Wallcraft, J. (1997). Psychiatric system survivors and emancipatory research: Issues, overlaps and differences. In C. Barnes & G. Mercer (Eds.), *Doing Disability Research.* Leeds: Disability Press.

Boyle, M. (2002). *Schizophrenia: A scientific delusion?* Brighton: Routledge.

Breggin, P. (1991). *Toxic Psychiatry.* New York: St. Martin's Press.

Campbell, P. (2009). The service user/survivor movement. In J. Reynolds, R. Muston, T. Heller, J. Leach, M. McCormick, J. Wallcraft & M. Walsh (Eds.), *Mental Health Still Matters.* Basingstoke: Palgrave.

Chamberlin, J. (1978). *On Our Own: Patient-controlled alternatives to the mental health system.* New York: McGraw-Hill.

Coldham, T., Russo, J., et al. (2009). Telling our truths, bringing about change. In A. Sweeney, P. Beresford, A. Faulkner, M. Nettle, & D. Rose (Eds.), *This is Survivor Research* (pp. 163–184). Ross-on-Wye: PCCS Books.

Coleman, R. (1999). *Recovery: An alien concept.* Gloucester: Handsell.

Coleman, R., & Smith, M. (2002). *Working with Voices.* Wellington, New Zealand: Keepwell.

Cordle, H., Fradgley, J., Carson, J., Holloway, F., & Richards, P. (Eds.). (2011). *Psychosis: Stories of recovery and hope.* London: Quay Books.

Curtis, T., Dellar, R., Leslie, E., Watson, B., & Monstersmith, C. (2000). *Mad Pride: A celebration of mad culture.* London: Spare Change Books.

Davidson, L., Stayner, D. A., Lambert, S., Smith, P., & Sledge, W. H. (1997). Phenomenological and participatory research on schizophrenia: Recovering the person in theory and practice. *Journal of Social Issues, 53,* 767–784.

Department of Health. (2010). *Equity and Excellence: Liberating the NHS.* London: The Stationery Office.

Fearon, P., & Morgan, C. (2006). Environmental factors in schizophrenia: The role of migrant studies. *Schizophrenia Bulletin, 32,* 405–408.

Fernando, S. (1988). *Race and Culture in Psychiatry.* London: Croom Helm.

Fernando, S. (1989). Schizophrenia in ethnic minorities. *Psychiatric Bulletin, 13,* 573–574.

Fleischmann, P. (2009). Literature reviews: An example of making traditional research methods user focused. In A. Sweeney, P. Beresford, A. Faulkner, M. Nettle, & D. Rose (Eds.), *This is Survivor Research* (pp. 82–97). Ross-on-Wye: PCCS Books.

Foucault, M. (1965). *Madness and Civilization.* New York: Random House.

Foucault, M. (1972). *The Archaeology of Knowledge.* New York: Pantheon.

Govers, L. (2011). *Healing from Schizophrenia.* Self-published, available from http://www.lulu.com

Gray, P. (Ed.). (2006). *The Madness of Our Lives.* London: Jessica Kingsley.

Greenhalgh, T. (1997). How to read a paper: Getting your bearings (deciding what the paper is about). *BMJ, 315,* 243.

IAGR-ICD-10. (2011). Mental and behavioural disorders: A conceptual framework for the revision of the ICD-10 classification of mental and behavioural disorders: International Advisory Group for the Revision of ICD-10. *World Psychiatry, 10,* 86–92.

James, A. (2001). *Raising Our Voices: An account of the Hearing Voices Movement.* Gloucester: Handsell.

Johnstone, L. (1989). *Users and Abusers of Psychiatry.* London: Routledge.

Kanani, N. (2011). Race and madness: Locating the experiences of racialized people with psychiatric histories in Canada and the United States. *Critical Disability Discourse/Discours Critiques dans le Champ du Handicap, 3,* 1–14.

Klafki, H. (2007). The voices accompany my life. In P. Statsny & P. Lehmann (Eds.), *Alternatives Beyond Psychiatry.* Berlin: Peter Lehmann Publishing.

Knight, T. (2006). *Beyond Belief: Alternative ways of working with delusions, obsessions and unusual experiences.* Available online as free download from www.peter-lehmann-publishing.com/beyond-belief.htm

Lehmann, P. (2005). *Coming Off Psychiatric Drugs.* Berlin: Peter Lehmann.

Leibrich, J. (1999). *A Gift of Stories: Discovering how to deal with mental illness.* Dunedin, New Zealand: University of Otago Press with the Mental Health Commission.

Lindow, V. (2001). Survivor research. In C. Newnes, G. Holmes & C. Dunn (Eds), *This Is Madness Too* (pp. 135–146). Ross-on-Wye: PCCS Books.

Mahone, I., Farrell, S., Hinton, I., Johnson, R., Moody, D., Rifkin, K., Moore, K., Becker, M., & Barker, M. (2011). Participatory action research in public mental health and the school of nursing: Qualitative findings from an academic-community partnership. *Journal of Participatory Medicine, 3,* e10, 23 February.

Mehta, N., Kassam, A., Leese, M., Butler, G., & Thornicroft, G. (2009). Public attitudes towards people with mental illness in England and Scotland, 1994–2003. *The British Journal of Psychiatry, 194,* 278–284.

MHRN. (2012). *Mental Health Research Network* [Online]. Retrieved 22nd October 2012 from: http://www.mhrn.info/pages/who-we-are-and-how-we-work.html

Minkowitz, T. (2011). Why mental health laws contravene the CRPD – An application of Article 14 with implications for the obligations of States Parties. *Social Science Research Network* [Online]. Retrieved 29 January 2012 from: http://papers.ssrn.com/sol3/papers.cfm?abstract_id=1928600

Moncrieff, J. (2003). *Is psychiatry for sale? An examination of the influence of the pharmaceutical industry on academic and practical psychiatry.* London: Institute of Psychiatry. Retrieved 29 January 2012 from, http://www.critpsynet.freeuk.com/pharmaceuticalindustry.htm

NICE. (2009). *Schizophrenia: Core interventions in the treatment and management of schizophrenia in adults in primary and secondary care.* London: National Institute for Clinical Excellence.

O'Hara, M. (2010). Fightback over claims on mental illness and its prevalence among black people. *The Guardian,* Wednesday, 3 February 2010.

Oliver, M. (1997). Emancipatory research: Realistic goal or impossible dream? In C. Barnes & G. Mercer (Eds.), *Doing Disability Research.* Leeds: Disability Press.

Palfy, R. R. (2011). *Psychiatry, Social Control, and Homosexuality:Clients' perceptions of therapeutic care in the decades following demedicalization.* University of Saskatchewan: Unpublished thesis.

Peck, E., & Parker, E. (1998). Mental health in the NHS: Policy and practice 1979–98. *Journal of Mental Health, 7,* 241–259.

Pennebaker, J. W., & Seagal, J. D. (1999). Forming a story: The health benefits of narrative. *Journal of Clinical Psychology, 55,* 1243–1254.

Porter, R. (1991). *The Faber Book of Madness.* London: Faber.

Read, J. (2004). The invention of 'schizophrenia'. In J. Read, L. R. Mosher & R. P. Bentall (Eds.), *Models of Madness: Psychological, social and biological approaches to schizophrenia* (pp. 21–34). London: Routledge.

Read, J. (2009). *Psychiatric Drugs: Key issues and service user perspectives.* Houndmills: Palgrave Macmillan.

Read, J., & Reynolds, J. (1996*). Speaking Our Minds: An anthology of personal experiences of mental distress and its consequences.* Basingstoke: Macmillan.

Roberts, G. A. (2000). Narrative and severe mental illness: What place do stories have in an evidence-based world? *Advances in Psychiatric Treatment, 6,* 432–441.

Romme, M., & Escher, S. (1993). *Accepting Voices.* London: MIND Publications.

Rose, D. (2009). Is collaborative research possible? In J. Wallcraft, B. Schrank & M. Amering (Eds.), *Handbook of Service User Involvement in Mental Health Research.* Chichester: Wiley-Blackwell.

Staley, K. (2012). *An Evaluation of Service User Involvement in Studies Adopted by the Mental Health Research Network.* London: National Institute for Health Research/Mental Health Research Network.

Susko, M. (1991). *Cry of the Invisible: Writings from the homeless and survivors of psychiatric hospitals.* Baltimore, MD: Conservatory Press.

Sweeney, A., Beresford, P., Faulkner, A., Nettle, M., & Rose, D. (Eds.). (2009). *This is Survivor Research.* Ross-on-Wye: PCCS Books.

Tew, J., Gould, N., Abankwa, D., et al. (2006). *Values and Methodologies for Social Research in Mental Health.* London: SPN/SCIE.

Thomas, P., & Bracken, P. (2004). Critical psychiatry in practice. *Advances in Psychiatric Treatment, 10,* 361–370.

United Nations. (2008). *Convention on the Rights of Persons with Disabilities.* United Nations Department of Economic and Social Affairs & Office of the United Nations High Commissioner For Human Rights. United Nations.

Wallcraft, J., Amering, M., & Schrank, B. (2009). *Handbook of Service User Involvement in Mental Health Research.* Chichester: Wiley-Blackwell.

Wallcraft, J., & Nettle, M. (2009). History, context and language. In J. Wallcraft, B. Schrank, & B. Amering (Eds.), *Handbook of Service User Involvement in Mental Health Research*. Chichester: Wiley-Blackwell.

Chapter 13

The Patient's Dilemma:
An analysis of users' experiences
of taking neuroleptic drugs

Joanna Moncrieff, David Cohen & John Mason

Since the 1950s, severe mental disturbance or disorganisation, known as psychosis or schizophrenia, has been treated with 'antipsychotic' or neuroleptic drugs. Nowadays, these drugs are generally claimed to work by reversing an underlying chemical imbalance, or some other sort of disease process that is thought to produce psychotic symptoms.

When neuroleptic drugs were first introduced into psychiatry, they were not regarded as having disease-specific effects, but were thought to consist of special sorts of sedatives, or tranquillisers. The psychiatrists who used them commented frequently on characteristic features that people displayed under the influence of these drugs. They reported how people became quiet without simply falling asleep, how their movement, initiative and motivation were reduced, and how their emotions were flattened. It was the drugs' ability to produce these abnormal effects that was thought to be the secret of their success. By suppressing mental and physical activity in general, they were able to reduce the intensity of psychotic beliefs and experiences.

Over the course of the 1950s through the 1970s, views about the nature of antipsychotic drugs, and other drugs used in psychiatry, changed fundamentally. In mainstream psychiatric thinking, they started to be presented more and more as specific treatments for particular diseases. By the present day, this way of thinking is so firmly embedded in psychiatric practice that most people have forgotten that there was ever any other way to understand these drugs and how they work. In the current chapter, we will go back to the early mode of understanding the nature of neuroleptic drugs and how they produce their effects, and we will present an analysis of data about the experience of taking these drugs from a website for users of medications, which supports this earlier view. We will formulate an alternative approach to using these drugs that presents their effects more honestly, and allows users and prescribers to make more informed and democratic decisions about their use.

Models of drug action

In order to provide a clear way to think about the nature of psychiatric drugs, elsewhere we have outlined two alternative ways of understanding how they might affect people with psychiatric problems (Moncrieff, 2008; Moncrieff & Cohen, 2005). We have called these different 'models' of drug action the disease-centred model and the drug-centred model. Their contrasting features are summarised in Table 1. The disease-centred model is the standard view that psychiatric drugs work by correcting an underlying disease of the brain. According to this model, drug treatment makes your brain more normal by helping to rectify the underlying problem. The disease-centred model is based on the way most drugs work in physical medicine. Insulin, for example, compensates for the underlying deficiency of insulin in diabetes, antibiotics target bacteria, and anti-asthma drugs help to reverse the lung problems that cause wheezing. Even painkillers, although they do not target any underlying disease, work by acting on the biological pathways that give rise to pain.

Table 1. *Alternative Models of Drug Action*

Disease-centred model	Drug-centred model
Drugs help correct an abnormal brain state	Drugs create an abnormal brain state
Therapeutic effects of drugs derived from their effects on an underlying disease process	Therapeutic effects derived from the impact of the drug-induced state on behavioural and emotional problems
Paradigm: insulin for diabetes	Paradigm: alcohol for social anxiety

The disease-centred model presents all psychiatric drugs as working in the same way. This is reflected in the way psychiatric drugs are named: thus antidepressants are thought to help correct the disease process that leads to depression, antipsychotics are thought to rectify the abnormality that gives rise to the symptoms of schizophrenia or psychosis and mood stabilisers are believed to correct an underlying instability of mood.

In the alternative way of thinking about psychiatric drugs, the 'drug-centred' model, it is emphasised that these drugs are *drugs*, that is, extraneous chemical substances that modify the body's functioning. Moreover, psychiatric drugs are a special category of drug because they have outstanding psychoactive effects. Like all psychoactive substances, they distort the functioning of the nervous system and by doing so they produce altered mental states. When we think of recreational drugs we refer to these altered mental states as 'intoxication'. Psychiatric drugs also produce states of intoxication. The features of these states vary according to what sort of drug is taken. Just as the effects of cannabis differ from those of alcohol or heroin, so the effects produced by neuroleptics are different from those produced by benzodiazepines or antidepressants like Prozac, for example. The characteristic features of the intoxicated or drug-induced state depend on the chemical structure and nature of each drug. Of course, as with all psychoactive drugs, the user's psychology and temperament, as well as the circumstances and setting of drug use, also shape the features of the drug-induced state.

What the drug-centred model suggests is that drugs can sometimes be helpful because the features of the drug-induced state superimpose themselves onto the manifestations of the mental disturbance. The accepted example of this is the helpful effect of alcohol in people who are extremely shy and avoid social situations (sometimes labelled as social phobia or social anxiety). Alcohol is not thought to be helpful because it corrects a deficiency of alcohol within the brain, nor because it corrects another chemical imbalance. It is thought to help because one of the characteristic features of alcohol intoxication is that it weakens social inhibitions. When we know the drug-induced effects of psychiatric drugs we can start to understand how people with various types of personal difficulties can find these drugs useful, in the same way that we can understand how alcohol might help certain very shy people in social situations.

The drug-centred model of neuroleptic action

In 1952, the two French psychiatrists who started using chlorpromazine, the first neuroleptic drug, in psychiatric hospitals described its effects as follows:

> The apparent indifference, or delay in response to external stimuli, the emotional and affective neutrality, the decrease in both initiative and preoccupation without alteration of conscious awareness or in intellectual faculties, constitute the psychic syndrome due to treatment. (Delay & Deniker, 1952, p. 504)

One of these psychiatrists, Pierre Deniker, went on to elaborate how the drugs effectively replaced the symptoms of schizophrenia with the symptoms of a drug-induced neurological syndrome, which closely resembled Parkinson's disease (Deniker, 1960). German psychiatrist Hans Joachim Haase also proposed that the therapeutic effects of the new drugs consisted of a mild version of the Parkinson disease-like syndrome (Haase, 1956). Later he coined the term 'neuroleptic threshold' to indicate the dose of a drug which could achieve therapeutically useful, mild neurological suppression, without producing frank Parkinsonian symptoms (Haase & Janssen, 1965).

Similar views were proposed by American psychiatrist, F. A. Freyhan, speaking at a symposium held in Switzerland in 1957 (Freyhan, 1959). He stressed the belief that the effects of the new drugs were not specific to any diagnostic group, but acted on signs of over-arousal, excitement and abnormal preoccupations due to their ability to reduce movement and initiative and blunt emotions, which he also linked to their overt motor effects. Like Deniker and Haase, Freyhan suggested that the drugs' useful and therapeutic effects (judged within the environments of large psychiatric hospital wards in the 1950s) were on a continuum with their obvious extra-pyramidal or Parkinsonian effects:

> From the beginning it was evident that no lines of demarcation could be drawn between therapeutic degrees of reduced psychomotor activity and early symptoms of parkinsonism … What we witnessed were gradual transition from hypermotility to hypomotility, which, in a certain proportion of patients, progressed to the more pronounced degrees of parkinsonian rigidity. Clinical evidence therefore, indicated that the therapeutic function of chlorpromazine

and reserpine could not be separated from their modifying influence on the function of subcortical motor system in transacting volitional, affective and intentional functions. (Freyhan, 1959, p. 10)

The drug-centred model also stresses the fact that drugs are chemicals that alter the normal functioning of the body and thereby highlights the relationship between the physical and mental effects produced by drugs. Neuroleptic drugs affect numerous bodily systems through varied mechanisms we do not fully understand. Many of their characteristic neurological effects are due to their propensity to block dopamine receptors, which induces the characteristic Parkinsonian effects on movement and volition, and also affects sexual function via its effects on the hormone prolactin. The drugs also affect a range of other neurotransmitter systems however, and, like other drugs, they provoke the body to react in both predictable and unpredictable ways. Animal studies have shown, for example, that one week of treatment with haloperidol can induce rats to produce more dopamine receptors and to increase their sensitivity to dopamine (Samaha, Seeman, Stewart, Rajabi & Kapur, 2007). An overreaction of the dopamine system to the presence of a dopamine-blocking drug is one theory of the causation of tardive dyskinesia, the sometimes irreversible neurological complication of long-term neuroleptic treatment.

The experience of taking neuroleptic drugs

Apart from the descriptions provided in the early days of neuroleptic use, and a few subsequent accounts (Healy & Farquhar, 1998), there has been no attempt to explore systematically the nature of the altered state produced by neuroleptic drugs and how it might impact on psychological symptoms. We therefore undertook an analysis of the comments people made about their experiences with these drugs on a website designed for users of various types of medication, called *askapatient.com*. These comments are freely available on the Internet for everyone to view. Most are anonymous, although respondents have the option of leaving an email address, which a small minority do. We conducted a descriptive qualitative content analysis of comments on different antipsychotics, comparing comments made about two of the most widely prescribed newer antipsychotics, olanzapine and risperidone, and the older drugs. We also conducted a quantitative analysis to compare the frequency of different effects between the different sorts of drugs (Moncrieff, Cohen & Mason, 2009).

We analysed 439 comments in total, including 46 first-person accounts of the effects of the older drugs chlorpromazine, trifluoperazine and haloperidol, 170 accounts of taking olanzapine and 223 comments on risperidone. Just over half of the respondents were women, and the average age of respondents was in the 30s. On average, people had been taking the older neuroleptics for around 26 months, risperidone for 20 months, and olanzapine for approximately 16 months. About a third of people taking the older drugs and risperidone had a diagnosis of schizophrenia or psychosis, but only 23 per cent of those taking olanzapine. Other common diagnoses were depression, anxiety and bipolar disorder. Forty per cent of people taking olanzapine had a diagnosis of bipolar disorder. The profile of medication users was similar to findings from a United States survey of antipsychotic use, which also found that only a third of users of atypical antipsychotics were diagnosed with psychosis or schizophrenia. The dose of medication used was not frequently recorded in the current study, but where it was provided, average daily doses of all types of drug were towards the lower end of the therapeutic range.

In the analysis that we undertook from a drug-centred perspective, we identified all comments describing alterations of normal physical and mental functioning which people believed were produced by taking neuroleptic drugs. Table 2 lists the 15 most common drug-induced effects reported. Comparing the different types of drugs revealed that most physical effects varied in their frequency according to the type of drug that was taken. Parkinsonian symptoms, for example, and akathisia (mental and physical restlessness) were reported more commonly by people taking older antipsychotics. In contrast, weight gain was more frequently mentioned by people taking risperidone and olanzapine, and most frequently by those taking olanzapine. A new category of 'extreme weight gain' was added during the analysis, when we noticed that a large number of comments described unusually large weight gain. Twenty-nine per cent of people taking olanzapine gave comments fitting these criteria, with 14 per cent of people on risperidone reporting these levels of weight gain, and only 4 per cent of people on older neuroleptics. Risperidone was particularly strongly associated with hormonal effects such as breast growth and lactation, with 14 per cent of people on risperidone reporting this effect, compared to none on the other drug types. Sexual impairment, which included loss of libido and impotence, was mentioned by a quarter of people taking risperidone, compared to only 2 to 5 per cent of people on olanzapine or the older antipsychotics.

As far as mental effects were concerned, all three types of drug were commonly reported to produce sedative effects, but people taking olanzapine mentioned these effects more frequently than those on the other drugs. Feelings of impaired cognitive or mental processes were reported more commonly by people taking the older drugs. Emotional and motivational effects, on the other hand, were equally common with all three types of drug and were mentioned by around a fifth of respondents.

Older neuroleptics

Several respondents provided a general description of the effects of being under the influence of these drugs, which indicated that overall the drugs induce an experience of general physical and mental slowness or impairment. Four respondents used the term 'zombie' to describe these effects. One respondent taking haloperidol explained that 'I feel like a zombie, I can't think clear and my movement is slow'. A young man on this drug described how it was 'extremely hard to move, think, talk'. Another described a feeling of 'heavy mental and physical stagnance' and a man taking trifluoperazine also used the term 'stagnance' and added that taking the drug had resulted in a 'general retarded feeling'.

All three of the older drugs were experienced by some respondents as being strongly sedative. This was indicated by increased time spent asleep and feeling drowsy, fatigued or lethargic during the day. Someone who had been taking chlorpromazine for six months said, 'sleepy knocks you out for a long time which was good for me. Woke up unrefreshed though.' A long-term user of trifluoperazine (20 years) said, 'I'm still fatigued in the mornings and can barely get out of bed some days.' A respondent who had used haloperidol for five years reported that 'I used to sleep on this med from 4 in the afternoon until the next day at lunch time'.

Several respondents described how their feelings were suppressed while taking the drugs. 'I feel absolutely nothing!! No sadness, no joy, NOTHING' (capitals in original), said one man of being on haloperidol. Two respondents mentioned a loss of creativity while on the drugs. One of these added that trifluoperazine 'took away my sense of humour' and made her feel 'emotionally empty, dead inside'.

Nine respondents felt the medication had helped improve their psychological problems, and three of these described how they thought this was achieved. One man diagnosed with bipolar I disorder described how he thought haloperidol had 'decreased brain activity, slowed down

Table 2. Drug-induced Effects Reported by Respondents

Category of effect	Descriptions	Older anti-psychotics	Risperidone	Olanzapine
Sedative effects	increased sleep, daytime drowsiness, fatigue, lethargy, difficulty waking	44%	42%	56%
Cognitive effects	impaired concentration or memory, mental slowness	35%	18%	17%
Motivational and emotional effects	flattened emotions, indifference, loss of interest, change of personality, loss of creativity, feeling like a 'zombie'	20%	22%	22%
Parkinsonian effects	stiffness, slowness, heaviness	33%	10%	4%
Involuntary movements	twitching, jerking, tremor, lack of co-ordination	11%	8%	9%
Tardive dyskinesia	described by respondents as 'tardive dyskinesia'	4%	1%	4%
Akathisia	mental or physical restlessness, feeling of tension, sometimes described as 'akathisia'	24%	7%	5%
Anxiety/irritability	anxious, irritable, angry	9%	9%	5%

Depression	feeling depressed or low	6%	4%	4%
Drug-induced euphoria or relaxation	feeling 'high', or pleasant feelings of relaxation and calmness	5%	3%	2%
Sexual impairment	loss of libido, impotence	5%	27%	2%
Hormonal effects	breast growth in males, lactation	0	14%	0
Weight gain	any mention of weight gain	52%	37%	11%
Extreme weight gain	excessive, huge or extreme weight gain, or weight gain exceeding 2kgs a month, or 15kgs in total	29%	14%	4%
Increased appetite or food cravings	cravings for sugar rich or carbohydrate rich foods, or 'junk food'	25%	9%	0

racing thoughts'. A woman who had taken haloperidol for 'delerium [sic] and hallucination' described the suppression of interest caused by the drug and linked that with being more in contact with reality:

> *Although I felt very well, I felt as if I had absolutely nothing to talk about. I kept wondering about whatever [it] was that had been so interesting during most of my life that I had suddenly lost ... But I was very much in contact with reality and for that I was thankful.*

Another respondent taking haloperidol, who did not give a diagnosis, commented that 'my husband says I am much easier to get along with when I take it and I agree 100 per cent. I feel calm, normal "smoothed out" but NOT sedated or medicated.' She also reports increased sleep and says, 'I am a little slower than normal but hey, better than erratic.'

Respondents who described akathisia confirmed that it was an intensely unpleasant experience. They referred to 'horrible restlessness' or being unable to 'sit still, could not concentrate'. A male respondent described how taking chlorpromazine produced 'extreme physical agitation combined with a zombie-like mind state'.

People's responses to the older drugs varied and both extremes of liking and disliking the drugs' effects were represented. For example, one respondent who was convinced that taking trifluoperazine had kept her well was so grateful that she stated, 'I love this drug'. One respondent prescribed haloperidol for two days for a manic episode felt that the 'drug saved my life'. In contrast, comments such as 'This is the worst I have been exposed to' from a man who had taken haloperidol for a month for 'psychosis' were not uncommon. Chlorpromazine was described as 'horrible stuff. Got off it as soon as possible' by one recipient who had been treated for bipolar disorder. Two respondents who had been forced to take haloperidol felt that psychiatrists should be compelled to take it to appreciate how unpleasant it was.

Risperidone

Global descriptions of the experience of being on risperidone emphasised loss of interest and drives and emotional flattening. 'I lost my ability to feel emotions, I lost my libido, I lost my drives, I lost my ability to get an erection' was a typical comment by a young man who mentioned taking the drug for auditory hallucinations. He continued, 'no emotions, only a weird, spacey, empty feeling, no arousal, no excitement, no joy, nothing.' Another respondent said, 'I feel like a complete zombie' and described 'tiredness, lack of interest in everyday activities'. Another respondent being treated for anxiety and bipolar disorder complained, 'This medication has made me lifeless. I have no energy, and my zest for life is at an all-time low.' She went on to describe 'an emptiness and depression too hard to bear'. Other respondents described a 'total shut down of my outgoing personality', a feeling of 'mental nothingness, a numbness that was unsettling' and a feeling of having 'no thoughts or inner world'.

Slow or restricted movements were less often associated with this state than in the case of the older drugs, as reflected in lower rates of Parkinsonian symptoms. However, cognitive effects included descriptions of slowed-up or impaired thought processes. One respondent expressed the experience as a feeling of being in 'slow motion'. Several other people mentioned feelings of 'mental fogginess' or 'cloudiness'. One respondent, a woman with anxiety, linked this state to the occurrence of what she believed to be a drug-induced depression. She described how taking the drug had 'led to a severe depression that when I lowered it lightened up'.

Risperidone was also experienced as being strongly sedative by some respondents. One respondent who was prescribed risperidone for hallucinations described how 'I slept 23 hours a day and the one hour I was awake I spent crawling into the living room'. Another respondent who did not give a diagnosis commented, 'I felt tired all the time. Too tired to be depressed.'

As in comments on older antipsychotics, comments on risperidone included some vivid descriptions of the experience of akathisia. One woman prescribed risperidone for a psychotic disorder said, 'I felt like scratching my eyes out and my skin off and running into the walls' and a man with psychosis referred to a feeling of 'ineffable anxiety, which was sort of like restless leg syndrome'.

Several respondents described how the drugs' effects had helped to reduce racing, troubling or delusional thoughts. A man with a diagnosis of paranoid schizophrenia described how risperidone had 'numbed my brain from psychotic thoughts, flattened most of my emotions'. Another respondent with anxiety and paranoia described how it 'stops my negative thoughts and feeling being amplified and overwhelming me'. Several respondents commented that the drug had produced feelings of 'calm' or relief from anxiety. However, in contrast, one respondent who had been diagnosed with schizophrenia who experienced akathisia described an increase in 'intrusive thoughts'.

In common with the older antipsychotics there were also some very negative evaluations of the drugs' effects. Comments like the following typify such responses: 'Lack of interest in life, no will to carry on living. Constant need to go to the bathroom. Constant headache. Living hell.' 'BEWARE, BEWARE, BEWARE!!! This medication is Satan in a flipping pill.'

Olanzapine

From the general thrust of the comments on www.askapatient.com, the overall subjective state produced by olanzapine appeared to consist of profound sedation accompanied by emotional flattening and indifference, in association with a markedly increased appetite for food. The following comment by a person diagnosed with bipolar disorder typifies many:

> I've never been able to eat as much as I did when I was on Zyprexa. I gained 40 lbs in no time and my mind was in a constant fog of lethargy and indifference. I didn't care about anything. I just wanted to sit around and eat.

Another respondent with a diagnosis of schizophrenia put it this way: 'I was a humongous zombie on Zyprexa.' The increase in appetite was described vividly by many respondents using phrases such as 'ravenous, rapacious hunger that never quit'.

Disabling sedation was frequently mentioned. A woman with depression described how 'I was sleeping over 14 hours a night and was so hung over during the day I couldn't go about my normal routines. I couldn't even get myself dressed to go out to the store.' Another respondent with a diagnosis of bipolar disorder described how 'I keep eating and eating and sleeping and sleeping and sometimes I manage to do both at the same time'. She felt the drug had turned her into a 'foodaholic, sleepaholic zombie'.

Comments categorised as indicating cognitive effects consisted of descriptions of having difficulty thinking clearly and of being slowed down. One respondent said, 'I am not able to think properly and am experiencing the world at about half the normal pace ... Can't keep my mind focused and my eyes are slow.' Another respondent commented on a feeling of being 'two steps behind everyone else'. Another respondent described a 'mild inhibited feeling'.

Emotional and motivational effects consisted of feelings of emotions being flattened, creativity dampened or personality being changed for the worse. One young man described his moods as being 'too zoned, too robotic, emotion dead'. Another respondent described feeling 'emotionally flat, listless, loss of libido'. A woman described an 'inability to feel sexual – totally blank mind – moodless. No ups and downs – flattened creativity – inability to be in love' and she commented, 'I feel numb, like I've been brainwashed. There is more to life than eating and sleeping.' Another respondent described feeling that her 'personality is dampened'.

Despite the nature of these comments, several respondents described benefits of the drug for various distressing experiences. Several mentioned that the drug had 'stopped the psychosis and thoughts coming into my head' and some described benefits in terms of reducing anxiety, irritability and suicidal thoughts. 'It has a wonderful calming effect' was how one man who had been diagnosed with bipolar disorder put it. One man with a diagnosis of schizoaffective disorder commented that 'despite its extremely negative side effects, this medication does wonders for paranoia and delusional thinking … the anxiety is non-existent now, I am able to function as a normal human being.'

Other drugs examined

As for the other drugs examined here there were positive and negative evaluations of the effects. Many people felt the drug had helped them. One said, 'The drug saved my life by getting me sleep so my nervous system could rest.' Another said, 'It made me feel great, but the side effects were too intense.' Some had disliked it intensely. An older man with anxiety said: 'This is the most horrible drug I've ever used.' A woman commented, 'If you would not willingly undergo a lobotomy, then do not take this drug.' Others expressed the difficult process of weighing up the pros and cons of taking it, 'It makes me feel like a veggie, but that was better than what I was going through and it kept me out of the hospital', said a woman who described herself as suffering from 'psychosis'. Another respondent with a diagnosis of schizophrenia commented in the same vein, but in a more negative fashion, 'It makes you sane, but you're not much better off.'

The impact of neuroleptics

To summarise, the data from askapatient.com indicates that all neuroleptics appear to produce a state that is characterised by sedation, lethargy, flattening of emotional responses, indifference and feelings of impaired mental functioning. These mental or psychoactive effects are also linked to the physical effects the drugs produce. As in earlier descriptions of older neuroleptics, descriptions from askapatient.com illustrated the connection between the drugs' psychoactive effects and Parkinson's disease-like symptoms consisting of feelings of slowness, rigidity, and difficulty with movement. Parkinsonian symptoms were less prominent with both of the two newer drugs, olanzapine in particular. Risperidone, however, was strongly associated with sexual impairment, particularly loss of libido but also impotence, and with hormonal effects. Olanzapine was associated with marked increase in appetite and extreme weight gain.

All three drugs produced akathisia in some respondents, with fewer reports from people on the newer drugs. Akathisia was strongly associated with reporting suicidal thoughts, especially in people taking olanzapine. Some respondents specifically described how the intolerability of akathisia led to suicidal thoughts.

Several respondents identified that the mental effects produced by the drugs had exerted a beneficial effect on some of the symptoms they were experiencing. They mentioned how the drugs appeared to slow racing thoughts and suppress psychotic symptoms. Some indicated that the emotional flattening produced by the drugs was helpful.

Overall, these descriptions support a drug-centred account of the nature of neuroleptic drug action. They suggest that the typical psychoactive state produced by the drugs, with its characteristic sedation, and emotional and cognitive suppression, can help to suppress intrusive and overwhelming symptoms of mental disorder, including psychotic experiences. Yet we note that although some respondents found the effects of the drugs helpful, most people found the drug-induced state to be unpleasant, and some found it highly aversive. Even those who welcomed the drugs' ability to relieve or suppress symptoms sometimes found that the price of this relief was just too high. People often disliked the emotional suppression and mental clouding produced by the drugs, but they were also concerned about potentially dangerous and harmful physical effects, such as weight gain, diabetes and neurological complications like tardive dyskinesia.

A democratic approach to neuroleptic treatment

So what implications does this description of the nature of the effects of neuroleptic drugs have for the way these drugs are used and prescribed? The drug-centred model of drug action suggests that users and prescribers of such drugs should share and discuss information such as that provided here about the sort of drug-induced effects the drugs produce, and how these effects might impact on the symptoms of mental disturbances like psychosis. As far as possible, patients should be offered choices about whether and how they want to use drug treatment, based on this information.

Knowledge about the mind-altering effects of the drugs will help people in distress and those who are trying to help them, including mental health professionals, to assess whether the drugs are likely to have any benefits in a given situation, and to weigh possible benefits against the impairments associated with the drug-induced state. For people who are so overwhelmed by psychotic experiences like hallucinations, or so preoccupied by delusional beliefs that they are unable to function in, and connect with, the real world, the suppressant effects of the drugs may bring relief. Moreover, if intrusive psychotic experiences can be dampened down, the individual may be able to interact with the external world again, which will enable them to benefit from the care and support offered by other people. This care may, in turn, help people to regain their bearings. So antipsychotic drugs may bring a measure of relief to people experiencing an acute episode of psychosis; however, some people may prefer to endure such an episode without drug treatment. Unfortunately, it is difficult for people to make this choice in current mental health services, since drug treatment is the mainstay of standard inpatient and outpatient treatment regimes. Innovative projects such as the Soteria project have shown that it is possible for some people to recover from psychosis in a supportive environment without drug treatment, and it is to be hoped that such facilities will be developed again in the future (Bola & Mosher, 2003; Lehtinen, Aaltonen, Koffert, Rakkolainen & Syvalahti, 2000).

Long-term treatment poses further problems. Although many people recover from episodes of psychosis, some remain disturbed for long periods of time. Neuroleptic drugs can sometimes help people in this situation to improve enough to have some measure of independence. The costs of long-term treatment are considerable however, including the impact of the drugs on intellectual and emotional functioning and physical consequences such as tardive dyskinesia, weight gain, diabetes, sexual dysfunction and increased risk of sudden cardiac death (Ray, Chung, Murray, Hall & Stein, 2009). Again, mental health professionals should support people with ongoing symptoms to consider the pros and cons of long-term drug treatment, and to make their own individual decisions based on this process. For some people with severe symptoms, the adverse effects of long-term drug treatment may be less severe than the impact of the mental disorder. For others, however, living with the symptoms of the disorder may be preferable.

People who experience persistent difficulties are not the only people recommended to take neuroleptics on a long-term basis, however. People who have recovered from an episode of psychosis are also routinely prescribed long-term neuroleptic treatment on the basis that it is thought to reduce their chances of relapse. Although numerous trials show that people who are converted to placebo treatment are more likely to relapse, there is evidence that withdrawal itself may precipitate deterioration or relapse and it is likely that the benefits of long-term treatment in preventing relapse have therefore been exaggerated by the methodology of clinical trials of long-term treatment (Moncrieff, 2006). Enabling people to make their own decisions about treatment in this situation means helping people to weigh up the benefits of the possible reduction in the risk of relapse that long-term drug treatment may confer, against its disadvantages and dangers. There are some people who would wish to avoid relapse at all costs, and any small reduction of that risk that drugs can offer would be worth taking. For others, the unpleasant effects of taking neuroleptics, combined with the hazards of long-term use, make drug treatment an unattractive option. Many people who become what services describe as 'non-compliant' with drug treatment are making this evaluation. Their decision is logical and rational, and based on the evidence of their own aversive experience of drug therapy, an experience which is not only unpleasant in own right, but signals the damage the drugs might do at a physical level.

As far as possible therefore, mental health professionals should support people with psychosis to use neuroleptic drugs in ways in which they themselves find useful, and in ways which reduce the impairments associated with drug treatment. In order to do this, professionals need to share and discuss information about the wide range of effects that psychiatric drugs produce, and help patients to weigh up the pros and cons of taking drugs for different situations. Since, according to the drug-centred model, psychiatric drug treatment does not cure an underlying disease, but produces drug-induced effects that might relieve symptoms, it is the patient's experience of these effects that should determine whether the drugs are useful or not, not some professional or technical assessment. Yet we know that professionals often dismiss or ignore patients' complaints about the unpleasant nature of neuroleptic effects (Seale, Chaplin, Lelliott & Quirk, 2007). This discrepancy will hinder the development of a therapeutic relationship in which patients and prescribers can work together to find ways of using drugs that maximise their potential benefits and minimise their unwanted effects, as well as exploring alternative ways of coping with symptoms.

Forced drug treatment

Although some people accept drug treatment willingly, neuroleptics are often forced on people against their wishes under the Mental Health Act. The introduction of enforced community treatment via community treatment orders has extended this involuntary use of drugs, and means that people who have recovered from an episode of mental disturbance can be forced to continue taking drug treatment against their wishes long after they have recovered, and even indefinitely. The disease-centred model of drug action makes forced treatment easy to justify because it disguises it as medical treatment, obscuring the social control that is actually involved in restricting someone's behaviour by chemical or any other means. A drug-centred understanding of the action of neuroleptic drugs makes the social purposes of forced drug treatment harder to conceal. As Thomas Szasz pointed out in 1957, the 'chief alterations in the patient produced by these drugs pertain to making his behaviour more socially acceptable' (Szasz, 1957, p. 88).

It may not be possible to stop forced drug treatment in this risk-aversive and chemically dependent society in which we live, but the drug-centred model at least reveals forced drug treatment for what it is: the compulsory modification of socially undesirable behaviour. Forcing someone to have drug treatment by infringing their biological integrity is, in some ways, a greater curtailment of liberty and autonomy than putting them in a straitjacket or a padded cell. It may make the professionals feel better; giving someone an injection or a tablet involves less direct force and violence than tying someone up, but it can be used to achieve the same results nevertheless. The drug-centred model therefore underlines the need for an open and democratic debate about when it is justified to subject someone to chemical control. If the practice is deemed acceptable at all, it would surely need to be subject to rigorous independent legal scrutiny, maybe through some sort of tribunal system. At present, incarceration under the Mental Health Act is subject to legal review, but drug treatment is mostly assumed to be medical treatment that is in the interests of the patient, and is, therefore, rarely questioned. If drug treatment is recognised to constitute, on occasions, a form of social control, then those advocating such 'treatment' would need to be explicit about its purpose, would need to provide evidence of its efficacy for this purpose, and would need to demonstrate that these benefits outweighed the physical harms the patient would be likely to incur, as well as the infringement of their biological and personal autonomy. Alternative forms of control would need to be considered, and one can imagine that it would be, as it rightfully should be, a difficult process to adjust someone's personality and behaviour through chemical means.

The view of neuroleptic drugs as a disease-centred treatment, or a 'chemical cure', has lead to massive and indiscriminate over-prescription of these drugs, with prescriptions in the United Kingdom rising by more than 60 per cent over the last 13 years (Ilyas & Moncrieff, 2012). They are increasingly prescribed to many people who will never derive any benefit from them, often for long periods of time. In this chapter we have argued that neuroleptic drugs are better viewed according to a drug-centred model, which highlights that they are psychoactive substances that induce a neurological state characterised by sedation, emotional flattening and mental impairment. Although most people find this state unpleasant, it can sometimes be useful in suppressing psychotic symptoms and other intrusive experiences and emotions. Understanding the drugs as a type of psychoactive neurological suppressant helps to highlight the relation between their physical and psychoactive effects, and helps us to negotiate the complex relationship between what may be useful about them, and what is undoubtedly harmful. Listening to what people have to say about the effects induced by these drugs and how they impact on their lives is an important source of information that has previously been neglected. We need to take people's views more seriously, and we should not trivialise the negative effect the drugs can have upon people's mental and emotional functioning. Using these drugs democratically means supporting people to make informed choices about whether to use them, and if so, how. It also means exposing circumstances in which the drugs are forced on people against their wishes for the purpose of social control, and advocating for a system in which drugs are only used in this way, if at all, with intense and independent scrutiny. Understanding the drugs as a type of psychoactive neurological suppressant helps to highlight the relation between their physical and psychoactive effects, and helps us to negotiate the complex relationship between what may be useful about them, and what is undoubtedly harmful.

References

Bola, J. R., & Mosher, L. R. (2003). Treatment of acute psychosis without neuroleptics: Two-year outcomes from the Soteria project. *Journal of Nervous & Mental Disease, 191,* 219–229.

Delay, J., & Deniker, P. (1952). 38 cas de psychoses traites par la cure prolongee et continue de 4560 R.P. *Compte Rendu du Congress des Medicine Alien et Neurologie France, 50,* 503–513.

Deniker, P. (1960). Experimental neurological syndromes and the new drug therapies in psychiatry. *Compehensive Psychiatry, 1,* 92–102.

Freyhan, F. A. (1959). Clinical and investigative aspects. In N. S. Kline (Ed.), *Psychopharmacology Frontiers. Second International Congress of Psychiatry Psychopharmacology Symposium.* London: J & A Churchill Ltd.

Haase, H. J. (1956). Definition and mode of action of the psychomotor Parkinson syndrome therapeutically induced by serpasil and largactil. *Monatsschrift fur Psychiatrie und Neurologie, 131,* 201–214.

Haase, H. J., & Janssen, P. A. J. (1965). *The Action of Neuroleptic Drugs.* Chicago: Yearbook Medical Publishers.

Healy, D., & Farquhar, G. (1998). Immediate effects of droperidol. *Human Psychopharmacology, 13,* 113–120.

Ilyas, S., & Moncrieff, J. (2012). Trends in prescriptions and costs of drugs for mental disorders in England, 1998–2010. *British Journal of Psychiatry, 200*(5), 393–398.

Lehtinen, V., Aaltonen, J., Koffert, T., Rakkolainen, V., & Syvalahti, E. (2000). Two-year outcome in first-episode psychosis treated according to an integrated model. Is immediate neuroleptisation always needed? *European Psychiatry, 15,* 312–320.

Moncrieff, J. (2006). Does antipsychotic withdrawal provoke psychosis? Review of the literature on rapid onset psychosis (supersensitivity psychosis) and withdrawal-related relapse. *Acta Psychiatrica Scandinavia, 114,* 3–13.

Moncrieff, J. (2008). *The Myth of the Chemical Cure: A critique of psychiatric drug treatment.* Houndmills: Palgrave Macmillan.

Moncrieff, J., & Cohen, D. (2005). Rethinking models of psychotropic drug action. *Psychotherapy & Psychosomatics, 74,* 145–153.

Moncrieff, J., Cohen, D., & Mason, J. P. (2009). The subjective experience of taking antipsychotic medication: A content analysis of Internet data. *Acta Psychiatrica Scandinavia, 120,* 102–111.

Ray, W. A., Chung, C. P., Murray, K. T., Hall, K., & Stein, C. M. (2009). Atypical antipsychotic drugs and the risk of sudden cardiac death. *New England Journal of Medicine, 360,* 225–235.

Samaha, A. N., Seeman, P., Stewart, J., Rajabi, H., & Kapur, S. (2007). 'Breakthrough' dopamine supersensitivity during ongoing antipsychotic treatment leads to treatment failure over time. *Journal of Neuroscience, 27,* 2979–2986.

Seale, C., Chaplin, R., Lelliott, P., & Quirk, A. (2007). Antipsychotic medication, sedation and mental clouding: An observational study of psychiatric consultations. *Social Science & Medicine, 65,* 698–711.

Szasz, T. S. (1957). Some observations on the use of tranquilizing drugs. *American Medical Association's Archives of Neurology & Psychiatry, 77,* 86–92.

Chapter 14

Speaking Out Against the Apartheid Approach to Our Minds

Rufus May, Rebecca Smith, Sophie Ashton, Ivan Fontaine, Chris Rushworth & Pete Bull

This chapter attempts to understand the experience of discrimination towards people experiencing states of confusion and distress. Apartheid comes from the Afrikaans language and means separation. It was a policy developed to divide people by racial categories in South Africa from the 1930s with Black people being given significantly fewer rights and deprived of citizenship. We feel this separateness also applies to how people with mental health problems are treated as an underclass with fewer rights and responsibilities. An important way to change this apartheid style of behaviour is to create spaces where we listen to the voices that are not usually listened to. This chapter will be introduced by Rufus and will be followed by a number of personal stories of dealing with mental health services and wider society. It highlights the effects of discriminative practices and the importance of speaking out about these experiences. We will also describe the benefit of coming together to create relationships that are free from societal prejudices towards mental distress and confusion.

Introduction

We don't get taught about emotional problems in school. We don't get taught about relationships, parenting and how to deal with loss. We don't get taught about how to support a friend who is sad or lonely or frightened. We don't get taught about how understandable sadness and confusion are in hard times. Because of that we fear what is not talked about, we call it weird and when we come across emotional pain and fear we seek to control it or to shun it away. The more we shun it the worse the pain and fear become. We have an apartheid approach to our emotional discontent. So it is no wonder families distance themselves from suffering relatives, and employers fail to support their workers when they have breakdowns. We could be recruiting people with lived experience of mental health problems to go into schools to share understanding and hope. We could be recruiting people with that same expertise to participate in the NHS mental health workforce to create respect for emotional turmoil, but largely we don't. The myth that the 'mentally ill', a term denoted by psychiatry, and the 'mentally well' are fundamentally different groups of people is perpetuated. We are encouraged to divide ourselves from each other and from ourselves.

Medicine offers society what the asylum previously did, a fantasy that we can hide away madness and sadness. This time it is with a pill rather than behind closed doors. Doctors are the high priests of our secular society and largely they go about their business of trying to control pain unchallenged. It's all well intentioned but by trying to get rid of mental health problems we can throw the baby out with the bath water. Mental health problems need to be respected; they are powerful messengers that give us big clues about what social and relationship tragedies people need to heal from.

So how do we change this, how do we speak out about this dynamic? The media cannot be relied upon. We cannot wait for Radio 4's *Today* programme to address this or the Sun or Sky news. The BBC is remarkable in how medical its coverage of social and emotional distress is. It is supposed to be quality journalism but rarely do we get to hear first hand people's accounts of their experiences. It ignores the 'expertise of experience'. Our society is in love with technological answers so we ignore people's personal stories of overcoming social adversity and psychological distress.

We have to create our own media, coming together as like-minded individuals sharing our commonalities, and respecting and celebrating our differences. We have been trying to exclude different experiences from our consciousness for generations; the 'them and us' divide is deeply held in our minds. We have to support each other to go beyond what medical experts have told us, to go to the heart of our experience, to speak of truths. We have to build emancipatory communities where we freely listen to the hidden truths and realities experienced on the journey of understanding and overcoming our confused minds.

At 18 I was a psychiatric patient labelled with schizophrenia. I did not find being labelled and drugged a helpful way to approach my confusion. It was through friendship, creative expression and social opportunities to work that I was able to rebuild my confidence and wellbeing. Then seven years later I entered the NHS as a trainee psychologist determined to try to change the psychiatric system from within. That was 17 years ago. Over this time period I have discovered the process of trying to change psychiatry from within is flawed, because workers are too identified with interests of the corporate institution. Over the last 10 years I have found that my work outside the psychiatric system in public meetings and self-help groups has tended to be more effective in initiating change. One of the projects I have been involved with is Evolving Minds, a monthly public meeting that looks at different approaches to emotional wellbeing. It has been meeting now for over seven years. It creates a space where people can learn from each other and build social connections. Over the next few years I will put more and more of my energy into these kinds of independent projects. The other contributors to this chapter, all of them, are people I have met in the last 10 years working in West Yorkshire. They all inspire me in their fire, their enthusiasm for speaking out against judgemental attitudes and behaviour.

Rebecca Smith

Rebecca volunteers for the Soteria Network which is trying to create alternative resources for people in psychological crisis. She tells us about how her emotional crisis as a young woman was handled by services so that for eight years she was isolated from both her family and the opportunity to make sense of her experiences. The fear that surrounded her mental confusion seemed to lead to professionals both writing her off and not helping her reconcile with her biggest resource, the people who loved her. She has now reconnected with her family and been given the space to process her visions and voices. Like all of the authors, she is using her experiences to connect with others and inspire them to move forward in their lives.

'Being treated like a naughty little girl'
My experience of the mental health system has been one of tears, heartache and loss. My family started to notice a change in me when I was 15. I started to self-harm on occasion and go out drinking with the wrong crowd. I lost my sense of boundaries with people and communication became increasingly difficult with my family. This went on for a period of two years until I finally broke down and developed a psychosis.

I was first admitted into hospital at the young age of 17, after a psychiatrist wrote something down in a file which neither my loved ones nor I was allowed to see. The staff put me on 'antipsychotic medications' even though when I asked them 'what is wrong with me?' they didn't answer. I noticed the looks they gave each other when I was around and the looks they gave me individually. These looks were not pleasant smiles or cheery glances but scornful and authoritarian, as if I was a naughty little girl. I was a funny, sunny girl by nature but as the years went by the system changed this.

During my first hospital admission when I finally met with my psychiatrist, I was hoping he would be able to help me and explain to me what was going on. I was scared and paranoid, so I told him what I was thinking. This was a bad move and he immediately told me I had schizophrenia. The irony: the only person I was speaking to about my problems was not listening to me. I told him that I thought my mother was taking my thoughts out of my head. Thinking about it now, I realise this was my imagination. It symbolised that deep down I wanted someone to take my psychological distress away from me. I wish someone had tried to make sense of this with me. My mother was trying her best to get me some psychological help; the care team I had been given were telling her that there was nothing they could do for me. I had had flashbacks before my first admission. These terrifying memories led me to having false memories of my family sexually abusing me so I lost all trust in them. Because of these false memories, the community psychiatric nurse I had at that time, refused to liaise with my family, telling them that I would have to give permission before they could talk about me.

Nobody in the mental health system tried to help me understand these beliefs about my family. When we have post-traumatic memories they can sometimes be accompanied with false memories. Nobody tried to collaborate with me and inform me about this and help me work out what was real and what was false. On the one hand, they treated my family as if they were abusers and cut them out of any discussions about my care; on the other hand, I was treated as psychotic and not given any counselling for the abusive memories and flashbacks I was experiencing. They wrote me off as a schizophrenic and this led to damaging circumstances. I left my family, told them I didn't want to see them again, that I hated them. The staff at the hospital encouraged me rather than challenging me and I had no contact with my family for eight years. After my family were out of the picture, mental health professionals persuaded me to go on a range of drugs that sedated me, suppressed emotion and thought processes and the real reasons I became psychotic. When I was distressed and angry the nurses held me to the floor heightening my distress, fear and anxiety. When I wanted to talk to somebody I was ignored or told I would be seen to later. If I didn't do as I was told I was warned that I would be put in a locked room or given a depot injection.

I was in and out of hospital for nearly 10 years and told I would never recover. In the end the medication nearly killed me. I took my normal dose of clozapine after not taking it for a few days and I fell unconscious and my heart stopped. If I had not been found by a support worker I would have died. I am still trying to find out exactly what happened because I have been told different things by different health workers. It was after this near-death experience I decided to make contact with my family. They have been a great resource to me since then and it has been great to be part of a family again. After 10 years of being isolated, with my family's assistance I finally got psychological help, but this was not from the care team I had, in fact they tried to stop me from getting help. The guilty feelings I feel for saying what I said about my family have no words. The anger I feel towards the services for not helping me realise that I was wrong about my family and encouraging me into thinking I would be ill for the rest of my life is huge. I feel a deep need to help people who have had psychological distress. Presently I contribute to Soteria meetings which in the long run plan to establish a Soteria House (which will be an alternative to psychiatric hospitalisation).

Rebecca Smith

Sophie Ashton

Sophie tells us about her five years of psychiatric treatment and how people inside and outside the psychiatric system wrote her off as second rate and hopeless. Sophie has experienced a lot of trauma and abuse in her life that, like Rebecca, psychiatry never tried to address. Her memories of treatment are very fresh due to the fact that she has been going back to different ages in dissociative states. This is part of a healing process she is going through that has only been made possible now that she has come off psychotropic medication. Working therapeutically on post-traumatic experiences that have psychotic features should be a right for anyone who wants to make sense of their 'madness'.

'People assume you are happy with a second-rate life'

I've just arrived back home after an invigorating walk in the West Yorkshire countryside. It has been the first walk I have had for four days. It has been the first time I have left the house for two days. Before going on the walk I was feeling very despairing. I felt trapped, stuck, tired, fed up. One of my voices was starting to turn from his recently new and improved, helpful self to his older ways of tracking me down and telling me to give up. After a walk he has returned to motivating me to pick myself up, speak my truth and write this piece on discrimination.

I have been struggling a lot over the last month, just like everyone does at points in their lives. I know it will pass because I am in a supportive and accepting environment, one in which my distress is not jumped upon and seen as an illness that must be stopped or controlled. But this hasn't always been the case. I spent five years in exactly the opposite environment, psychiatry. A system that, very quickly, assumed I was genetically flawed and had to be dumbed down and stupefied before anyone deemed me safe.

Recently I have been regressing to different ages. I have been 12, 17, 19, 23 and 5 years old. When I regress to these ages I have only the memories I had at that age. I talk as I did then, I hold myself as I did then and even my handwriting becomes how it was at that age. I suppose my regressions to 23 years old have really opened my eyes again to the things that I want to talk about here. At 23, I was at the lowest point in my life. I had been a psychiatric patient for almost four years. Four years previously, I had naively assumed that I would be able to talk about my life experiences that had been causing me such distress. I thought I would be met with listening ears and plenty of understanding and support. But now, at 23, I was a medicated zombie, truly stupefied. I had been given diagnosis after diagnosis and medicated up to my eyeballs. I had been written off, essentially, as a treatment-resistant freak. I had a severe mental illness, one they couldn't cure. I had given up because everyone around me had given up.

I am told by others around me that when I become 23, I am hunched over, eyes looking down at the floor. I don't give anyone any eye contact. I am, essentially, apologising for myself. This demeanour makes sense to me given how I remember feeling at the time. I felt invisible, useless, a waste of oxygen, a pain in the neck to society. I didn't dream any more. I'm a big dreamer. Sometimes I dream too big and, even in the darkest moments of my life, I believed that things would get better. I guess that is how I managed to get to 23 and not commit suicide, because somewhere inside, a part of me was saying, 'You can do this, keep going, you deserve something better and you will get it'. But as life went on, that hope slowly dwindled, as things didn't get better but continued to get slowly worse. By the time I came into contact with psychiatry the 'you can do it' flame was almost out completely. I needed an injection of oxygen to get it going again. I needed non-judgemental guidance to explore what was going on for me. But I didn't get that. I was bombarded with messages that I was doomed and by 23, the flame had been snuffed out completely. I had resigned myself to a second-class citizen status. I had decided that trying to fight to be respected was a complete waste of time. I saw no way out of this doomed existence of just having to be happy with second-class treatment. Rather than finding the support I needed from a mental health system, they had driven me to a decision to end my life.

I had worked in Boots the Chemist for a year previously. I had completed their in-house training as a healthcare assistant and was ready to take the next set of qualifications so that I could work as an accuracy-checking technician in the dispensary and earn a higher salary. However, I had to take time off due to an admission into hospital. On my return to work, I was told I had to speak to their occupational health therapist. It was standard procedure. However, I had now been diagnosed with schizo-affective disorder and, apparently, this meant that I was now incapable of training to work in the dispensary and earning a higher salary. I was told it was too dangerous for me to be working with medications and that I was not responsible enough to put the correct number of tablets into a bottle. I wasn't allowed to do the training anymore, even though, before having that label, I was being heavily encouraged by my boss and team to do the training. So now I was to stay a healthcare assistant and be grateful that they were letting me work at the pharmacy counter at all. I was fast learning that if you are seen as having a 'mental illness', people assume you are happy with a second-rate life.

Whilst in hospital, my psychiatrist frequently brought student doctors to see me. I would sit there and he would describe my symptoms as though I was not even in the room. I wasn't a human being but a 'case'. I felt like a monkey in a cage at a zoo, being pondered over. He would tell these students 'she is an unusual case, two diagnoses, a tough nut to crack'. When you are on the receiving end of this kind of treatment on a constant basis, you begin to believe them. Disagreeing and fighting your corner only caused more of the same treatment. Until you submit to your lunatic status, you are not considered to have insight into your 'condition' and you will not be listened to. It becomes easier and at times the only option was to admit defeat: 'Yes I should be very grateful for this second-rate life I am now living.'

I was lucky to find a psychologist who managed to give me my hope back. He helped me to rekindle my belief in myself so that I could dream again. He didn't do anything magical to achieve that. What he did was treat me as an equal, listen to me and help me to reintegrate myself back into society. Through connecting with people again, I began to learn that I was not sporting purple skin, three eyes and eight arms but that I was just the same as everyone else in this world. I have had tough times just like everyone else and the experiences I have are just a creative way of dealing with the trauma I have experienced throughout my life. I learned that there are a whole host of people out there who hear voices just like me. These people live just as normal a life as the next person. People react to stress and trauma in different ways. No one is genetically flawed because they feel depressed, anxious or paranoid. Stressful life events and our reactions to them should not signal a life of discrimination. It should signal a supportive, accepting environment to help that person out of crisis. I refuse to be seen as a second-class citizen just because I hear voices or because I see things that others do not see. Anyone could suffer a traumatic event and anyone could end up 'crazy', even Mr Psychiatrist. I'm certain that he wouldn't settle for such treatment.
    Sophie Ashton

Ivan Fontaine

Ivan tells us about what it is like to be written off as a person. He takes us inside the institutions and describes the boredom and the lack of respect that is found there. Ivan has been using services for over 25 years. He is a valuable witness to the fact that while some things have improved, many things have got worse. Ivan's story about the separate and inferior toilets for patients reminds me of the 2012 film *The Help* which describes the campaign by white supremacists in the 1960s in Mississippi to enforce homes to have separate toilets for their black servants. Separate toilets are a sign of the 'them and us' atmosphere that continues in society's attitude towards people with confusion and distress.

'Treated as a second-class citizen'
As a patient in a mental hospital, you are treated as a second-class citizen. Not everywhere I have been is so bad, but in many places I have been you are not treated as an equal. In the 1990s I was really poorly and was admitted to a secure hospital. At first when I was really tired and kept falling asleep because

I didn't go to activities, they came in and pinned me down and gave me an injection. This made me very dizzy and I was put in a padded cell for not going to activities. But no one explained to me the importance of going to activities. It was the first day and no one had explained the rules and regulations. But in some ways it was better in the 1990s because there were activities going on.

In the last 20 years I have lived in Bradford. I have worked, had my own car and I have had my own home. I have got involved in Mind and another organisation, Sharing Voices. From time to time I have gone into psychiatric hospital. There are fewer activities than there used to be, making it extremely boring. Also there seems to be more force used these days.

On one occasion a couple of years ago I was an inpatient and got into conflict with the staff. I wanted to clean the toilets and shower, the staff refused to give me equipment. The toilets were filthy; there were separate toilets for the staff. The staff ignored my need for a clean bathroom, so I said I would do a dirty protest. Then I got restrained by four nurses, although I wasn't being violent. They injected me by force and took me to my room and tried to force-feed me tablets as well.

When they eventually released me I had to take their tablets and my wrist had swollen up double the size. It turned out my wrist was fractured. I left hospital that week. I put on five stone in weight soon after due to the amount of medication I was given. I tried to make a complaint about what happened to my wrist. It was a really long-winded affair. When I saw the notes I didn't agree with how staff described me in the notes. Now at the end of each visit, I ask my community workers to give me a copy of notes they make about me, so I know what is being written about me.

When I was recently in a private hospital, there were many problems: filthy bathrooms, restrictions to your room at night and disrespectful staff. Even if you just wanted fruit you had to wait outside the office where they kept it. When you knocked on the window you could be asked to wait for ages or even ignored. Once you have been classed as having a mental health problem, a lot of people try to take advantage of your vulnerability when you are living in the community. It seems like people see you differently if they think you have mental illness. They write you off, they put you on the scrap heap. It's alright if you've got money like Britney Spears, Maria Carey, Robbie Williams or Peter Andre but if you haven't got money people treat you like somebody to be avoided.

How do I resist this? I try to be strong and let other people's prejudices go over my head. My interest in sport helps me, watching it and cycling. I'm also interested in art and photography. Having a close relationship with my family has helped me also. I make an effort to connect with people even if they don't come to see me. You've got to get out there and not sit at home stewing on things.

   Ivan Fontaine

Chris Rushworth

Chris describes how his treatment and the lack of understanding he has been shown have been alienating. He has had a lot of physical problems caused by neuroleptic medication. These have become more manageable since he gradually reduced his neuroleptic medication and has now come off it. Until relatively recently no one was willing to support him to reduce his medication.

   Chris is justifiably angry at the lack of respect and understanding he has experienced from many working in the mental health system and how unhelpful medication has been.

'I had to try and fight to stay awake'

When I first came to the attention of mental health services 30 years ago, I was given a label of paranoid schizophrenia. The doctors talked to my family telling them that because of my diagnosis I would always need strong medication, that I could be very dangerous and unpredictable. After this talk a lot of my family members were very frightened of me and pulled away. The medication made me very sleepy and slow. My family thought I was being lazy and did not understand that the medication was causing me to be lethargic and slowed up. It took a lot of effort to do little things. I had to fight to stay awake as I kept nodding off. I did not understand the effects of the medication I was prescribed. For example, after going swimming my whole body seized up. This was caused by the neuroleptic medication.

   I found it extremely frightening getting on a bus after being in hospital. I felt very disconnected from my normal self. I felt lost, I felt helpless. I never knew what caused this. I am sure medication played an important part in this confusion I experienced.

   I believe people stopped seeing me as a person and started seeing me as being stupid and not able to think for myself. I have had to deal with support workers, nurses and doctors treating me like I'm a seven-year-old. I've been fobbed off with excuses for 30 years about why I need to keep taking medication that has been bad for me in a number of ways. One permanent effect I have is restless legs or akathisia that keeps me awake at night and can be very painful. It is only in the last three years with the support of my psychologist that I have been able to negotiate gradual reductions in my neuroleptic medication. When I was heavily sedated I couldn't think through thoughts of wanting to self-harm. But on lower doses I can think through self-destructive ideas. If you are intoxicated you do things more on the spur of the moment.

Before I had a mental breakdown I was a heavy drinker and this drove me to a certain kind of mental isolation. But I have been a lot more lonely on psychiatric medication because on medication you tend to be left to your own devices. Nevertheless over the last 10 years I have started to get my confidence back, doing voluntary work, cooking, going to college, being part of a running club and having a girlfriend. It is doing these things that has made people see me as a person and value me. Without a low dosage I wouldn't have been able to do these things. Over the last three years I have started seeing my daughter again. Again, mental health professionals did not encourage me to make contact with her. She chose to come to see me when she was old enough to make this decision.

I get very angry about the type of support I have had from mental health services. I have channelled this anger into training as an advocate to help others have more of a say over their lives. I don't understand why people have to have training to care, I care naturally. I have done a lot of caring for my Mum as she got older. She also gave me a lot of care and believed that I could recover. There should be more opportunities for people like me to work in mental health services. We should not be treated as second-class citizens. Somebody tried to pay me in hospital the other day, but unlike the psychiatrists I don't deal in dope!

Chris Rushworth

Pete Bull

To finish, Pete gives us a rap poem called *Subject to* that describes the entrapment people get caught within. People's mental escape strategies are framed in scientific terms that dehumanise the process of breakdown and prevent us from really listening to each other's dreams and pain. Pete has been a recipient of mental health services and has trained as a psychotherapist and as a mental health professional.

Subject to

Now that I'm 30
What have I made from this dirty, fucked up hurting place where I
have learned
There is a journey
No arrival
Where being has no meaning but survival
It's a stressor
Becoming any kind of transgressor
It'll mess you up cos you ain't greater
You're the lesser
Then they'll tell you you're ill when your better

Fuck the system
Fuck the system
It's no good cos it can't fucking listen.
Make you go to work in some pointless abusive task
Wear a mask for the mission
What is missing?
Slash your wrists then?
Pain is part of the human condition
I need an admission that life in a man can't be measured by some
mathematician.

Chorus
Subject to whatever they want to make you subject to (x 2)

Rules they applied to me and my dreams
Altered the means to my schemas and themes
Words they defined me they license, they kill,
When the whole of my culture dictates 'He is ill'.
Brainwash completed I learned to be still
With the thought it is they who decide what is real
No truth in the speech of disease and disorder
I paid the price for the rupture in order

Family and friends could all say 'He's insane –
Everything's pain? Something's wrong with his brain!

We can't be blamed for what he became!
Leave him with those who are trained to restrain
Safe in the knowledge what he is, we ain't'
Descry his claim, bloody his name
Encompass what's Other into the same
A kid is on fire but who lit the flame?

Chorus
Subject to whatever they want to make you subject to (x 4)

Now the anger in me has respect
For what I did in retrospect
The troubles in mind that I speak of are ending
I want you to know of the lies I'm transcending
The label
The mind-fuck
The shame-on exclusion
Robbed of a future by your kind collusion
How much do you care for how I feel?
When you know there's no such thing as ill?

   Pete Bull

Conclusion

Fear and discrimination go hand in hand. Society fears what it does not want to understand. We live in a world where science is used to justify the control of those who are in extreme states of confusion. We try to control what we are too afraid of or unfamiliar with to understand. Confusion only happens when people experience violence and/or loss and isolation. But we are encouraged to ignore these social roots if we take a technological approach to their difficulties. Medical language confirms people's 'otherness' and cements the divide between 'them and us'. We can only break this down by promoting the stories of those who have been written off. This means speaking out about our apartheid approach to the mind. Rebecca, Sophie, Ivan, Chris and Pete all describe being treated as if they were invisible. They all describe how their humanity was ignored. We need to find ways to speak up about this and show how confusion is a reasonable response to difficult circumstances. This apartheid approach to people's turbulence happens both within the psychiatric system and within the wider society we live in. Through listening to these stories of resistance we learn that what we thought of as 'other' is part of ourselves. We all act in crazy ways and we all fail to hear each other properly. We realise that confusion and distress are understandable parts of being human and that using the dualistic concept of health and illness may actually add to our problems. To create a healing community we need to be prepared to really learn from what does not work and do the opposite: assume we are all worth of respect as equals. This means that we should always be looking for opportunities in all parts of our lives to dialogue, negotiate, be transparent, trustworthy and share decision-making. We need to be creative and learn together to explore our vulnerabilities and face our fears rather than push them away.

Chapter 15

Toxic Mental Environments and Other *Psychology in the Real World* Groups

Guy Holmes

Introduction

This chapter initially gives an overview of community-based groupwork as exemplified by *Psychology in the Real World* groups (see Holmes, 2010). Such groups have been seen as an alternative to the interventions and philosophies that characterise most mental health services. This is followed by a more in-depth description of one group of this ilk: *Toxic Mental Environments*. The chapter then looks at how *Psychology in the Real World* groups help people move from analysis of individual and social causes of distress to social action aimed at helping people reduce that distress for themselves and other people in their communities. The final section describes how such groups can serve to counter the effects of social devaluation and stigma that characterise the lives of many people who have had long-term involvement with psychiatric services.

In the chapter I have tried to avoid the word *psychosis* as, alongside psychiatric diagnoses such as schizophrenia, I do not find such words convey much useful information – people labelled psychotic can be so different that they share nothing in common. However, *Psychology in the Real World* groups have included many people, as group members and facilitators, who have been described as psychotic, schizophrenic, as suffering from bipolar, etc.

Psychology in the Real World groups

Psychology in the Real World is an umbrella term under which, with the support and involvement of many other people, I have set up a number of groups, courses and ventures in Shropshire since the late 1990s. Rather than bringing people together because they have a shared problem or

---

Parts of this chapter are based on extracts from Holmes, G. (2010). *Psychology in the Real World: Community-based groupwork*. Ross-on-Wye: PCCS Books.

diagnosis, *Psychology in the Real World* groups bring people together who have a shared interest. For example:

- *Understanding Ourselves and Others* provides people with opportunities to explore a range of theories that might help us understand various aspects of our lives (e.g., What leads us to be angry; violent; depressed? What helps people feel safe and secure? Why are we so afraid of mental illness?).

- *This is Madness* brings people together from various backgrounds (including people who identify themselves as service users, people who identify themselves as mental health professionals, and people who identify themselves as both) in order to critique mental health services and set up joint projects aimed at reducing the impacts of stigma.

- *The Black Dog* enables people to collectively critique modern conceptualisations of depression and explore a wide variety of theories and research on what leads us to become depressed (e.g., looking at whether depression might be one way we react to oppression).

- *Thinking about Medication* enables wide-ranging discussions between people who take psychiatric drugs and various professionals who prescribe and help people come off medication.

- *Out of the Box* helps people trying to come off psychiatric drugs to support each other.

- *Bipolar Explorers* brings people together to explore what might be fuelling the rise in numbers of people receiving this diagnosis and to pool ideas from a variety of sources about what might help when people get very high or low.

- *The Writing Group* helps those of us who feel we gain much from writing about personal experiences to meet up, share and discuss our written work.

- *Walk and Talk* assists people who have an interest in walking along the riverside to connect with nature and connect with others in their locality.

- *Toxic Mental Environments* provides people with opportunities to analyse aspects of the world we live in that might be detrimental to our wellbeing, and link up with others with the aim of bringing about some changes in these environments.

Although each group is different, they share some characteristics. They all occur in non-mental health settings, such as arts and education centres, libraries, along river paths and in local pubs. People are not formally referred to the groups – the groups are open to all and are advertised locally in non-mental health settings as well as within services. When advertising the groups, attempts are made to get as broad a mix of people as possible in terms of age, class, gender, sexuality, race and, particularly, mental health service involvement. Roughly a third of participants in most groups tend to have had no previous mental health service involvement, a third have had some primary care service (e.g., taken psychiatric drugs prescribed by a GP or received counselling) and a third tend to be accessing secondary services such as community mental health or assertive outreach teams. The age of participants has ranged from 4 to 84 – from a young child who regularly joined in *Walk and Talk* alongside his parents to an octogenarian who, during *Thinking about Medication,* described herself as a 'carer and psychiatric system survivor who was damaged by ECT over 30 years ago'. This mix of participants contrasts sharply with most mental health services which tend to categorise people in terms of some attribute or presenting problem and exclude people who do not fit certain criteria.

The groups tend to be time limited and are often inspired, planned and co-facilitated by people who have previously attended other *Psychology in the Real World* courses, being frequently based on ideas that came out of these groups. For example, *Toxic Mental Environments* and *Thinking about Medication* led to explorations of the importance of accessing the countryside as a way of people detoxifying reactions to contemporary culture and as an alternative to taking psychiatric drugs. This led to Anna Hughes and me jointly setting up *Walk and Talk* in 2007. Anna, as well as being a mum and a marathon runner, describes herself as a mental health service user. *Walk and Talk* has subsequently been run and organised by a collective of people, some of whom have a long-term history of mental health service involvement and multiple hospital admissions, some of whom do not, but all of whom initially came along as members of the group.

The groups are not 'skills for ills' groups – they respect the fact that, as one participant put it, 'there are as many recoveries as there are people'. There is a recognition that each person's reactions to their life experiences are unique and complex, there are a myriad of causes of distress, and sharing our experiences and thoughts with others enables a collective wisdom to arise that often outweighs the wisdom of any expert (see Surowiecki, 2004).

Participants are not seen as empty vessels needing to be filled up with knowledge passed on by the group leader, but rather as people who can develop their own ways of critiquing the world that they live in and its impacts on them and others (see Freire, 1996). Group members may learn *how to think* but are not taught *what to think*. As one participant put it, 'I expected to be told the answers, but this is much more liberating!'

In the groups, research findings are discussed and critiqued (e.g., how much might pharmaceutical company research be compromised by the companies having a financial interest in obtaining favourable results?). When assessing the evidence base, NICE guidelines rate randomised controlled trials as the gold standard and demote service user testimony to the category of least persuasive form of evidence. *Psychology in the Real World* groups, however, give just as much weight to group members' lived experiences, and reflections on those experiences, as other forms of evidence. Evidence from group members' collective experience is also held up for critique (e.g., to what extent are such insights applicable to others?). Through this process we not only explore theories and research relating to the causes of distress, but look beyond immediate factors to the causes of causes, for example, aspects of twenty-first century society that perhaps damage us all. Participants are encouraged and assisted to move from critique and analysis to social action during and on ending participation in the groups.

The groups, and skills needed to facilitate such groups, are described in detail in *Psychology in the Real World: Community-based groupwork* (Holmes, 2010). People with long-term involvement with psychiatric services, who have attracted diagnoses that might label them as psychotic, wrote chapters in the book and have published papers and given conference presentations detailing their experiences of being members and facilitators of *Psychology in the Real World* groups (e.g., Clare, 2006; Elisabeth X, 2010; Holmes & Evans, 2011). Evaluations of the groups are also available online (www.psychologyintherealworld.co.uk) and in the published literature (e.g., Holmes & Gahan, 2007).

Toxic Mental Environments

Toxic Mental Environments was a group run in 2006 (see Holmes, 2010). The name of the group was inspired by Kalle Lasn and *Adbusters: The Journal of the Mental Environment*, as was the literature advertising it:

Thirty years ago, people became worried that the physical environment was becoming toxic and making people sick. This anxiety led to the green movement. In the West (but also increasingly globally) we have been able to consume enormous amounts of consumer goods which we were led to believe would make our lives easier and happier, but we live in a time when people are experiencing great levels of dis-ease, describe themselves increasingly as stressed, are diagnosed with mood disorders and mental health problems on unprecedented scales, and are prescribed ever-increasing amounts of psychiatric drugs. Business cultures and the $450 billion a year advertising industry appear to have infiltrated everything, and perhaps infect our thinking and behaviour in ways that human beings might not have evolved to cope with. The media is owned by a small number of people with agendas to get us think in ways that make corporate profits soar but may not be good for us as human beings. Pharmaceutical companies make billions of pounds selling products that purport to cure mental health problems but the numbers of people being treated for so-called mental illnesses continues to rise and increasing numbers of people report the drugs are making them ill. Is it time to clean up our mental as well as physical environment? (from Holmes, 2010, p. 144; see also www.adbusters. org)

Orford (1998) stated that the task of community clinical psychology was to help people:

(i)   understand the connection between the social and economic reality of their lives and their states of health and wellbeing,

(ii) join with others with similar realities in order to give voice to this understanding, and

(iii) engage in collective action to change these realities. This ethos has guided the facilitation of *Toxic Mental Environments* and other *Psychology in the Real World* groups.

Group members have found the Power Horizon diagram (see Fig. 1) helpful as it shines light on why we are all drawn to focusing on changing aspects of ourselves as individuals rather than the world we inhabit. For example, it is our feelings and bodily sensations that burn brightest for us and therefore attract much of our attention. The Power Horizon also helps us understand why personal change is often much more difficult than we, or our therapists, envisage: our individual thoughts, feelings and behaviours are perhaps overwhelmingly shaped by the actions of powerful institutions over which as individuals we have little power to change. For example, one of the most consistent findings in the research literature is the association between poverty and mental health (Friedli, 2009). Poverty levels are largely affected by government policies (e.g., on spending and taxation) and business practices (e.g., on wages and recruitment) rather than mental health interventions. As people cannot think themselves richer, or think themselves into having qualifications that provide gateways into decently paid jobs, the interventions of cognitive therapy, positive psychology and many talking therapies may not be powerful agents of change for people damaged by the impacts of poverty.

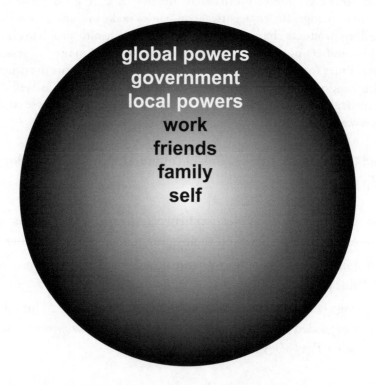

Figure 1. The Power Horizon (from Smail, 2005, p. 33)

During *Toxic Mental Environments* and other *Psychology in the Real World* groups we often use a different form of laddering from that used in cognitive therapy. Cognitive therapists start with one thought and get people to discover links in the ladder until they arrive at an underlying, often unconscious, internal core belief that people hold about themselves. We try and take the ladder outwards rather than inwards, taking the analysis to outer regions of the Power Horizon, to things people might be unconscious of in a different way from that which therapists usually mean. For example, as people on *Bipolar Explorers* have identified, when entering manic states many people feel drawn to high stimulation environments, feel overwhelmed by grandiose ideas that artificially inflate self-esteem and feel driven to spend money irrespective of financial problems that might accrue. Psychiatry, through the *ICD* and *DSM*, categorises these experiences as symptoms of the mental illness 'bipolar disorder'. Such drives can be experienced as overwhelming and outside control through will power alone, whilst family and friends often also struggle to help someone rein in such drives. Yet as many people on *Toxic Mental Environments* and other *Psychology in the Real World* courses have noted, twenty-first-century consumer capitalist culture, rather than helping people to rein in such impulses, often pushes people in that direction.

We are all exposed to thousands of advertising images every day that make a direct appeal to, and stimulate, our senses. Each fights for our attention. Such advertising is aimed at getting us to spend money on things we rarely need. Such consumption at best produces fleeting amounts of pleasure, which we subsequently feel needs replenishing once it diminishes, fuelling greater consumption. We live in a high stimulation, speeded-up, manic society (see DeGrandpre, 2000) that pushes many of us in the direction of taking increasing quantities of stimulant drugs just to keep up. Little wonder society's intake of caffeine, legal and illegal stimulants, SSRIs and Ritalin keeps increasing. Governments focus on economic growth and are wedded with corporate interests that are geared around ever-increasing amounts of consumption. As with the individual experience of mania, people seem blind to the consequences of this. For example, the inevitable period of bust after boom when the economic cycle turns and the bubble bursts – succinctly summarised by Engels as long ago as 1882 (1882/1986) – is shut out from awareness, mirroring the manic person's blindness to the debt problems caused by spending beyond one's means. Similarly, public relations lies, spin, positive psychology and business cultures try and artificially inflate the esteem of governments, corporations, public bodies and people who work in them (e.g., by removing from conscious awareness things that do not create a positive image): this mirrors the fragile grandiosity many manic people experience before reality plunges them into depression. Modern capitalism's ruthless and destructive exploitation of the earth's natural resources risks creating planetary conditions that will struggle to sustain human life: this appears to mirror the manic person's defences against the destructive consequences of their actions. Whilst pharmaceutical companies suggest bipolar disorder is under-diagnosed in individual people, one might more fruitfully ask whether such a diagnosis is under-applied to modern Western society as a whole.

During *Psychology in the Real World* groups, when we examine the research literature and participants' accounts of their own life experiences regarding the causes of problems, it is not difficult to see that social, economic and political systems further from the centre of the Power Horizon (Fig. 1) are important in creating the conditions in which individual problems arise. Again, taking the literature on manic depression/bipolar disorder as an example, high levels of criticism (sometimes called high expressed emotion or EE) is associated with increased problems and poorer outcomes (Miklowitz, Goldstein, Nuechterlein, Snyder & Mintz, 1988). Yet as occupational psychologists have often shown (e.g., Cooper & Payne, 1994), work cultures seem to be increasingly infused with criticism of workers at all levels. This is often aimed at pushing workers into making systems more efficient (to reduce costs), which leads to increases in working hours and often a sense of personal inadequacy in staff who cannot meet what objective analysis tends to rate as unrealistic demands. As if such stress is not enough to make people disturbed, workplace stress is known to increase stress in the home (thus creating another high EE environment).

It is very difficult to engage in such analyses alone; one of the advantages of *Psychology in the Real World* ventures is that people with a great divergence of opinion and experience are often brought together. In Watkins and Shulman's words, this enables a democratisation of the truth and psychic spaces to be opened up where we can collectively critique a great range of aspects of the world we inhabit (Watkins & Shulman, 2008).

What little research there has been into the kinds of social and physical environments that assist people's recovery from severe mental health problems has highlighted the importance of things such as people living and spending time in places that enable them to feel safe and secure; being members of socially valued and supportive groups; and having access to green spaces and other environments that detoxify the stress of modern living (see Yates, Holmes & Priest, 2011, 2012). *Psychology in the Real World* groups have not only embraced such analyses, they have sought to assist people to access such places and engage in social action to bring about such things for other members of the community.

Social action

It often seems very difficult to change distal factors that are embedded in our society. We perhaps need to spend more time, energy and resources on this, rather than trying, sometimes valiantly, sometimes vainly, to change our personal reactions to life events that we experience ultimately because of some of the decisions made by organisations and people at the outer reaches of our power horizon. The enormity of the challenge of bringing about radical change in embedded aspects of our culture and society can overwhelm us and we sometimes need to 'think small' (see Boxes 1 and 2), do what we can at any one moment, and seek out allies.

When I began critiquing pharmaceutical company research over 20 years ago, it appeared that the only people interested were people taking psychiatric drugs (whose experiences had inspired the critiques). Very few psychologists, even though we are trained in research methodology, seemed to see this as relevant. At times I felt that bringing this up in team meetings, giving lectures, publishing research and running groups that explore the whole power horizon regarding medication was a pointless exercise next to the wealth, power and sophisticated marketing machine of the pharmaceutical industry. But 20 years on, things seem to be changing. As one *Toxic Mental Environments* member said: 'When it came to psychiatric drugs, in the past we were told nothing and we knew nothing.' Nowadays information is readily available and informed consent is seen as a core part of services that provide medication. I have attended many conferences where both service users and professionals, whilst being able to recognise benefits of medication, also openly talk about damaging aspects of these drugs and how the discourse regarding drugs has not given sufficient credence to their toxicity. Newspapers print stories of pharmaceutical industry cover-ups akin to those of the tobacco industry. Websites buzz with people exchanging personal experiences whilst campaigning for change (e.g., the Seroxat User Group and APRIL). A small number of initially isolated people speaking out about such issues now form part of a loosely connected group that, with powerful allies in the media as well as

Box 1. On Smallness: An overhead used in *Psychology in the Real World* groups

On Smallness

1. Small is beautiful

2. Small is effective

3. Small is tolerable

4. Small is manageable

5. Small is knowable

6. Small is usual

The bottom line ... Small is normalising.

(adapted from Mosher & Burti, 1994, p. 105)

professional and voluntary sector organisations, have become a formidable force for change in this area.

'On Smallness', initially written by psychiatrist Loren Mosher regarding the policies of the small but highly successful Soteria Project which helped people who had been classified as 'psychotic' (see Mosher & Burti, 1994), often leads to discussions about the advantages small projects can have over large ones. Box 1 is also aimed at helping people counteract the negative impacts of feeling helpless triggered by the fact that some social problems seem overwhelming in magnitude. For example, there is considerable evidence that inequality is psychologically and physically unhealthy for people in all strata in society, with people in poverty suffering the most (e.g., Friedli, 2009). But how do you bring about change in such an ingrained aspect of society?

During *Toxic Mental Environments* people raised the possibility that it suits certain vested interests to ensure that vast numbers of people feel unable to change the status quo. Learned helplessness does ensue when people struggle to change inequitable systems without success. But there is also mystification. When people think of the anti-war protests about Vietnam they tend to envisage students and then the wider population protesting in ever-increasing numbers until the American Government pulled out. But if you listen to accounts from people involved in the protests from their inception, it is clear that for many years only a small number of people protested, these people were mostly met with indifference and hostility, even on university campuses, and it took years of commitment and resilience to keep protesting until the movement started to grow and eventually snowball.

Box 2. Think Small: An overhead used on *Toxic Mental Environments*

What next? *Think Small* ...

How can you ...

- spend less time in toxic mental environments and more time in healthy mental environments?

- work collaboratively with others towards changing embedded toxic elements in our local community and wider society?

- set up and help others set up a mentally healthy environment?

At the end of each session of *Toxic Mental Environments* participants were encouraged to try and bring about some change in the environments that they and others inhabited (see Box 2). People attending this and other groups subsequently set up, or helped other people set up, several projects. For example, a number of *Walk and Talk* and *Thinking about Medication* groups have been set up in Shropshire and other parts of the UK by *Psychology in the Real World* members and by people who consulted with members about how to get such groups going. Participants have also been involved in local and national campaigns. For example, by lobbying to have tablets available in small enough doses to enable tapered withdrawal from psychiatric drugs, and by campaigning to have 'wild' areas of the countryside not turned into managed parks or opened up for urban development. Group members have also gone on to set up their own informal support groups. For example, 'Amongst Friends', a group open to anyone who has recently been bereaved, was set up by an *Understanding Ourselves and Others* group member who said she was inspired by coming to see her own depression as relating to loss rather than biochemical imbalances. Further examples of social action are detailed in Holmes (2010) and in the following section.

The potential for *Psychology in the Real World* groups to counter the effects of social devaluation and stigma

> *It was so good to realise that in spite of or because of all our faults and failings we are all mortal and members of the human race and it's OK not to be scared of those who live and express themselves differently.*
> (Participant on a *Psychology in the Real World* course)

i. The process of social devaluation

As Wolfensberger (1992) pointed out, powerful groups tend to treat people who do not fit what society at that time has defined as desired norms as 'other' and start to classify them as members of a socially devalued group. Modern phrases such as 'the mentally ill' and 'people with psychosis' might seem more acceptable than older terms such as 'lunatics' and 'idiots' which were used to legally categorise people in the past, but in many ways attitudes and behaviours to people assigned to these groups have changed little over the years, with people still often seen as a 'charitable burden' or 'threat'. The media, government policies and mental health services still emphasise risk regarding people deemed to be psychotic despite the evidence that, if factors such as alcohol and drug abuse are controlled for, people with diagnoses such as schizophrenia are at higher risk than the general population of being harmed by others, but are not a greater risk of harming others (Fazel, Langstrom, Hjern, Grann & Lichtenstein, 2009). Opportunities to take up certain roles in life available to members of socially valued groups may be subtly or brutally denied to people deemed to 'suffer from psychosis' – roles such as 'breadwinner' or 'therapist'. They often become embedded in roles such as 'patient' and have limited access to opportunities to learn skills needed to take on more socially valued roles.

Socially devalued people have historically been grouped together and have suffered what Wolfensberger calls *wounds*. Such wounds include branding with stigmatising labels (e.g., schizophrenia), congregation with other branded people and separation from non-labelled people (e.g., through living in hospitals or group homes). Similarly, people often suffer relegation to low status and low power positions (e.g., service user). People often experience impoverishment in terms of their relationships, which might be largely limited to relationships with paid workers who are in roles that are more highly socially valued (such as a psychologist). People suffer impoverishment in terms of material resources (e.g., suffer the impacts of poverty and insults of receiving benefits where qualification for that benefit involves acceptance of devaluing labels) and impoverishment of experiences (e.g., through social exclusion). Other wounds can include a loss of control over major and minor decisions regarding what happens (e.g., institutions are inevitably run in ways that meet institutional and staff needs rather than individual needs which are so varied they cannot be met in such settings).

Some of the people who get involved in *Psychology in the Real World* ventures have for years been involved in Community Mental Health Team (CMHT) services that are aimed at helping 'people with severe and enduring mental health problems'; some have had periods in psychiatric hospital; some have diagnoses such as schizophrenia, manic depression and personality disorder; some until recently lived on long-stay hospital wards receiving years of rehabilitation that was based on token economies (a recent conversation on *Walk and Talk* led to us renaming this as 'earning the right to get your fags back'). Such people are at high risk of social devaluation and stigma. In most groups I have facilitated over the past 15 years, the wounds listed by Wolfensberger (1992) have consistently been identified by people with long-term involvement in mental health services as just as, or more debilitating than, their so-called symptoms.

Treat people badly and they soon learn how to treat themselves badly. The devaluing process leads people to devalue themselves. Some come to feel that their life has been wasted. One man who had been involved with psychiatric services for over 25 years said to me that the only point of his life seemed to be to provide work and therefore pleasure and meaning to staff who were paid to help him. Little wonder that therapists providing cognitive and other form of talking therapy often find that their interventions struggle, despite all efforts, to have much impact when so many things ingrained in our society weigh down negatively on people in terms of their sense of self-worth.

Through similar processes, when alienated and treated as alien, people can start to feel alien. As Laing (1965) showed, this can become part of a person's core identity and can manifest itself in behaviours that get labelled psychotic, leading to greater labelling and stigmatisation. Some may develop fantasy relationships or live in a fantasy world where their self-worth is protected, whilst others find all sorts of ways of displaying the resentment and rage they feel about the devaluing process and life in general. Some people may withdraw from life, whilst others might become manically driven

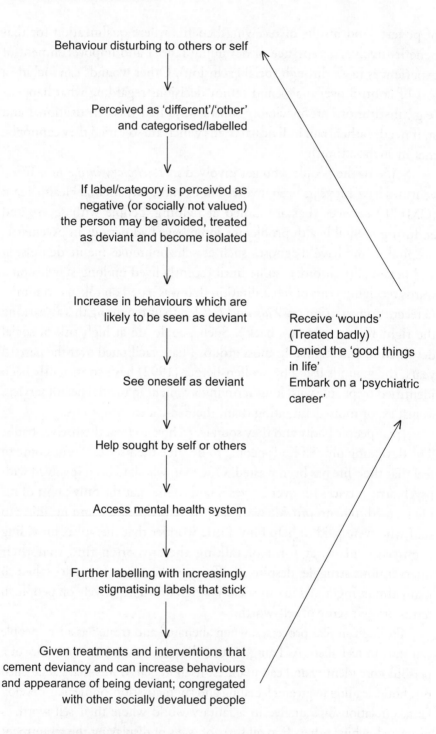

Behaviour disturbing to others or self

Perceived as 'different'/'other'
and categorised/labelled

If label/category is perceived as
negative (or socially not valued)
the person may be avoided, treated
as deviant and become isolated

Increase in behaviours which are
likely to be seen as deviant

Receive 'wounds'
(Treated badly)
Denied the 'good things
in life'
Embark on a 'psychiatric
career'

See oneself as deviant

Help sought by self or others

Access mental health system

Further labelling with increasingly
stigmatising labels that stick

Given treatments and interventions that
cement deviancy and can increase behaviours
and appearance of being deviant; congregated
with other socially devalued people

Figure 2. A Stigma Cycle (developed from the ideas of Goffman, 1963 and
Wolfensberger, 1992)

to try and inflate their self-worth, engaging in grandiose schemes that are likely to fail. All of these and a myriad of other reactions can be labelled as psychotic symptoms and can serve to fuel a stigma cycle (see Fig. 2).

ii. Overcoming the effects of social devaluation and stigma

Over several decades John O'Brien has written not just about the harm that services can do but also about *what is worth working for?* (O'Brien, 1990). He identifies five closely linked service accomplishments that do not prescribe how staff working with people assigned to socially devalued groups should

Box 3. The Five Service Accomplishments (adapted from O'Brien, 1990)

1. *Community presence*
Countering the risks or effects of social devaluation involves people: (i) sharing the ordinary places and engaging in the ordinary activities that define community life; (ii) avoiding segregated services that increase the process of social devaluation and the risks of being treated badly because of that process; (iii) increasing the number and variety of places a person knows and accesses.

2. *Community participation*
This emphasises the importance of people being part of a network of personal relationships that includes a variety of people, not just those that one is congregated with as a requirement of receiving help.

3. *Having valued social roles*
This points to the importance of people: (i) engaging in activities and taking on roles that bring about a sense of dignity and respect; (ii) having a place among a network of valued people; (iii) avoiding being entrenched in low-status activities.

4. *Making choices*
People should have as great autonomy as possible (and much greater than they are often permitted) in: (i) small everyday matters (e.g. what to do); and (ii) large life-defining matters (e.g., who to live with).

5. *Increasing competence and contributing*
This involves people skilfully performing meaningful activities (with training and assistance when required) and contributing as fully as possible (e.g., to other's welfare).

behave but identify outcomes worth struggling for. These are: community presence, community participation, having valued social roles, making choices, and increasing competence and contributing (see Box 3).

There are many chapters in Holmes (2010), including chapters written by participants in the groups who have long histories of involvement with psychiatric services, that detail how O'Brien's service accomplishments can be achieved. For example, people attend the groups as participants, students, writers or walkers not as patients or clients. Participants chose to come having seen the flyers (on notice boards in as diverse places as GP clinics, mental health services, cafes, shops and pubs) rather than being referred in letters detailing their problems and deficits or forced to attend as part of a community treatment order. The venues are free of the stigmatising signs and messages that characterise many mental health settings and tend to be full of people attending courses (or drinking) rather than people who are being assessed or receiving treatments. The groups occur in the ordinary places of life not places where socially devalued people are congregated in order to receive help and be efficiently processed through systems by (socially valued) professionals. Participants are treated as autonomous individuals, as equal members of the group, whatever their background.

Through the *Psychology in the Real World* groups, people with long histories of involvement with mental health services mix with people with no involvement with these services. This not only enables community presence and participation, it lessens stigmatising attitudes in the wider population. For example, people who have attended mental health services often disclose this fact at some point during the groups. Participants who have not had this experience are often surprised to discover that group members they have got to know as people have been in the local psychiatric hospital, hear voices, have been diagnosed with schizophrenia, and so on. As a consequence they come to have some of their stereotypes and prejudices challenged (see Holmes & Gahan, 2007). The groups offer people from all walks of life opportunities to become friends and feedback shows that this often occurs, assisted by the fact that we have breaks which enable more informal contact between people, and participants often lunch together after the main activity has taken place in the venues' cafes or in local pubs (e.g., after *Walk and Talk*).

As well as making friends, people on the courses have gone on to set up formal and informal groups aimed at supporting each other and other people. For example, one *Black Dog* participant set up a *Changes* group, initially with a membership made up of several people who had come on the course, but later with a much wider membership, which ran for several years with people meeting on a weekly basis. One mental health professional and a long-term mental health service user, who met on *This is Madness*, set up a *Medication Group* which helped people on antipsychotic medication to find out more about medication and consider the pros and cons of taking and coming off psychiatric drugs. Another member, who was diagnosed as manic-depressive, contacted me to help him set up *Bipolar Explorers*, a group where people initially came together to critique the diagnosis and learn from each other's experiences, but which has developed into a group that through the Internet service 'Dropbox' and regular follow-ups continues to enable members to inform and support each other. This has helped participants to not only avoid any further hospital admissions but has led several people to successfully apply for jobs. Group members are currently planning to devise ways of passing on the expertise that they have developed to newly diagnosed people in the hope that they might avoid some of the mistakes they felt they made (e.g., avoid getting entrenched in unhelpful systems and roles such as that of 'long-term psychiatric patient').

Social roles are crucial to our psychological wellbeing. Some members of *Psychology in the Real World* groups have subsequently taken on a variety of socially valued roles regarding projects connected with *Psychology in the Real World*. These include: consultant and contributor to the planning of other groups and projects; group leader/facilitator; researcher; sole or co-author of articles in peer-reviewed journals; chapter writer; lecturer at universities; trainer of staff; conference presenter; campaigner; committee member on a local authority committee; consultant to other people wanting to set up similar groups. The majority of people who have taken up these roles have had long histories of involvement with psychiatric services and have suffered many wounds to their status associated with being seen as psychotic at some point in their life. Some have needed help to attain specific competencies in these roles, for example, assistance preparing talks given to staff teams and at conferences (including role-play preparation and psychological support on the day); training in facilitation skills; training in research skills; editorial help regarding writing in an academic style. In providing encouragement and the minimum necessary support to people in these areas I have followed the maxim 'There can be no real freedom without the freedom to fail' (Fromm, 1996). No one, however, has failed in these roles. People's inner critics have often lambasted them after they have, for example, given a talk about one of the groups, but the actual feedback from listeners has tended to highlight their contribution rather than mine when it has been a joint endeavour. Some who have gone on from being a participant in a group to taking up other roles have been naturally gifted in these areas, or re-acquainted themselves with skills not utilised since perhaps having a breakdown. Others have been keen but at the outset did not appear so well suited to such roles. Yet perhaps through being relied upon, they have become reliable, and through being depended on, they have become dependable. Similarly, through being trusted and respected they have perhaps grown to trust and respect themselves.

One evaluation of *Psychology in the Real World* groups specifically looked at stigma and social inclusion (see Holmes & Gahan, 2007). Based on questionnaires sent to people who had in the past attended *Understanding Ourselves and Others* groups run over a two-year period, the research indicated that members of the groups appeared to have more understanding and acceptance of people who have been diagnosed as mentally ill. For example, one person commented: 'I feel a lot less fearful of people with mental health problems. I see mental health now as a scale that we are all on somewhere rather than "them and us".' This reduction in 'us and them' thinking seemed to apply to people who had never been involved with mental health services *and* to the people who had. An ethos 'that we are all people who can and will struggle when life overwhelms us' appeared to replace ways of thinking that can be seen as a core part of the stigmatising process, that is, categorising and differentiating between people – the 'well' and the 'ill', the 'sane' and the 'psychotic', the 'depressed' and the 'clinically depressed'.

This fits with an ideological belief that permeates many *Psychology in the Real World* ventures: if we all see each other as part of the human race then categorisations such as these will lose their power, and prejudice against people who have been assigned to socially devalued groups such as the 'mentally ill' may lessen. The groups are aimed at helping us notice similarities between people whilst accepting individual differences, and seeing those differences as characteristic of the individual rather than general characteristics that are emblematic and symptomatic of a socially devalued group they might have been assigned to. This fits with research conducted by Gordon Allport whose contact hypothesis stated that prejudice can be lessened by people who have prejudiced views about each other meeting together in groups where four conditions are present: mutual inter-dependence, a common goal, equal status of group members, and social norms that promote equality (Allport, 1954). Facilitators of *Psychology in the Real World* groups work hard to bring about norms and group cultures that mirror these conditions (see Holmes, 2010). And when we feel overwhelmed by the scale of the task of reducing stigma and discrimination and creating less toxic mental environments for all, we remind ourselves again of Margaret Mead's inspiring words:

> We should never doubt that a small group of thoughtful, committed citizens can change the world; indeed, it is the only thing that ever does.

References

Allport, G. (1954). *The Nature of Prejudice.* Reading, MA: Addison-Wesley.

Clare, J. (2006). Psychology in the Real World: A participant's response. *The Journal of Critical Psychology, Counselling and Psychotherapy, 6*(2), 107–109.

Cooper, C., & Payne, R. (1994). *Causes and Consequences of Stress at Work.* Oxford: Wiley.

DeGrandpre, R. (2000). *Ritalin Nation.* New York: Norton.

Elisabeth X. (2010). Reflections of Psychology in the Real World groups. *The Journal of Critical Psychology, Counselling and Psychotherapy, 10*(3), 141–145.

Engels, F. (1986). *The Condition of the Working Class in England.* London: Grafton Books. (Original work published 1882)

Fazel, S., Langstrom, N., Hjern, A., Grann, M., & Lichtenstein P. (2009). Schizophrenia, substance abuse, and violent crime. *JAMA, 301,* 2016–2023.

Freire, P. (1996). *Pedagogy of the Oppressed.* London: Penguin.

Friedli, L. (2009). *Mental Health, Resilience and Inequalities.* Copenhagen: World Health Organization.

Fromm, E. (1996). *To Have or To Be?* London: Continuum.

Goffman, E. (1963). *Stigma: Notes on the management of a spoiled identity.* Englewood Cliffs, NJ: Prentice Hall.

Holmes, G. (2010). *Psychology in the Real World: Community-based groupwork.* Ross-on-Wye: PCCS Books.

Holmes, G., & Evans, N. (2011). *Walk and Talk.* Paper presented at 1st International Well-being Conference, Aston University, July 2011. Retrieved 2nd December 2012 from, http://www.biad.bcu.ac.uk/research/wellbeing2011/

Holmes, G., & Gahan, L. (2007). The Psychology in the Real World – Understanding Yourself and Others course: An attempt to have an impact on stigma and social inclusion. *Groupwork, 16*(3), 9–25.

Laing, R. D. (1965). *The Divided Self.* Harmondsworth: Penguin.

Miklowitz, D., Goldstein, M., Nuechterlein, K., Snyder, K., & Mintz, J. (1988). Family factors and the course of bipolar affective disorder. *Archives of General Psychiatry, 45*, 225–231.

Mosher, L. R., & Burti, L. (1994). *Community Mental Health.* London: Norton.

O'Brien, J. (1990). What's worth working for? In V. J. Bradley & H. A. Bersani (Eds.), *Quality Assurance for Individuals with Developmental Disabilities: It's everyone's business.* Baltimore, MD: Paul H. Brookes Publishing. (Original work published 1989)

Orford, J. (1998). Have we a theory of community psychology? *Clinical Psychology Forum, 122,* 6–10.

Smail, D. (2005). *Power, Interest and Psychology: Elements of a social materialist understanding of distress.* Ross-on-Wye: PCCS Books.

Surowiecki, J. (2004). *The Wisdom of Crowds: Why the many are smarter than the few.* London: Abacus.

Watkins, M., & Shulman, H. (2008). *Towards Psychologies of Liberation.* Basingstoke: Palgrave Macmillan.

Wolfensberger, W. (1992). *A Brief Introduction to Social Role Valorization as a High-Order Concept for Structuring Human Services.* Syracuse, NY: Training Institute for Human Service Planning, Leadership and Change Agency (Syracuse University).

Yates, I., Holmes, G., & Priest, H. (2011). There seems no place for place: A gap analysis of the recovery literature. *Journal of Public Mental Health, 10*(3), 140–151.

Yates, I., Holmes, G., & Priest, H. (2012). Recovery, place and community mental health. *Journal of Mental Health, 21,* 104–113.

Chapter 16

Redressing the Balance of Power: Psychiatric medication in Nottingham

Nottingham Mind Medication Group

It was only on being sectioned that I realised that the whole of the 'system' is topsy-turvy, and something needed to happen to redress the balance of power. (Anonymous group member)

The Nottingham Mind Medication Group was set up in response to the anger and frustration felt by many people who use mental health services in Nottingham. It provides a forum for peer support and allows members to access knowledge about psychiatric medication. The group also aims to challenge the power imbalance between us and the psychiatric system through outreach to the wider community, for example, explaining the ethos of the group at conferences. The group began with the help and support from similar groups in Shropshire and Leicester and similarly we hope that this chapter will provide others with some ideas about how to set up their own groups. This chapter outlines how we set up the group and highlights why we think our group is essential. We also talk about how psychiatric medication is used and abused within the mental health system and some of the attempts that we have made to redress this balance of power. Each of us has contributed in some way, some of us choosing to express ourselves through poetry, editing, writing sections for the chapter or contributing to debates about how it should read.

The beginning

The Nottingham Mind Medication Group was established in 2008 following a public meeting at which there were presentations from two

This chapter is written and influenced by the Nottingham Mind Medication Group (Clare Metushi, Peter Broadhurst, Peter Young, Sarah, Sarah Keenan, Will Duke, and others who would like to remain anonymous).

other established medication groups, these were the Shropshire 'Thinking about Psychiatric Medication Group' and the Leicester 'Living with Psychiatric Medication Group'. Approximately 60 people attended this meeting, the majority of whom were either mental health service users or members of the general public; several members of mental health service staff also attended. Following the presentations there was an opportunity for open discussion about psychiatric medication and the psychiatric system. The majority of comments reflected a great deal of anger, frustration and powerlessness about how people had been treated within the psychiatric system. There was particular anger about the speed and ease at which they were put on psychiatric medication and the difficulties and barriers that they faced in trying to reduce or come off medication or find out about alternatives. Two members of staff were interested in whether it would be possible to set up a regular meeting to allow people to meet and discuss the impact of psychiatric medication. Several people from the general meeting agreed to meet and form a new group.

Group structure

Whilst there was an awareness of the goals and structure implemented by other medication groups, there was an open platform for this group to be as its members determined. Initially we met every fortnight at a mental health day centre; more recently we have moved to a self-help centre located within Nottingham city centre. The group has alternated between being a social support meeting and a meeting which is addressed by a speaker of our choosing. We were keen to create a space where everyone felt accepted and able to contribute and therefore some general ground rules were agreed. These included ideas such as confidentiality, mutual respect and keeping to time.

The role of mental health worker support

The group is supported by two mental health workers (a clinical psychologist and a social worker). These roles have changed over the years partly in response to the changing support needs of the group and partly due to mental health service time pressures. Importantly the ethos of the group has always given equal status to every member, and every member of the group has an equal voice. It is for this reason that the group continues to run regardless of whether the mental health workers involved attend. We continue to reflect on how mental health workers are involved and whether they are helpful or whether on occasion they may hamper discussion. The mental health workers also reflect on their position within the group and have observed that this changes depending on group dynamics, sometimes feeling a central part of the group, and other times feeling outside the group. Furthermore, mental health workers are aware that they are part of the psychiatric system and therefore cannot truly take a position of neutrality when involved in group discussions that critique mental health services.

Our group is peer led, which makes it different to many other support groups which are often staff led. This is important for a number of reasons. Mainly this means that we own our agenda rather than having an 'expert' agenda imposed on us. Therefore we can evaluate the group and change it flexibly depending on how successful particular group structures or projects have been. This also means that the mental health workers involved can stand aside from some of the bureaucracy that is implicit within their roles, for example, the need to record group members' personal details. Rather, the group can assume its own identity and ground rules and accept responsibility for one another. For example, sometimes people are distressed within the group and we take it in turns to support people, whether this be a phone call during the week, meeting for a coffee or supporting each other when visiting the psychiatrist.

Why is the group important?

The group is important because it provides a forum for people to connect with each other, both within the group and between the group and the wider community. Mental health problems attract prejudices from society as a whole, and sometimes sadly from closer to home. Prejudice in society, family and mental health services can be very damaging. The mental health system is often found to be intimidating and can make us feel as if we are somehow second class. A sense of powerlessness can result from people who use mental health systems feeling that they are in the minority and are in some way different to the norm. The Mind Medication Group is one place, and one network, where we can be ourselves without feeling ashamed and can feel part of a supportive collective.

Mind medication poem
Will Duke

What the mind medication group means to me,
A supportive environment, most especially,
In which issues various one can explore,
From side effects to biscuits and more.
My confidence and self-esteem,
Have risen gently thanks to this team,
Of friends, that I, a founder member of,
Have expressed myself to and not been rejected.
At times I laugh or cry but not alone, always respected,
For my point of view,
This my friends was something new,
For prior to this I never felt that I was really listened to.
Now sometimes with a salient point to make,
A gritty topic to argue,
I find that I can hold my own,
In conversation with a crowd.
Without being derided or mocked,
Or having my peers laugh out loud,
At some faux pas I might have made,
No more a figure of fun and reproach,
I feel respect for who I am,
No scum or worm, simply a man.
You ask me if I mind medication,
Sometimes 'yes' and sometimes 'no',
I've come off it a few times,
Never successfully though.
This new stuff that I'm on,
Is making me right fat,
I am slightly concerned about that,
But I will really worry when the doctor says to me,
Take this pill for the rest of your life, and he only gives me three.
Mind medication has helped me to grow,
In self-respect and love,
Yet we have another help,
It comes down from above.
God created everything,
Even little pink pills,
He makes a man, healthy, wise,
He makes one weak and ill.
He brings happiness and sorrow,

And I will love him still,
For yesterday, today, tomorrow,
In poverty and sickness I,
Can still be happy here on earth,
Until at last I die.

We feel that the group has helped us discover new ways of coping and has helped us feel less dependent on psychiatric medication. Being less dependent on psychiatric drugs means we have somewhat more power and feel less intimidated:

> *I've had a tendency in the past to depend on the mental health services. I saw myself very much a victim of bipolar and would look to professionals and drugs to overcome my difficulties.* (Sarah, group member)

It's acknowledged that to challenge such a dominant and powerful system is daunting and we recognise that this is easier when we support each other, for example, we have gone together to discuss medication with psychiatrists, rather than going alone. We have also created a space where we can share stories and feel less alone and alienated by problems:

> *When I entered the room I felt at ease, I finally found harmony, I finally found where I feel safe, now I am in a better place.* (Clare Metushi, group member)

Group members also say that they respect each other for their achievements in battling with psychiatric medication, and they recognise that support from each other can be very important in trying to make changes to their medication:

> *In the Mind Medication Group I have met people who are on no medication at all and this is inspiring to me. I've always wanted to take more and more medication to stop the depression and mania but on reflection my rapid-cycling mixed affective mood disorder has not been stabilised by psychiatric medication … With the support of the group I believe that eventually I could lose my psychological dependency on medication and even my prior dependency on the mental health services per se.* (Sarah, group member)

One group member commented that they had felt like a 'prisoner' within the psychiatric system. In contrast, often through conversations within the group, problems that have previously been seen as symptoms of an 'illness' are translated as being understandable reactions to difficult environments and life events. For example, when someone loses their job, social connections, power and worth it seems understandable that they might struggle; this does not mean that they are ill, but rather they may need extra support that may or may not include medication.

How does medication link with our experiences and environment?

So often when someone is referred to a psychiatrist that person is in a crisis. Many people's first experiences of hospitals, psychiatrists, mental health workers and medication arise from the bleakest times in their lives. This is usually due to a culmination of difficult and traumatic experiences. Often by the time people have entered the psychiatric system they are already experiencing feelings of extreme powerlessness. Unfortunately, because of these experiences they can be viewed as either a threat to themselves or to others, and this initiates a series of events over which people also have no control and which can be extremely distressing. In such a situation the system can take over a person's life. A person can be sectioned, which is the ultimate loss of control. However, even if not sectioned, the psychiatrist has considerable power given the person's distressed and often desperate state. At these times medication is often prescribed as an 'emergency' measure. The upshot is that the person is now less of a problem because they cannot actually function as an autonomous individual. Many in the group have found that once on a medication regime, which was prescribed at a time of intense distress, it can be difficult to change or come off at a later date. Indeed, the mental health system (in contrast with the substance misuse services) does not appear to have a clear procedure to help people come off or reduce their medication. Our view is that medication should be the last resort, not the first. The problems with psychotropic medication are sedation, lack of energy and drive, and a dulling of emotions. It leads to merely existing and not a full and bountiful life. Moreover, we feel that by taking such medication major life events, such as having a career, long-term relationships and a family, are put in jeopardy and do not occur as often as without medication.

The power of linking with others

A Ditty
Anonymous

A chance to unwind, let it all hang out,
You're not alone, of that there's no doubt.
It's the camaraderie that does it for me,
The empathy and equality.
It's your cup of tea (that'll be 30p).
No need to get fraught, there's mutual support,
Every view is respected, yours won't be rejected.

Linking with others has helped to lift feelings of powerlessness and allowed us the opportunity to make social networks and gain social support. One member of the group commented that it has helped them 'get their life back', another said 'a sense of solidarity tends to arise, people feel accepted and supported, they feel helped and are helped'. Just belonging to a group where people feel they have a connection with others helps group members cope. Sometimes this means a physical connection in the sense of having a regular place to go, and at other times this is about the experience of feeling comfortable enough with a group to share hopes, fears and experiences. We feel that being of help to others has also increased our sense of self-worth and confidence.

The group has also valued being part of a wider network of people who question the current psychiatric system. The Nottingham Mind Medication Group linked with the Leicester Living with Psychiatric Medication Group to present their work at two national conferences. We also joined forces with the Leicester group to host a public debate about child psychiatric medication, in which two psychiatrists debated the pros and cons of medication for children. The result of this was an overwhelming majority of people supporting the motion that 'it is wrong to prescribe psychiatric drugs to control children's behaviour'.

The search for answers

Whilst psychiatric services represent medication as some form of cure or 'quick fix', we believe that it only (at times) alters symptoms and does not treat the cause – it is no more than palliative care. Sometimes we feel that mental health workers just do not listen when we ask to change or reduce our medication. At other times it can be difficult to know whether we should ask questions or we can feel under pressure from other people in our lives, like our families, to stay on medication. This uncertainty is compounded by the fact that the medication that we are on often makes it hard to think. Many people find it difficult even if not on 'intoxicating' medication to challenge a doctor – it is a part, so to speak, of a person's social conditioning. We are brought up to think that doctors are authority figures whose word cannot be questioned and whose power is absolute. Society dictates that we should trust our doctors, although we often feel that they do not trust us or our judgements. One way the group helps challenge some of these barriers is to team up and visit psychiatrists together. For example, one group member did not feel able to challenge her prescribed medication even though it caused extreme drowsiness which was making it impossible for her to have any quality of life. This lady discussed the situation at the group, wrote a list of questions to take with her and took someone else from the group with her. As a result her psychiatrist changed her prescription which resulted in a dramatic improvement.

As previously discussed, one function of the group is a more private search for answers which takes place confidentially between group members. Another function is the more public search for answers. We try to raise awareness about what it is like to take psychiatric medication, and also in return try to make sense of why the psychiatric system is the way it is. For this reason we often invite speakers to help us find some answers to our questions. Speakers have included: a drug representative talking about the marketing and ethics of the pharmaceutical industry; a psychiatrist and pharmacist, speaking about diagnosis and the side effects of medication; the Nottingham Involvement team talking about their medication project; speakers from a local service user organisation 'Making Waves'; an Introduction to Homeopathy; and a representative from the 'Expert Patient' Programme. We found that we felt much more empowered to ask questions when we were part of a group rather than when we are on our own. This might be because we were asking questions in a place where we feel comfortable (rather than a hospital), or because we have the support of other group members, or because the speakers were not directly related to our care. For example, when a psychiatrist came to speak to the group he was not in charge of our medication, and therefore had less power over our lives. Interestingly, we noted that it seemed easier for the presenters to speak more openly than they were able when within the confines of NHS buildings and expectations. We wondered about how much power and control mental health workers have to work in the way that they feel is therapeutic and how much this is compromised due to the demands of the wider system?

Through asking questions and listening to others, many of us now believe that psychiatric medication can help you cope at certain very specific times of life. We believe that psychiatric medication can undoubtedly save life, but the quality of life it provides is often greatly diminished by the negative effects. We have learned that when provided within a supportive relationship that emphasises choice, medication can be helpful for a brief period of time. We recognise that some psychiatrists support people to make informed choices and that many people value this relationship. However, we do not believe psychiatric medication to be a cure and we do believe that some undesirable effects can be irreversible such as inhibiting emotions, slowing down your thinking and metabolic effects that increase the risk of, for example, diabetes, obesity and muscle spasms. In short you can end up more 'ill' than before contact with the psychiatric system.

So what does psychiatric medication do?

Joanna Moncrieff's work has helped us understand the effects of psychiatric medication differently (Moncrieff, 2007, 2008). It has helped us challenge some of the dominant understandings of medication; particularly that it is a cure for an 'illness'. We know that one commonly held belief is that psychiatric medication corrects some form of chemical imbalance in the brain rather like the way that insulin corrects for an insulin imbalance in diabetic patients. Some people believe that mental distress is the result of a brain malfunction brought about by too much or too little of something, a view that could be seen as going back to pre-modern times when all difficulties were interpreted as due to an imbalance of humours. There is no convincing evidence for the chemical imbalance theory (Moncrieff, 2007). This does not mean, however, that giving drugs to people cannot make a positive difference to their behaviour, but this is not proof of 'illness', any more than giving alcohol to someone with social anxiety cures them by correcting an alcohol imbalance (Moncrieff, 2007). Once we start to erode the credibility of whether mental illness exists then questions naturally arise as to what psychiatric medication does. We have come to the conclusion that medications have a myriad of challenging effects, some of which, depending on circumstances, can be positive (e.g., sedating effects can mean that voices can feel less intrusive), or negative (e.g., sedating effects can mean that you struggle to maintain a conversation or go to work).

We also know how important it is to acknowledge the 'rebound effect', which can be a real challenge in trying to come off psychiatric medication, as it is often assumed that our 'symptoms' are worsening and therefore medication is increased again. We know, however, that this is a natural response that will pass, but it is important that when going through this stage we have access to support systems like our group. It can be very powerful at this time to talk to others who have also been through this process and realise that it is an understandable reaction rather than a crisis. We feel that there should be a lot more emphasis within mental health services on supporting people to come off medication. In contrast, the psychiatric system is very focused on medication compliance. It can also be helpful to have access to knowledge (e.g., The Harm Reduction Guide to Coming Off Psychiatric Drugs by the Icarus Project, 2007) that can add to our understanding and therefore our means of negotiation with our psychiatrists at this time.

Making informed decisions

The group's aim was not to advocate that people should never take psychiatric medication or that they should necessarily change their medication. We are, however, interested in accessing information about medication. We feel that through learning more we could be more central in decision making. Often we ask questions about stopping medication, for example, understanding the rebound effect, the consequences of staying on medication, and whether there might be alternatives to medication or different, more suitable, medications. Other important topics we have discussed are advance statements or crisis plans; protective factors and stressors, for example, finances and past traumas; and ways in which we could feel like we had more control over our medication.

The future

A group like ours provides a conduit for information and influence between mental health service users and providers. The group connects psychiatry, service users, alternative therapies, the community and wider society. We are about change and the potential for change. Each of us in the group has been changed by the group and have changed the group, and we continue to evolve in this way. It is not necessarily about being 'well' or 'ill' but rather about being together and gaining a sense of solidarity with others. We have wondered together about whether groups like ours will become even more important given the cuts to mental health services and support. It seems vital at times when services cannot provide stability and care that we are able to support each other.

What we all want, whatever our mental state of health, is a life that is worth living; a life that has meaning, which is not just existence. We want autonomy, to be able to take charge of our lives and to feel that our lives matter. Drugs can alter the mind in a way that makes existence easier or more bearable either for those taking them, for others in the person's world, for mental heath services or for wider society. As a group we want to help each other make decisions that are right for us. The Mind Medication Group offers advice and support. It also allows us to gain knowledge and power through accessing speakers who give us ideas about alternative therapies and more insight into the mental health services. Importantly we also provide friendly faces to welcome people in from the 'mental health desert'. Our group offers peer support which we feel is the essential component in our success. We hope that others might also be inspired to develop similar groups and that eventually these groups will join together and form a powerful network that challenges the abuses within the psychiatric system from a service user perspective.

References

Icarus Project and Freedom Centre. (2007). *Harm Reduction Guide to Coming Off Psychiatric Drugs.* New York: Icarus Project and Freedom Centre. Retrieved 5 December 2012 from, http://theicarusproject.net/downloads/ComingOffPsychDrugsHarmReductGuide1Edonline.pdf

Moncrieff, J. (2007). Diagnosis and drug treatment. *The Psychologist, 20,* 5.

Moncrieff, J. (2008). *The Myth of the Chemical Cure: A critique of psychiatric drug treatment.* Basingstoke: Palgrave Macmillan.

Chapter 17

Ordinary and Extraordinary People, Acting to Make a Difference

Leicester Living with Psychiatric Medication Group

Introduction

We are the 'Living with Psychiatric Medication' (LWPM) group; a community group in Leicester with an interest in the relationship our society has with psychiatric drugs. Since 2006 we have achieved a staggering amount and are continuing to evolve as an active, informed and supportive collective. We will describe how and why we formed the LWPM group, how we have evolved and the work we engage in. We would also like to encourage the formation of similar groups and so we will go into some detail about the working of our group, the roles each member takes on and how we situate ourselves in the wider society. One of the most important aspects of our group is that while we are a group of individuals, with different experiences and views, there is something vital which unites us – the aim of creating a space that is liberating, democratic, respectful and useful.

There are many different voices in our group and we hope that as many of these as possible are heard as we write this chapter together. An important theme in our critical understanding of the world is power, and the structures within which it is withheld or asserted. Language is one such structure and we want to draw attention to words that we find potentially problematic, words such as 'patient', for example, are therefore put in quotation marks. We use the terms 'medication' and 'drugs' interchangeably as, while we are supportive of Moncrieff's model of understanding psychiatric drugs (Moncrieff, 2009), we also acknowledge that the term 'medication' is more widely used. We hope this invites readers to think about words we tend to associate with distress and how they might impact on our understanding, experience and identity.

How and why the group formed

Our group came into being in 2006 after founder members were inspired by a public discussion evening led by Judy Harvey and Guy Holmes, two members of the 'Thinking about Medication' group from Shropshire. A significant number of people attending felt that there was a lack of information about psychiatric medication available to people taking it, even during personal medical consultations. We wanted a space to think about alternatives to medication and other activities that can be life improving that do not involve medication, for example, university, work and hobbies. It was also important for us to create somewhere to challenge and question taken-for-granted knowledge about drugs. We wanted to share experiences about taking psychiatric medications and ensure that we are not just taking medication without question.

We established an overall aim to create a much-needed space for people in Leicester to think, talk and take action on issues surrounding psychiatric medication. When we became independently constituted, in 2009, we developed our mission statement:

> The aims of the group shall be to gain knowledge, ask questions, find answers, challenge assumptions and spread awareness about psychiatric medication in a supportive, relaxed atmosphere. We provide a safe environment which promotes us to make our own choices, decisions and thinking critically about living with psychiatric medication.

Who are we?

We are a group of ordinary and extraordinary people with an interest in psychiatric medication. No one is referred to the group and meetings are open to anyone; people choose to come because they are interested. The group is always open to new members and we believe that all of us live with psychiatric medication in some way (whether as people who take or prescribe medication, care for, or work alongside someone who does). We each hold different experiences of psychiatric medication; some of us used to take psychiatric drugs but no longer do, some have never taken them, some hope to come off, some have been taking them since childhood. While everyone is welcome in our group it is necessary to acknowledge that many of our group have been prescribed psychiatric drugs for many years and have some very important knowledge to share. We have around 10 members who attend regularly and who are involved in the group activities. Our collective has a fluid membership, with some people coming for only a few meetings or who keep in touch with us indirectly and it feels important to maintain this openness.

What do we do?

We want our meetings to find a balance between being structured and flexible and, crucially, to provide a forum for open debate where differences of opinion are welcomed and respected. This is something which we have found to be lacking in many formal mental health services. For example, in the relationship between 'prescriber' and 'patient' we have found that many topics are not up for discussion. We are seen as 'patients' whether or not we wish to take on this identity because we are being seen in a clinical context by someone who has been assigned the identity of 'expert.' In this supposed protection of our best interests, we are denied opportunities to explore really important issues, such as why the leaflet that comes with some of our medications lists death as a possible 'side effect'. Perhaps because there are no easy answers to some of the difficult questions we have, we have experienced a lack of space in which to think critically as adults in an equal relationship with those that prescribe to us. Our group then becomes a vital opportunity for us to have freedom to talk about these issues and to reclaim power by seeking knowledge and solidarity with others. The group is not exclusively about coming off psychiatric drugs, yet similarly we do not suggest that drugs are an answer to our distress; we aim not to prescribe knowledge, but to provoke critical reflection. The group gives all of us an opportunity to explore the complexities of the relationship between distress and the medical model, and to be mindful of the social and political issues surrounding a society that gives such weight to pharmaceutical solutions to human problems.

Sometimes our meetings include a speaker who talks about their role in relation to psychiatric medications and offers a question-and-answer session. We have invited psychiatrists, pharmacists, psychologists, community psychiatric nurses and solicitors, for example. This gives us greater access to mental health professionals. Meeting on our territory makes a powerful difference to the kinds of dialogues we can have. We feel able to ask more questions, to be more open and reflectively critical of aspects of psychiatric medications and the process of prescribing that concern us. We see that the professionals who come to our group also react differently in the context of our meetings, seeming more comfortable with these types of conversation. Perhaps this is because they feel less responsible for us as 'patients' in a group setting; they may have more time to listen to our views or feel safer talking to us in a forum where the distribution of power is shared. Importantly, the support and knowledge we develop as a group stays with us as individuals outside of group meetings. For example, we feel more confident in asking questions and expressing a difference of opinion during an appointment with our psychiatrist; there is something about being part of such a strong collective that legitimises our voice as an individual. We have developed good relationships with speakers we have invited to the group, some of whom come back regularly. We have also developed strong links with the Leicestershire Partnership NHS Trust and Network For Change – a local voluntary sector mental health project in Leicester.

Over time our group has changed and seems to have taken a similar journey to that described by bell hooks in relation to the feminist consciousness-raising groups of the 1960s and 1970s (hooks, 2000). In the beginning the group provided a forum within which we could share experiences and learn about psychiatric drugs and the pharmaceutical industry. Concurrently we became aware of the multiple ways psychiatric drugs influence our everyday lives. Whilst doing this was crucial, in those early days there was 'little or no focus on strategies of intervention and transformation' (hooks, 2000, p. 7). Like the consciousness-raising groups, our initial focus of inviting open communication and doing this in a non-hierarchical way 'created a context for engaged dialogue' (hooks, 2000, p. 8). Navigating through agreements and disagreements gave us a 'realistic standpoint' (hooks, 2000, p. 8) from which to understand the complexity of what it means to live with psychiatric medication, and in turn led us to social and political action.

We feel strongly that our individual experiences and work together should have a wider impact. With this in mind, we have consulted with people around the UK about the setting up of similar groups, we have presented at national conferences, published articles and booklets about the group, held a drug company marketing amnesty and related art exhibition, organised a debate about prescribing psychiatric medication to children and have plans to organise a national meeting about psychiatric medication. We have also forged important links and relationships with other community groups, e.g., 'Brightsparks Arts in Mental Health' group, 'Seroxat User Group', the medication groups in Shropshire and Bradford, and the 'Nottingham Mind Medication Group'. We all encourage and support each other and it feels important to be part of a growing network of allies.

Consciousness raising is an important aim of our group and we try to engage in actions that will encourage others to think critically about important issues. The public debate about prescribing psychiatric medication to children, organised alongside the Nottingham-based Mind Medication Group, became important to us after we had spent some time thinking about the implications of prescribing psychiatric medications to children and whether this should be acceptable. We had discussed and shared our fears and recognised how important it was to keep open channels of dialogue. Organising a debate was our way of responding to our concerns. We wanted to encourage critical reflection on the lack of alternatives in understanding and alleviating a child's distress. We wanted to explore what this might say about our society and how else we could respond. It was empowering on many levels to organise such an event; we as a group had to learn many new skills as it was the first time we had had the opportunity to be part of such a project. We also received positive feedback from the speakers we invited to present at the debate and those who participated in the discussion:

> *The debate finished five hours ago now, and I still feel like I am buzzing from being there ... It has left me wondering about the powerful influence that open public mental health debates (like this one) could have on perceptions of mental health in our society. It would be fantastic if they were to become more regular events.* (Debate attendee)

How we run our group

We created some 'ground rules' at the very first meeting of the group and these have since evolved into a 'group framework' which makes the ground rules feel more democratic and less dogmatic. The group framework helps everyone (group members, new and old, as well as speakers) to know what to expect in the group. The framework is read out at the beginning of each group and is sent to speakers in advance of the meetings. It also ensures that the speaker and group are not disturbed and keeps the group on track with its ethos. We found that developing our own framework for working together was and continues to be a major part of the evolution of the group. It can be hard to navigate, for example, the dynamics of a difference of opinion, particularly in a context where we are sharing personal and often distressing experiences. The framework grows out of the challenges we come across as the group progresses and gives us a process through which we can sort out the disagreements we may have.

A good example of how our group framework helps us to manage group dynamics is the evolution of one of our agreements. For a long time we maintained that members could not join in the group session if they were late. This was so that we were not interrupted when discussing personal stories or listening to an invited speaker. However, we often found it difficult to balance the tension between respecting the conversations that were already going on and the passion of latecomers to join the discussion. We spoke at length about how this made us feel and agreed to allow existing members (who were well acquainted with our framework) to come in late if they agreed to be quiet and not disrupt the discussion. This felt a frustrating and difficult situation for us and we all had different opinions on how to solve the problem. We needed to balance conflicting concerns such as respecting the rules we had all previously agreed to; we also did not want to unwittingly become gatekeepers of knowledge. Appointments with a psychiatrist, for example, cannot easily be changed and often run late. While compromising has produced tensions (and could quite easily have led members to leave the group) we are proud of the way we have managed the situation. There have been positive outcomes from the conflict; for example, it has led us to think about ways in which we structure the room layout so that speakers are not interrupted when we need to pop out and, importantly, it has led us to learn a little about ourselves. One group member, for example, was surprised at how rule-bound they were and felt it was powerful to think of ways in which they could be more flexible.

We regularly identify particular roles within our group meetings that are important in maintaining our ethos and focus. We feel it is important to share these jobs and for group members to participate in any way they feel comfortable. This may mean taking on a particular job on a regular basis (such as minute taking, updating the website or reading the group framework) but it is also important that we feel comfortable in saying 'no' to taking on a named role and we recognise that this does not detract from the value of our participation as a group member. This has led us to become more democratic in the way we uphold our group framework; for example, the whole group takes responsibility for not speaking over each other. We have a lot of aspirations that are not easily fulfilled in the two hours every fortnight that we meet. Some work needs to take place outside of the group and we each share this. As we only do as much as we can or want to this does not feel like a burden, in fact some of us thrive on it!

To be more specific, some of the interventions that a group facilitator might make that we try to take responsibility for as a group (without allocating them to one person) are:

• inviting other group members to respond to something someone has said

• offering information as material to be questioned, debated and discussed rather than accepted

• respectfully disagreeing

• encouraging group members to take on roles that might make the most of their talents or offer them a structure for their contributions

• reminding people of their own commitment to say 'no' to taking on tasks for the group.

When we do not have a speaker booked, we either use sessions to share our own experiences, or we work on one of our projects. For example, this might mean jointly writing presentations, adding to our website or responding to emails. Since we became independently constituted, we have been able to apply for small grants which have allowed us to cover the costs of the projects and buy resources such as a laptop, phone and books.

It can be very difficult to find out information about psychiatric medications and we have found it empowering to build up a collection of resources. Our collection of books, articles and general resources is now fairly extensive and we find these useful to refer to during our meetings. Group members and speakers also bring and share articles, views and experiences with each other during the session. Holmes refers to this as the 'democratisation of truth' (Holmes, 2010; see also Diamond, 2008; Watkins & Shulman, 2008); information about psychiatric medication in Leicester is no longer in the hands of one dominant group.

Balancing different roles

> *It is important to go to conferences because I hear about medication from professionals in a way they would not usually discuss with us. I hope the group can create a society where we don't need medication. We lack the opportunity to study psychology etc. at a professional level. The group gives me a chance to look at this and learn.* (Group member)

Some of us attending the group also work in mental health services (two in the voluntary sector, one in the NHS). Two of us have psychology backgrounds and have been involved since the group's inception, sharing and developing an enthusiasm in community and critical psychology (see, for example, Kagan, 2007; Kagan, Burton & Siddiquee, 2007) and liberatory group work (Holmes, 2010).

Developing independence as a community group has been important for all of us. We periodically talk as a group about whether it is the responsibility of those of us who also work in services to withdraw from the group; to offer facilitation only to the point where the group can continue to evolve without workers being directly involved. This feels like an ongoing process. Members of the group who work in services certainly take less of a lead now than they used to and it feels less as though they are essential for the group to run. Nevertheless, we are not sure that we are aiming for a position where workers do not attend the group at all and we wonder whether our experience may call into question the notion that it is always more empowering for paid workers to disengage with groups once a collective has been achieved. Those of us who have paid positions in the mental health services continually reflect on their stake in the group and the extra dynamics their roles may bring, for example, acknowledging how it might feel for someone accessing mental health services to join a group which includes people who work in those services.

Often we talk of those in professions as though they are at the end point of their learning while, actually, they have much still to learn. Working alongside community groups can be a rich source of education and liberation for those who work in services and it is vital to acknowledge and appreciate this. While we feel we meet as equals in our group we also need to be aware that our work is situated in a context that is inherently unequal; acknowledging this together can at times feel challenging and confusing. We are used to talking about power in terms of 'them and us' and we can find it harder to locate and name the powers that are structurally embedded, particularly in forums which manage to achieve democracy.

These differences need to be reflected on, regardless of how much we enjoy working together, and doing this has helped us to witness the shift from paid workers being needed in the group to simply being welcome. It has been important for paid workers involved in the group to manage the power they are afforded within their working roles via discussion rather than being tempted to simply make their roles invisible. At the same time Holmes (2010) warns workers participating in community group work that because of their position of relative power their perceived opinions carry a lot of weight.

In providing a critique of the particular ways in which some of our roles need to be considered we are in danger of expressing a simplistic and false dichotomy between those who work in and those who seek support from mental health services. Some of our group have the opportunity to take on voluntary roles within local statutory mental health services, developing inpatient services for example, and many of us have positions within service-user forums. This is vital in building links, publicising our projects and working collaboratively with others in our community; we benefit collectively from the work we do as individuals outside of the group. It feels important to acknowledge the benefits that can be achieved when people with different roles work together and reminds us of the concept of 'edge effects' in community psychology whereby alliances between different communities (or those with different roles in the community) provide a 'phenomenon of enrichment ... energy, excitement and commitment' (Kagan, 2007, p. 225). By redistributing, sharing and encouraging each other to make the most of our personal resources, we find ourselves investing in something much larger than what we could achieve as individuals, a collective effort which has the potential to engage in transformative change (Kagan et al., 2007).

Why we value the group

We were recently asked, at a teaching session, how we have managed to keep talking about psychiatric medication for five years, yet the topic is so pervasive and broad that we have never run out of ideas and projects. We regularly hold reviews and evaluations to make sure that we continue to evolve in ways that are meaningful and useful to us all.

Individually, we feel motivated to attend because:

- it's friendly
- we discuss a common interest
- we feel involved
- it encourages a sense of purpose
- it's a place where we can be heard by professionals or get feedback from them
- we spend a lot of time listening to and learning from others and have gained a lot from other people's experiences; sometimes just listening to other people's ideas can help validate your thoughts or encourage you to think in a slightly different way – in this sense we are encouraging a 'listening therapy' as well as 'talking therapy'!
- the group is continually evolving.

We also have support from individuals, organisations outside of the group, and speakers who tell us that our work is very important and they urge us to carry on. We appreciate the support we offer to each other by having respect in the experiences and opinions each of us share and the knowledge that we are all meeting with a common aim. It is important our meeting environment is free of vested interests, in particular around whether each of us takes or does not take medication.

It always feels like an optimistic group, even as we uncover more questions than answers and talk about some very deep and troubling themes. We are a proactive group and this sense of momentum feels important; we identify themes that concern us and then we try and do something about them, even if all we can do is to raise consciousness amongst ourselves and others so that some of this knowledge is no longer hidden. It is a positive place to get involved; we love the way it buzzes with ideas and we value exploring these in a space in which we don't impose our judgements on each other or dictate how others should act.

The LWPM group is important because it gives us a space where we are validated and listened to and, for many of us, this is not something we have regular access to. Some of us have been in the psychiatric system for many years and this is disempowering in a number of complex ways. We can find ourselves disenfranchised, for example, by being prevented from entering the job market or higher education. The medication we take can leave us with physical health problems. We feel like we do not always have an equal place in society, that we are shoved to one side and others can find it difficult to understand us or, at times, do not want to know about our distress or label us as 'hard to cope with'. We acknowledge that the mental health system is unique from other frameworks in our society in that we can be subjected to a loss of our human rights as legally legitimised by the state in the name of our best interests. Some of us have had powerful experiences of being coerced into continuing or starting medication regimes we do not agree with because of the possibility of being sectioned under the Mental Health Act. Some of us have memories of the lack of dignity and basic human rights we were offered while we were at our most distressed and in hospital. We also face being perceived by society as a discrete section of the population rather than as diverse individuals. The current rhetoric of the government can feel like a harsh indictment of the many of us who are entitled to welfare and we are subject to the negative stereotypes perpetuated by the media regarding mental health. Experiences like these, and the many more we share with each other, can have lasting legacies. Being in the group can offer a refreshing alternative to this.

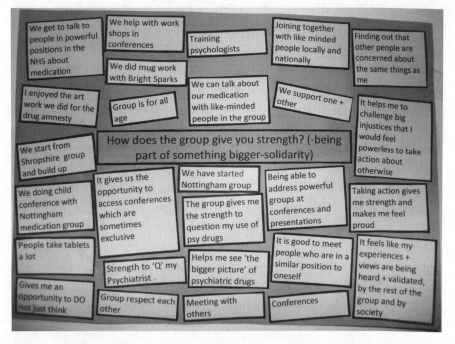

Figure 1. Photo showing how 'the group gives us strength' from a recent group evaluation

It is important to us that we can be comfortable amongst others who have experiences of psychiatric medication; in other contexts our ideas have been perceived as radical or maverick, but here they are accepted. We all feel proud to be part of the group and to work on the projects we initiate. We have been able to represent and promote Leicester at a national level and have had many people say that they now think of Leicester as progressive and inspirational.

Challenges we face as a group

Today talking is difficult; my mind feels like treacle. (Group member)

It is difficult to write exclusively about the challenges we have experienced because we have almost always managed to transform them into an area of growth for the group that is a powerful positive experience (for us as a group and as individuals). We recently worked alongside a trainee clinical psychologist to evaluate our group; one specific area we considered was what made attending or contributing in the group difficult sometimes. We identified a few themes. Past experiences (such as being put down, punished, bullied or called names) can interfere with our capacity to contribute as much as we would like to the group. Sometimes our experiences are just too painful to talk about. Some days, although we want to attend the group because we find it valuable, we don't really feel like contributing. It can be difficult when feeling fragile or in a bad state or when we are suffering from the effects of medication.

We think we need to continue to work hard to make the group an easy space for new people to join. Several of us have been involved for a long time and this helps maintain a collective identity but we do not want this to exclude newcomers. It can feel daunting for someone to come into our group for the first time and it can take a while for new members to feel comfortable. It is easier when an existing member knows the new member and can introduce them to the rest of us. We make our group framework and a list of our hopes and fears for the group available to new members and this can help give people some idea of what to expect from a meeting. Despite this there are times when our group meetings are quite busy and intense as we might have deadlines to work towards for our projects. This can be intimidating for new members. For this reason we take turns in the role of 'hospitality and greeter' so that new members feel welcome and included. Some people only come to our group once or twice and it is not always easy to find out why. This feels OK though and we have several members who only come every now and then and who have told us that it is important to them to know that the group is there. There is security in the knowing that debate occurs even when they are not directly involved.

It can feel empowering to be engaged in so many projects but this can leave us with little time to talk about our experiences and concerns about our own medication. Our diverse group aims (taking action, inviting speakers to the group, sharing personal experiences) sometimes compete for time and we need to try and achieve a balance. This can be a fertile conflict though; it can keep us motivated, passionate, structured and ever mindful of the need to question what we are doing and why.

There is also the careful balance that all of us have to strike between silence (which can itself be difficult) and talking too much. We recognise that, despite the current fashion for 'talking therapies', talking is sometimes unhelpful, especially if we do not feel listened to or understood and it is not always possible to put into the words the complex and intangible experiences we have. It can be retraumatising to bring the things that disempower us into a space that is limited in power. While we are proud of our achievements as a group, we should not ignore that there are things that we cannot change and wrongs that we cannot right. For example, one of our concerns is the long-term effects of taking psychiatric drugs. For those of us who have taken these drugs for several decades and those of us who do not have an alternative this can be terrifying to think about. It is important that we are all mindful of each other's right to not want to talk about ourselves or our experiences so that each of us consents to the information we share.

When we first started the group, we feared that professionals would feel it too risky to talk openly with us about our concerns; however, on the whole, this has not been the case. One notable exception arose when we invited drug company representatives to come and talk with us about their role within the industry and how it was located within mental health services. Two major drug companies were approached, both of whom declined to come and speak with us, referring to the code of practice for their industry. They acknowledged the role of drug company representation as promotional and refused to reply even in writing to some of our questions stating that '... plentiful opinion exists in the public domain' (private correspondence). We acknowledged that it would not be right for a representative to come and market their drugs to us, but felt angered that we needed to be 'protected' in this way. The drug companies acknowledged they would have come to talk to us if we were a body of healthcare professionals. We wondered why it was not acceptable to come and talk to us as adults, but it was OK to advertise to us on the pens our doctors write our prescriptions with and the clocks on the psychiatrist's wall. This frustrating barrier led us to become involved in a drug-advertising amnesty. We worked alongside a local arts collective gathering pieces of marketing paraphernalia left by drug reps in the services we use and turning them into works of art. These were then exhibited locally and at a national conference as a consciousness-raising exercise.

All of these challenges to contributing and being involved have over the years been addressed by our group framework, and because these are read and discussed at every meeting and reviewed regularly they are always at the forefront of any work that the group does together and this helps us to openly and collaboratively tackle difficulties that we come across.

The future of 'social action' groups

Perhaps it is too early to call our work part of a movement, but there are now groups in Bradford, Leicester, Nottingham and Shropshire. It is interesting how the groups vary; for example, the Leicester group seems to concentrate on the ways each of us in our society lives with psychiatric medication, whereas the Shropshire group has developed a focus more on coming off medication.

A pivotal point for our group's growth was becoming independently constituted. However, this also brought with it challenges, especially those arising from group's growing need to apply for funding as an evolution towards independence and action. Applying for funding, receiving it, spending it, and accounting for it are all skills we found very difficult and in some ways we resent the time it takes away from the more important work the group does, even though in many other ways it facilitates us being able to do them. It can impose structures on the group that feel less meaningful than the time we spend listening to each other and acting on issues that are important to us.

There is something especially important about being together that we worry is undermined by society's push towards the formalisation of community groups as social enterprises. There is currently much political rhetoric about supporting community groups to have more control over community resources and to have more say about how local issues are addressed. We are fully aware that our views sometimes situate us outside of a mainstream consensus and we wonder whether this can preclude us from accessing some funding pools. This highlights the potential barriers to achieving radical change. There is something very fundamental about the need for us to come together in our communities that is, perhaps, lost by the formal structures encouraged/foisted on grass-roots groups.

We are proud of how we have developed as a group and it can be staggering to think of all that we have been able to achieve together over this time. We often surprise ourselves at how much we have achieved and how much we still want to do. Much of what we do is new to us and it is important to acknowledge our gradual and organic evolution from developing a tentative meeting space to becoming an active, empowered group with a growing sense of agency. Writing this chapter has been useful to remind ourselves of just what is possible; ordinary people really can achieve extraordinary things.

For more information about our group (and a longer version of this chapter) please visit our website: www.livingwithpsychiatricmedication.co.uk

References

Diamond, B. (2008). Opening up space for dissension. In A. Morgan (Ed.), *Being Human: Reflections on mental distress in society* (pp. 174–189). Ross-on-Wye: PCCS Books.

Holmes, G. (2010). *Psychology in the Real World: Community-based groupwork.* Ross-on-Wye: PCCS Books.

hooks, b. (2000). *Feminism Is for Everybody: Passionate politics.* Cambridge, MA: South End Press.

Kagan, C. (2007). Working at the 'edge'. *The Psychologist, 20*(4), 224–227.

Kagan, C., Burton, M., & Siddiquee, A. (2007). Action research. In C. Willig & A. Stainton-Rogers (Eds.), *Handbook of Qualitative Research in Psychology* (pp. 32–53). London: Sage.

Moncrieff, J. (2009). *The Myth of the Chemical Cure.* London: Palgrave Macmillan.

Watkins, M., & Shulman, H. (2008). *Towards Psychologies of Liberation.* Basingstoke: Palgrave Macmillan.

Chapter 18

Peer Support

Becky Shaw

When I was in hospital I received all my help from the other patients and not from the staff which you might have expected. Other patients knew the level of my distress, I could be open about how I felt, and they could help because they were going through similar things. When I came out I had no friends and no one who understood. I thought that there must be others like myself going through similar stuff and founded a small peer support group. There were far more people than I initially expected. People who had been through similar distressing experiences could get together in a safe, supportive group to offer and receive support from each other. People who came needed to talk about what they had been through, often stating that even family and close friends couldn't understand. The important bit for me has always been that it is two-way, no one judges, people are often honest and can say things health care staff members wouldn't dream of saying, they challenge me when needed and other members accept the way you are. I literally wouldn't be here today without it. I can talk about the hallucinations and depression without fear of being judged, having my medication increased or being sectioned. It has been my main support in my recovery. (Author's personal experience of peer support)[1]

Self-help and peer support in the past has often been underrated, being seen as an 'extra' alongside other health care services. The reason peer support survives and thrives, even with little money or resources, is that it seems to work for a lot of people with many never needing to access health care services at all. This chapter examines what peer support is, what it does, and the differing types, before using one example to highlight the benefits and hurdles of peer-run groups and areas to think about when setting one up. The final part of the chapter focuses on the role in which

---

1 See Shaw (2009) and Rushcliffe Support Group (2009) for further accounts of experiences of peer support.

peer-led initiatives can support people in the broader context and the wider impact for society.

Peer support in practice

Peers naturally gather together to discuss experiences. Ideas shared about ways to cope are based on everyday life, tried and tested in the real world. The way we view experiences is often diverse, but sharing these experiences can prove useful to find our own personal understanding and coping mechanisms. Peer support occurs in all walks of life and peer support within mental health is no different to any other peer group. You might recognise this from your own life. Who do you get together with to receive and give support? This might be at the school gate with other parents, to talk about your children, swap advice, ideas, and share difficulties. It is quite human for us all to do this. It is beneficial to know we are not going through life on our own and that we have some connection with others in a similar position. Peer support in mental health is no different. It is not a new or alien concept; humankind has been doing this in one form or another since its beginning. The difference in mental health support networks is that it is becoming more organised. A significant aspect of having a mental health difficulty is that we feel alone. People with mental difficulties can feel misunderstood, stigmatised, vulnerable and have low self-worth; this means that it is harder to find people to give and receive peer support from when we really need it. Therefore, having groups that are set up specifically for peer mental health support means getting this much-needed support is easier.

In Western culture having a mental health problem is stigmatising; it is not openly talked about even though it is one of the most common difficulties someone might have in their lifetime, thought to affect one in four people in any year (www.1in4.org.uk). Discrimination can be one of the most distressing symptoms of having a mental health problem, the stigma that comes with living with a label. Peer support groups can help lower this sense of stigma and the feeling of being marginalised in society. Challenging discrimination and stigma is also very difficult to do on our own. Peer support can help by challenging discrimination as a group or supporting individuals with their particular circumstances (see also the Time to Change anti-stigma campaign: www.time-to-change.org.uk).

Different types of groups

There are many different types of peer support groups. The common themes running throughout all these groups is that they are run by people who have or are currently going through similar experiences. Within the area of mental health this means that the people running the group have personal experience of having mental health difficulties. For some, groups can offer a safe space to be ourselves without the need to hide how we're feeling. There are a variety of groups: structured and formal through to groups which are very informal. All the groups give the opportunity for each member to share their difficulties and for others to offer ideas that they may have tried themselves that may be helpful.

Formal groups offer a forum in a more structured and controlled way. Members commit to join and there are often strict rules, for example, members only share first names and are asked not to share contact details or meet outside of the group. The meeting may be run by a chair who manages the meeting, allowing everyone to have a turn. These meetings can feel a safer option for some. At the other extreme there are groups which are run in a very relaxed manner with few rules if any, where anyone can drop in, and are more like a social group than a formal meeting. Members might be encouraged to meet outside the group as friends. There are, of course, groups which fall anywhere between these two extremes. Whichever group a person benefits from will always depend on personal preferences. There will never be one type of group that suits everyone.

There are other groups which are based around activities e.g., art, walking, reading etc.; these are still peer support groups. Groups which are based around an activity are useful because members have another common area to discuss besides their mental health. These can be easier for those who may find it difficult to share their feelings with others straight away and it can be relaxing sharing something that has nothing to do with mental health, but at the same time being with people who understand our difficulties and are there when we need to talk. Peer support groups are also helpful for those who take on a caring role.

The Rushcliffe Mental Health Support Group

The Rushcliffe Mental Health Support Group has been running successfully in Nottinghamshire for 16 years and runs on a semi-formal basis. It is a useful example of how a group can work in practice. The group has been allowed to evolve over the years. This is the main reason it has succeeded and survived for so long. It is very different now to when it was first formed. It was initially a more formal type of group. Meetings were held in a hired meeting room with free hot drinks, meeting fortnightly in an evening. Members came by self-referring and never met outside the group meeting.

The changes we made helped us succeed, and these successful factors included:

- *Maintaining consistency* – same venue, time and day. This meant that people would know when and where we met even if they could not make it every week.

- *How we viewed success* – in health services the success of groups is often measured by the numbers attending. Without sufficient numbers, funding would be lost and the groups would close. We did not have to be tied by this and therefore numbers didn't matter. We decided the success of the group should be measured by the benefits members got from attending, whether three members or thirty.

- *Meeting every week* – meeting fortnightly was confusing. Members often turned up on the wrong week, wasting a journey, and then stopped coming completely.

- *Meeting at lunchtime* – initially we met in an evening in order to provide a group when there were no other services and allowing those who worked in the day to attend. However, people did not like venturing out in an evening and this became very apparent in the winter.

- *Venue choice* – we started with a very small pot of money from the Nottinghamshire Voluntary Sector Liaison Service and this helped cover meeting room costs and advertising for the first few years. This funding ended and we had to rethink how we were going to run with no money. As many were now benefiting from the group we needed to keep running. We decided to try meeting in a quiet pub even if this was a temporary measure. The venue was a more social, relaxed and friendlier environment than the stark meeting room had been and was a good move.

- *Social outings* – the group also started having a few social activities. In the fifth year we started making these social activities more regular. It was what the group wanted. We could do activities and things that we would never do on our own. We started the newsletter to let group members know what activities were on. We even went on holiday, now a yearly event, and sometimes we had short breaks.

- *Funding* – We have only ever had a small amount of funding. We can last at least six months without any income before we struggle. We had considered a small subscription to cover costs but selling a few books has meant we could avoid this.

The group has always had a written set of aims and ground rules, uncomplicated and clear. At first we did not see their importance, but although we have had few problems, having these aims and ground rules means we have direction, focus, and clarity. Problems have been resolved through talking and addressing issues early rather than allowing them to fester. We actively ask people to let us know if they have any concerns and ensure that they can talk away from the main group. We get to know people so well that we can tell when something is wrong.

The group was also constituted as a not-for-profit voluntary community group. We have gone from strength to strength but always take our direction from what the group members want. This has been through questionnaires, discussion and actively being open to all ideas even if they seem crazy at the time. Some of the craziest suggestions have been the best. This has always been the key to the group's success – not staying trapped in old ways but allowing the group to adapt and change to the different membership, taking on new ideas and trying new things. Change has kept the group fresh and alive, with any difficulties talked through as a whole group as part of the decision-making process. In doing this we have published four books, conducted research, delivered some training, provided weekly group meetings, social activities, holidays, had information stalls at events, provided an information bank and developed a website.

Tips for starting and running a peer support group

Where to begin

When you are thinking about starting a group you need to decide why you want to start it. What is its purpose? What will people get from it? Who will benefit from it and who will help you run it? This last point is one of the most important as it is inadvisable to run a group on your own – you will risk running out of energy very quickly. If you are the key

Box 1. The Rushcliffe Mental Health Support Group: Aims and ground rules

Aims of the group

- To provide a peer social support and information group, run by its members for its members, for anyone affected by mental health difficulties primarily in the Rushcliffe and Nottinghamshire areas

- To collaborate with other organisations to improve the delivery of mental health services including training and research

- To provide a mental health information bank for anybody affected by mental health issues

Group ground rules for meetings

- Members will respect each other and be considerate about the fact that other members may be vulnerable/experiencing difficulties

- Members will offer emotional support when they are able and will encourage/offer support to those who are new or find it harder to be involved at meetings to do so and be welcoming to all

- Members will respect the privacy of others

- Every member will respect that we meet in a premises that serves alcohol and agree not to abuse alcohol whilst we are meeting, arrive sober and not have any more than 3 units of alcohol

- Members will not use or be under the influence of illicit drugs at any meeting

- The group rules can change if agreed by a majority of its members and amendments will be circulated to all current members

- If anyone is having difficulties with any part of the group or other members they should speak with one of the facilitators

person and you start to struggle or become unwell, the group can quickly fold. Advertising the fact that you are thinking of starting a group and inviting other interested people to join you is a good way of finding like-minded people to help. The core group of people then need to sit down to work through the ideas and work out initial logistics. There are usually two to four facilitators, also peers, who help run the group, organise trips, sort finances and support newcomers. Facilitators are also key in helping to resolve any difficulties within the group.

Aims

The aim of the group and its purpose, who it is for and how they will join all need to be worked out in advance, written down and agreed.

Ask yourself the following:

- Who is the group for? – women, men or mixed, a specific area like self-harm, hallucinations, paranoia or based on an activity like walking or art?

- How will people join? – self-referral, drop in, recommendation? Will you use a dedicated mobile? Will you have adverts, flyers, or will people hear of you via word of mouth or through a community team or day service? Will you have a membership form, meet people prior to coming or do they just turn up?

- What ground rules do you want? Who decides what the ground rules are? How open are the rules to change? How can they be amended?

- Do you need a vulnerable adults or equality policy? Should the facilitator do anything if someone describes currently being at risk of harm? If so, what should they do? How will the facilitator deal with someone expressing prejudicial views? Is the group attracting members from a range of sections of the local community?

None of this should be written in stone and, as membership changes, these aims should be reviewed as a group. The group aims and rules should reflect the group membership. It is worthwhile evaluating the group from time to time. An informal questionnaire, survey, feedback session, ideas sessions etc. can all help inform the facilitators of what is working well and what members want. It is worth remembering that if you stay flexible to the needs and wishes of the membership then you will survive, but if you are rigid and get stuck in old ways, the group will quickly sink.

Choosing a venue

This does not have to be a paid meeting room. Thge venue could be a cafe, pub or even a free room or area offered by other voluntary organisations, especially if using their services. Is it a relaxing environment? Do you have enough privacy? We were even offered a gym once as a venue which would have been good publicity for them and we would have bought their refreshments. We decided not to take up the offer because of the location, and this is another big factor to consider. Who will come and where will they be travelling from? Will everyone drive or does it need to be on a good bus route? Does it need to be central in the area, in a very specific area or doesn't it matter? Don't forget factors like access for disabilities, childcare/crèche and refreshments. Meeting at a regular time, place and day will help membership grow. We have had members drop in after a year's gap because they knew when we would be meeting.

Advertising

Advertising for members can take a while. It can be useful to laminate your posters as they last longer. The group has had posters up after six years, whereas paper posters last only weeks. Hand delivering posters and leaflets gives you an opportunity to let people know who you are and what you do. We asked local people to take posters and leaflets to their library or doctors' surgeries where they already knew staff. Posting out leaflets was not as successful. Word of mouth seems to be the most effective method. If your group is of benefit to its members, news of this will spread and numbers will build up. The community know who we are now and what we do and will let others know if they think the group might be helpful. Don't be disheartened if numbers are low, ask yourselves whether those who are currently coming are benefiting, and if they are, then it is worth it. If not, think again about how the group works, adapt it and try something different, but don't give up.

Funding

Funding doesn't have to be a barrier and a group can run on very little money. Subscriptions can be used to cover basic costs. Having a reliance on regular funding can be problematic. Funders may require the group to have particular attendance numbers, to hit targets or to be run in a certain way. They may need monitoring forms to be completed and reports returned. It can cause unnecessary stress. If the funding is then lost a group which is reliant on it to survive will suffer or even close.

Running the group

As mentioned you need a core membership of ideally three people to run the group. Tasks will include keeping a membership list and contact details, distributing newsletters, advertising, facilitating meetings, organising the venue, keeping the petty cash and finances in order, producing accounts, organising outings and many more items on top of these.

For enquiries to the group, it is best not to give out your home phone number but perhaps use a dedicated group mobile instead. The other option is to use a self-help organisation (many exist around the UK, such as Self Help Nottingham – www. selfhelp.org.uk), which directs enquiries about self-help groups to the most suitable group in their area. They may also help with obtaining funding, getting started, finding a venue, and often advertising your group for free too.

Referral to the group

There are some peer groups which do meet potential members in advance to make sure the group is right for them. It can be difficult to come to a group only to find it is not what you are expecting or wanting and it might put you off trying another one. Meeting potential members gives an opportunity to signpost people to a different group when yours is not for them. It also gives an opportunity to discuss what the group is about, who it is for, talk through the ground rules and answer any questions. It can be frightening attending a group for the first time and getting to know one member can make joining less daunting.

Involvement

Members are responsible for themselves and autonomy is encouraged, at the same time as being supported to do as much as they can when they can for the group. New members can find the experience of making decisions and having a say uncomfortable. This is usually due to people having had little power or control in other areas of their lives, particularly in mental health services. One of the challenges a group often faces is breaking down this perception. Members may start by being involved in decisions on outings and later become involved in organising trips, sorting the accounts, supporting new members or facilitating the group. The confidence that grows within each person is huge when they realise they can help someone else and that what they are doing is not a token gesture but is actually essential to the group's running. When members gain self-esteem, confidence and autonomy they then become less reliant on the need for services.

Concerns and difficult decisions as facilitators

Facilitating a group can be very rewarding but it is not always easy. It is worth having a think in advance about what you would do if someone was a danger to themselves or others. The Rushcliffe Support group have agreed that only in exceptional circumstances will they contact outside agencies. This is one of the most difficult decisions to make and it definitely helps when there is more than one facilitator to discuss this with. The reason this is such a difficult decision is because people who come to the group can be open without fear of what they say getting back to their workers within the health service. Group members will naturally keep information confidential because they too are sharing information that they want to be kept confidential. Having to make the decision to let someone outside the group know that someone is experiencing acute difficulties and that we have major concerns breaks this confidence. You have to take into account a huge range of factors before doing this because the group may be someone's main support and breaking confidence could mean they feel uncomfortable about returning or feel less able to be open at future meetings.

Health care staff support

Health care staff can be of great benefit to peer-led groups helping with:

- obtaining funding
- printing posters/leaflets and distribution
- an initial launch event to gather a core group of people
- a venue
- a friendly ear – emotional support
- raising awareness of peer support and the group.

With a peer-led groups, whilst a staff members can usefully offer support from a distance, direct input encroaches on the autonomy and self-sufficiency of such groups.

Staff-run groups

There is a distinction between peer-led groups and staff-run groups, but both have a place in providing support. In my opinion the presence of staff members changes the very nature of a group. It is very difficult to be open with a member of staff in the room no matter how nice or understanding they might be. I do not believe a staff-led group can successfully become a peer support group and it is important to be clear about what kind of group you want. However, the situation is more complex as some staff live in both worlds, being both a staff member and service user.

Power, knowledge and influence

Peer advocates

An important factor for a peer support group is the power balance. Though there might be someone or a small group of people who organise the group, essentially everyone within the group is equal. Decisions are made as a group. This is very different to a doctor–patient relationship. The doctor has far more power than the patient. A doctor can section someone under the Mental Health Act and detain them in hospital, they can increase medication and ultimately, although decisions are discussed, a doctor has the overriding say. It can be hard, if not impossible, to challenge these decisions if you feel they are not right, especially when feeling unwell. However many years of training a doctor has, the individual often knows best what support they need, whether this is talking therapies, practical help or something to help take the edge of the symptoms for a while. Appointments may be very short and infrequent and it can be easy to accept what you are being told, even when it goes against your gut feeling. Knowledge equals power. A peer support group can help by enabling someone state what they believe, redressing this power imbalance to some extent. Just knowing what support is available through the health service can help an individual take more control. In all other parts of the NHS you are given the information necessary to make a fully informed choice. There is often a lack of such information and choice in mental health services.

Group members sometimes act as peer advocates and attend meetings to offer support. This could mean going to a doctor's appointment or to the council with housing or benefits concerns or numerous other scenarios. Peers are more likely to know what anxieties you may be facing (as they will have faced similar), be more likely to know how to help (because they know what has helped them) and what to say or ask on your behalf (because they know you). Peer advocacy is often reciprocal – on some occasions one person is the advocate and at other times they are being supported themselves. Being able to help others builds confidence and self-esteem and makes receiving support less stigmatising.

Influencing and linking with other groups and organisations

Peer support groups, whilst remaining independent, will often link with other organisations including the NHS and social services. Remaining independent is important for groups because it gives them the freedom to speak openly. When peer groups link with similar groups their power base increases due to larger member numbers and shared knowledge. I believe that sharing knowledge has been the key reason behind the service user-led movement becoming stronger. The aim of all the groups is the same: to raise the voices of the people who are struggling with their mental health and address their difficulties. Disagreement and debate stimulate ideas and challenge concepts, which can then grow and become more robust. Groups that work alongside each other share knowledge and ideas, and give and receive support.

When groups link with organisations such as the local community mental health team or the NHS they have the opportunity to be part of a larger collective voice. Peer groups often challenge the way services are run and thereby help to inform improvements. The collective voice of a group has more power than an individual voice, saying what needs to be said without fear of personal reprisal. Staff members often want to express similar concerns but fear losing their job or not getting promoted. Furthermore, problems might not be seen by those working in services and little things that can be suggested by groups can have a big impact. This can help shape services, tailoring them to their clientele, thus creating a more effective service. Working together can help improve understanding of the difficulties faced by both the health services and those using them, and therefore erode barriers.

Peer support groups can also influence organisations through service user-led research and training. Groups and networks coming together can lead to research being undertaken that is generated from personal experience, which can lead to results that are directly relevant and useful to the health care services (Shaw & Stapleton, 2011). Peer-led training (with trainers who have direct experience of mental health difficulties) can be relevant and insightful for nursing students, doctors, health professionals, other peers and groups, businesses and carers on numerous topics. Peer support groups can also help train and support each other to be able to develop and deliver training, which increases the confidence and self-esteem of everyone involved.

Sharing knowledge and resources

Peer support and self-help don't only happen within groups. Peer support is far broader and includes books and the Internet. There are many people who, for a variety of reasons, struggle to venture out or find meeting people face to face overwhelming. The Internet can be a useful resource for sharing ideas and finding out about alternative concepts in mental health. Publications of all sorts can provide valuable information, expanding knowledge around mental health issues and giving a much-needed alternative viewpoint based on real-life experiences. Workbooks written by peers can be an alternative way to work through complex issues in your own time, at your own pace and in privacy. For example, the Rushcliffe Support Group have just published a workbook on advance statements (Shaw & Smith, 2011). Advance statements were seen by the support group as a useful tool and it was thought that others might also benefit. Producing a workbook was a way to share this knowledge. They have also written a group book collating individual experiences (Rushcliffe Support Group, 2009).

Publishing is just one of the many creative ways that peer support can reach further afield. The use of art and video is another. Films aired on television and in the cinema can have a huge impact and are a good way of putting information across to a wider audience. Sharing, creating and disseminating knowledge and providing an alternative viewpoint to the medical model, which is predominant in mental health care, are always needed. It can be very distressing when an individual's experience doesn't fit within the model which is being thrust upon them. Having alternative viewpoints available enables individuals to find the model that suits them and explore all the information and options for support and recovery. Groups often help to normalise situations and feelings, recognising that it is OK to feel angry, happy or sad at certain times. Once you have a diagnosis, services often then start to label everything you do or say as a symptom of your mental ill health.

Knowledge ultimately results in an increase in power and choice. If you do not know that certain services are available for support, how can you know to ask to access them? If you are unaware that certain symptoms may be the side effects of a drug you are taking, would you even think about asking for a change or reduction in medication? If you don't know you should have a copy of your care plan, how can you know to request one? If you don't know you can take someone with you to appointments, would you? Just knowing the breadth and variety of support available gives you choice and control over the decisions you make. Often groups provide information on support services not available on the NHS. Knowledge increases power and choice, and ultimately increases the control you have over the decisions that are made.

Conclusion

This chapter highlights what peer support can achieve with a very limited budget and a lot of passion. I have a hope for a future where peer support is more than just an add-on to health care services, but has become an integral part of providing support for those suffering with mental health difficulties. If the health care services really did take heed of what service users are saying they want and need, the services would be shaped very differently. I can envision peer-led respite centres, cafes, training groups, publications and services of all types. Some of these already exist but more are needed. People travel to the Rushcliffe Support Group from four different counties because they don't have a group like it locally.

If peer-led initiatives can achieve what they have done so far on so little, just imagine what they could achieve with more. Peer initiatives happen not because people want to earn huge profits or because of government directives, they happen because people believe and value the support they give, and they survive because they work.

References [2]
Rushcliffe Support Group. (2009). *Discovering Recovery.* UK: Rebecca Shaw in conjunction with Writersworld.
Shaw, B. (2009). *Wonderfully Strange.* UK: Rebecca Shaw in conjunction with Writersworld.
Shaw, B., & Smith, R. (2011). *Advance Statements Workbook.* UK: Rebecca Shaw.
Shaw, B., & Stapleton, V. (2011). *Reality of Crisis.* UK: Rebecca Shaw.

---

2 The referenced books are available through RSG Books – www.rsgbooks.co.uk

Chapter 19

A Critical Journey from Involvement to Emancipation: A narrative account

Theo Stickley

Introduction

The following is a narrative of my journey from a belief in the power of service user involvement to bring about significant change in mental health practice, to a more questioning and critical perspective on notions of involvement. When I came into nurse education at the University of Nottingham 12 years ago, I was immediately introduced to the possibilities of service user involvement in nurse education. There were a handful of lecturers in the mental health branch who were keen to progress this agenda. At the time, the English National Board for Nursing (ENB) had earlier expressed their desire to see service user and carer involvement incorporated into nurse education (ENB, 1996). I soon learnt that in the National Health Service (NHS) service-user involvement had become a key component of government health policy in the UK (DH, 1990, 1991, 1992). Furthermore, it became apparent that I had entered higher education at a time of significant change; the Department of Health (DH) outlined proposals for implementing the vision of a patient-centred care in the NHS Plan (DH, 2001).

Historically, there had been some evidence of service user involvement within our School of Nursing, but this was minimal and relied upon the contribution of one or two individuals who I perceived as 'professional' service users. It was clear that with the enthusiasm and initiative of colleagues, I too could help to bring about some meaningful change in the curricula. Together, we began to think of ways we could extend our research towards the involvement agenda. One way was through supervising dissertation students. One of these, a student on our undergraduate Master of Nursing course, interviewed mental health lecturers about their attitudes to service user involvement for her dissertation, I supervised this work and she went on to get this published (Felton & Stickley, 2004). This has become a widely cited paper in the involvement canon of literature.

Some early efforts

When I first started at the School of Nursing, I also worked part time in practice. I realised that a number of people I had worked with might well enjoy the opportunity to speak with student nurses in the classroom. There were four or five people in particular who worked with me over the first couple of years I was in the school and together we found ways that they could meaningfully contribute to taught sessions. I was proud of this initiative; I felt I was doing something original and inspiring. I had the necessary skills to work with the service users and to facilitate sessions that were meaningful and appropriate. At the same time, a conference was being organised by Pavilion Publishing called 'Crossing Boundaries: User Involvement in Nurse Education' and it was held in Brighton in September 2001. A group of us presented our developments. Although these felt rather tentative, it was evident that other institutions had not progressed as far as we had. Our presentation was written up and was published in *Mental Health Today* (Repper, Hanson, Felton, Stickley & Shaw, 2001). We felt we were on the 'crest of the wave' of contemporary development in this important area. Furthermore, there were other national developments that we could link up with, especially the Mental Health in Higher Education (mhhe) set up by the Higher Education Academy. One of their key themes was 'user and carer involvement'. From this initiative a number of publications, workshops and conferences have since emerged.

One of the organisers of the Pavilion conference, Thurstine Basset, had a background in mental health social work and he began to collaborate with me on books focusing on mental health teaching and learning, but with a strong service user orientation (Stickley & Basset, 2007, 2008). The significance of these texts was that both included chapters written by service users and, as such, became mental health educational textbooks that supported the philosophy of involvement.

The school where we worked was (and still is) extremely supportive of the innovations we were making. The School of Nursing Executive supported the group and in 2002 granted funds to conduct a consultation amongst service users regarding the qualities that service users value in nurses and how these might become priorities in mental health nurse education. It was thought that this consultation would have implications for curriculum development. The report from this consultation, *Carry on Nursing,* has informed subsequent developments in the school.

An overview of *Carry on Nursing*

Making Waves, an organisation whose members have had their own experiences of mental distress and who try to challenge current medicalised understandings of such experiences, were commissioned to hold five workshops/focus groups over a period of several months. There were 15 people at the first meeting and a regular group of between 8 and 10 people at the following meetings. People were paid for their attendance and were supported by the Making Waves co-ordinator. The findings from *Carry on Nursing* have never previously been published and an overview of the report is given below. All quotes below are excerpts from the *Carry on Nursing* report. The report was constructed around these main areas identified by the service user group:

1. Interpersonal skills and the role of nurses
2. Knowledge
3. Services.

Interpersonal skills and the role of nurses
One of the key themes highlighted by the report was around service users wanting to feel 'listened to' and staff 'getting alongside' them. The report noted that:

> It was felt that nurses seldom really listened and were just 'checking you out'; it was also felt that people's opinions, ideas and feelings were not often taken seriously.

The report also noted nuances in how service users viewed the life issues and mental health problems of nurses. The reported noted that:

> Some people came into nursing to try and resolve issues they had and that this sometimes led to nurses 'acting out'. It was felt that the course should assist nurses to examine their reasons for becoming nurses and to provide opportunities for them to deal with these issues.

Service users advocated for more 'explicit support given to staff struggling with mental health issues'. It was felt that employing nurses who had experienced mental health issues would be of benefit and 'would challenge some of the prejudice that sustained a "them and us" mentality'.

Knowledge

In terms of nurses' knowledge there were a number of areas which services users highlighted and critiqued – two key areas were psychiatric drugs and diagnosis. Regarding knowledge of psychiatric drugs:

> It was felt that nurses were often poorly informed about the effects of drugs … There is not enough recognition of the physical and mental ill effects created by different drugs. We also feel it is important that nurses understand the role drug companies play in the promotion of certain 'illnesses' and in shaping government policy.

The *Carry on Nursing* report reflected service users' concerns about diagnosis and questions over what the practice means in mental health. Service users noted that rather than focusing on diagnosis, other issues needed attending to. 'What is more important is that someone has suffered years of damage from powerful drugs, prejudice, institutionalisation, poor medical treatment etc.' The report advocated for 'a critical approach to the categorisation of symptoms'.

Services

There were a number of issues raised regarding the function of services, such as the unequal treatment of some groups in society, for example, older people. 'There was general agreement that older people got a poor service, and many ended up on a cocktail of drugs.' Services users wanted more information about how organisations functioned and decision making in these systems, as it was felt 'large statutory bodies tend to be undemocratic and a major barrier to any kind of user-centred philosophy'.

The consultation also highlighted that service users wanted more information on non-statutory services such as self-help groups (see Rose, 2001), but nurses 'showed very little knowledge about the range of services outside of the Trust'. This appeared to relate to the consulted service users advocating for support with meaningful activities.

The consultation was conducted in early 2003, before service user involvement had become mainstream in the curricula. The findings from the report enabled us to focus on funding applications to develop the work further. This consultation laid the foundations for the development of the Participation in Nurse Education (The PINE Project, 2004[1] to the present; see Roberts, Collier, Shaw & Cook, 2007). Much of this work was ahead of its time in terms of user involvement in nursing and still contains much to be proud of. Many of the above themes highlight ongoing difficulties in services and are clearly important to the development of services and the experience of service users; however, gradually over time I started to question the construction and practice of involvement.

A critical appraisal emerged

What became clear during our years of implementing service user involvement in nurse education was that there were many problems and we had made a number of mistakes. It seemed, however, that these elements were not always discussed in the literature or presented at conferences. I began to develop a critical edge to my thinking. I observed that although there was much policy development that promoted involvement, there was little cash to support it. My own institution was generous, but in the world of research funding there was little opportunity to access funding for nurse educational development (the one exception was The Burdett Trust for Nursing, a nursing research funder). I began to question policy and the discourses that contained the concept of involvement. I began to wonder if the tokenism that I had observed years previously had in fact been translated into policy, with a camouflage of genuineness. I also began to question the ethics of what I had organised years previously by inviting service users to speak in the classroom.

I thus began an inquiry into policy relating to involvement. I supervised a dissertation student (Hui & Stickley, 2007) who examined government policies on involvement, and by using a discourse analysis approach compared government policy language with that of papers written by service users on the same subject. The findings from the research identified concepts occurring within government discourse that revealed how power

1 Acknowledgements: The PINE project was funded by the University of Nottingham, Learning & Teaching Development fund; the SUSA project was funded by the Burdett Trust for Nursing in collaboration with the Nottinghamshire Healthcare NHS Trust. The staff of the University of Nottingham acknowledges the tremendous amount of work that has been delivered by the members of Making Waves. If you would like to contact this organisation please visit their home page: http://www.makingwaves.org/

is exerted through language relating to service users. Differences in perspectives were identified which distinguished government from service user discourses. Greater flexibility in ideas and perspectives was demonstrated by service users, with a seemingly greater range of theoretical underpinnings than government policy enshrined. We concluded that:

> ... greater awareness is needed of the significance of language, of how subtle inferences may be drawn from the rhetorical language of policies, of how these might affect the involvement of service users, and of the implications for the role of mental health nurses. Nurses need to be aware of these tensions and conflicts in managing their practice and in creating a mental health nursing philosophy of 'involvement'. If true 'involvement' is to ensue, nurses may also need to consider the transfer of power to service users. (Hui & Stickley, 2007, p. 416)

Around the same time, I began to study critical realism and wondered if this philosophy might be able to shed some light on the topic. I started by thinking about the language of the topic and whether the words 'service user involvement' themselves might indicate the inherent problems with the concept? I began to question how the concept had been constructed and subsequently construed in health discourse. Whilst it is clear that the concept has been widely accepted in mental health education, I wondered if the nature of this acceptance has resulted in a form of rhetorical assimilation rather than a radical transformation that many of us had once hoped for (Stickley, 2006).

When I set out on my journey of promoting service user involvement, I believed that together we could bring about institutional change for the good. Now however, I'm unsure that 'involvement' is the answer. The institution of psychiatry is, I have come to believe, too powerful, and the notion of service users ascending the power hierarchy is illusive and does not pay adequate regard to the institutional powers that exist within the wider society. If we continue to work within existing models of service user involvement, then the change that is wrought within mental health services will only ever be mediated by those in control of services, to comply with their agenda. In other words, by perpetuating the involvement agenda, I suggest we play into the hands of those who pull the strings. What I have called for is a new way of conceptualising the problem, away from 'involvement' and towards 'emancipation' through collaboration (Stickley,

2006). I suggest that service users establish a power position outside the traditional hierarchy of statutory mental health services. Therefore, rather than service users working in health service institutions, I proposed a more arms-length relationship where those who use services are commissioned as consultants and not in a servant–master relationship.

Mental health nurses are often the workers who have the most contact with service users. It is they who may be expected to implement strategies for involvement. It is essential that mental health nurses therefore give some consideration to the philosophies and approaches that underpin these models. There are opportunities to develop new models and approaches that go beyond involvement and that are genuinely emancipatory for people who use mental health services. These new approaches need to be based upon a more collaborative relationship rather than one of 'involvement' in an unmovable hierarchical system. These models may well provide the framework for consigning the current, inadequate model of service user involvement to history.

When I started working in Higher Education I was highly motivated to embrace the new agenda of involvement that implied emancipation and social justice. In retrospect I was maybe naive, visionary and idealistic. But why should I not be? At the heart of nursing and social work in particular are the values informed by ethics, rights, justice and liberty. I had believed in the philosophy of involvement, but over time, I have also become sceptical of the rhetoric that surrounded it.

Whilst we have achieved much in Nottingham and this is worth celebrating (see Stickley et al., 2009; Stickley et al., 2010, 2011) it is still all too easy to gloss over the difficulties. One example is that whilst the idea of students being assessed by service users sounds highly appropriate and desirable, in reality the research showed how fraught with complexity the idea is in practice. Nevertheless, this is called for by the Nursing and Midwifery Council (NMC) in spite of the lack of research. Furthermore, apart from discovering difficulties from research, there are many barriers to effective change in any organisation and the NHS is the largest employer in the UK; genuine transformation based upon ideas of emancipation is beginning to feel illusory for me. Whilst the notion of user involvement is well established in NHS discourse, I now believe this is largely rhetoric. In reality, systemic barriers exist that are apparently insurmountable. The most obvious barrier is getting access to adequate funds to enable professional practice to develop. For every project we have designed, it has been wholly reliant upon short-term funding. My school at the University of Nottingham has been very supportive and has paid for development work and teaching fees for service users, and more recently has engaged in a Service Level Agreement with Making Waves to provide teaching. However, there is no 'pot' of money from NHS commissioners anywhere, as far as I can make out, that will pay for what is called for in policy. Even the week prior to writing this chapter I was told not to include payments to service users in a Research Council application because it would be rejected.

Even if we were allocated adequate funds to pay for 'service user involvement' there is still the issue of the rigidity of the benefits system that appears to punish people for working part time or on a sessional basis. Huge amounts of money are spent by institutions developing staff, but there is often little money for developing service users and providing training and support for their role in teaching. It is not good enough to 'wheel in' a service user to 'tell their story' and wheel them out again. To tell a story of pain, suffering, loss and so on will take its toll. I would go as far as to say it is unethical to ask this of people. We need robust models of 'service user collaboration' that include training, development, support, supervision, evaluation and so on. But this needs investment and should not be done on the cheap. The NMC are preparing for a new curriculum for nursing and their guidelines are peppered with references to 'user and carer involvement' (note the language that lumps together very different agendas). I recently telephoned the NMC to ask if they would pay for research to provide evidence for the involvement of service users in student assessment (their negative response was inevitable).

Conclusion

This chapter has been one person's narrative of their experiences of trying to facilitate service user involvement. I have believed in the philosophy and ethos of the concept, but I have become sceptical of the practical implications for poorly informed policy. There is a need for robust research, but there appears to be a lack of funds to support such research. One of the beacons in the UK that has promoted the involvement agenda (mhhe) is currently being pared back because of cutbacks. If lack of adequate funding has been a problem in the past, it is set to become an even bigger problem in the future.

There is, I believe, an even bigger problem, and that is one of dominance and power. To retain the established model of involvement (directed by those in power), we reinforce the inferior position of service users in society. I would argue therefore, that instead of involvement, we should be developing emancipatory models of collaboration that not only address the pedagogical reasons for the inclusion of service user views into nurse education, but also address power imbalances inherent in the system (Stickley, 2006; Collier & Stickley, 2010). In practice, this might mean focusing less on service user teaching in classrooms, and more on delivering entire modules or courses or perhaps also reviewing students in practice (see Stickley et al., 2010). The last decade has focused on involvement in nurse education, but across the UK there is little evidence of any shift in power that might bring about significant change in the future.

References

Collier, R., & Stickley, T. (2010). From service user involvement to collaboration in mental health nurse education: Developing a practical philosophy for change. *Journal of Mental Health Training, Education and Practice, 5*(4), 4–11.

Department of Health. (1990). *The NHS and Community Care Act.* London: The Stationary Office.

Department of Health. (1991). *The Patient's Charter.* London: The Stationary Office.

Department of Health. (1992). *The Health of the Nation.* London: The Stationary Office.

Department of Health. (2001). *Involving Patients and the Public in Healthcare: A discussion document.* London: The Stationary Office.

English National Board. (1996). *Learning from Each Other.* London: ENB.

Felton, A., & Stickley, T. (2004). Pedagogy, power and service user involvement. *Journal of Psychiatric and Mental Health Nursing, 11,* 89–98.

Hui, A., & Stickley, T. (2007). Mental health policy and mental health service user perspectives on involvement: A discourse analysis. *Journal of Advanced Nursing, 59*(4), 416–426.

Repper, J., Hanson, B., Felton, A., Stickley, T., & Shaw, T. (2001). One small step towards equality. *Mental Health Today, December,* 24–26.

Roberts, S., Collier, R., Shaw, B., & Cook, J. (2007). Making Waves in nurse education: The PINE Project. In T. Stickley & T. Basset (Eds.), *Teaching Mental Health.* Wiley: Chichester.

Rose, D. (2001). *Users' Voices.* London: Sainsbury Centre for Mental Health.

Rush, B. (2008). Mental health service user involvement in nurse education: A catalyst for transformative learning. *Journal of Mental Health, 17*(5), 531–542.

Stickley, T. (2006). Should service user involvement be consigned to history? A critical realist perspective. *Journal of Psychiatric and Mental Health Nursing, 13*(5), 570–577.

Stickley, T., & Basset, T. (Eds.). (2007). *Teaching Mental Health.* Wiley: Chichester.

Stickley, T., & Basset, T. (Eds.). (2008). *Learning about Mental Health Practice.* Chichester: Wiley.

Stickley, T., Rush, B., Shaw, R., Smith, A., Collier, R., Cook, J., et al. (2009). Participation in nurse education: The PINE Project. *Journal of Mental Health Training, Education and Practice, 4*(1), 11–18.

Stickley, T., Stacey, G., Pollock, K., Smith, A., Betinis, J., & Fairbank, S. (2010). The practice assessment of student nurses by people who use mental health services. *Nurse Education Today, 30*(1), 20–25.

Stickley. T., Stacey, G., Pollock, K., Smith, A., Betinis, J., & Fairbank, S. (2011). Developing a service user designed tool for the assessment of student mental health nurses in practice: A collaborative process. *Nurse Education Today, 31*(1), 102–106.

Chapter 20

Rebuilding the House of
Mental Health Services with Home Truths

Bob Diamond

As citizens of a free society, we have a duty to look critically at our
world. But if we think we know what is wrong, we must *act* upon
that knowledge. (Judt, 2010, p. 237)

If I were to imagine mental health services (MHS)[1] to be a house, it
would look something like this: the foundations based on the science
and moral values of a reductionist empiricism and positivism, with the
structural central pillars constructed from medication and psychotherapy.
The furnishings would be the many different types of medication,
nursing, talking treatments and occupational therapies available. The
roof, aiming to provide a covering of benevolent, well-meaning care, is
also thatched with coercion and control. Finally, the history, location
and functions of the property are clearly demarcated and gated through
professional socio-judicial roles and duties. Throughout this chapter I
question the form, structures and functions of the existing house.
Drawing on the values and practice from critical community psychology,
I will illustrate how the house of MHS could be redesigned and utilised
very differently.

This chapter hopes to encourage more personally meaningful,
informative and supportive practice in MHS. Currently, services are not
as inclusive and reflective about distress as is possible; ultimately this
undermines the quality of care provided. MHS have become too dependent
on prescribed medication and psychotherapy protocols with staff deferring
to technical solutions proffered by experts. One consequence is a form of
dependency that makes staff feel less confident to engage meaningfully
with the very people seeking their help. This chapter is not about casting

---

1 The term 'mental health services' (MHS) refers primarily but not exclusively to the services
provided by the National Health Service.

blame at individuals or particular groups of staff working in MHS, equally, the opinions expressed here are open to critical reflection. Significant meaningful improvements to our practice require structural changes and will not be achieved by wallpapering over the cracks.

The history, location and functions of the existing house

We laugh in disbelief and sometimes cry at the ridiculous and life-threatening treatments enforced on people considered mad over the past 150 years. Supposed prophylactic care ranged from spinning people in revolving chairs, drenching them with water, to administering comatose-inducing injections of insulin. Currently the controversial treatment, electro-convulsive therapy, continues. All these interventions, misguided or not, were administered at the time within the sanctioned approval of a system that considered it was acting benevolently (Porter, 1991). Today, we criticise such actions with disdain and consider them inhuman. We assign such acts of cruelty and barbarity to the annals of history. The likelihood of reoccurrences is dismissed on the grounds that we know better now. It is all too easy from the armchair of historical reflection to appear wisely informed and to believe that we have learnt our lessons. Given that with each new generation of care providers, we have, in retrospect, become alarmed by the nature of care, what makes us any more certain that we are not currently unintentionally inflicting harm on one another? Imagine 50 years ahead, what will the new generation of care providers reflect on and stare in disbelief at in our current practice? Of course we cannot be sure in our predictions, but when our current practice is viewed through a critical constructive lens we are more sensitively informed to anticipate future concerns.

It appears, over time, that there have always been some people who act in more extreme ways. Over the last two millennia we have in one way or another termed some of this behaviour as mad. Yet it is only very recently, in the past 100 years or so, that MHS and most specifically, psychiatry, have offered their services as gatekeepers and custodians of the supposed welfare of madness. For the past 60 years we have had specific legislation to enforce such powers. Although it is now possible for other professions to undertake the role of responsible clinician, the role of enforcing mental health law and removing people's civil liberties through detention currently remains more or less with the profession of psychiatry.

There may always be a role required by society for intervening in extreme behaviours. However, whilst this role remains within the same profession, essentially psychiatry, as a society we must recognise that the role of carer is at the same time contradicted and any provision of treatment and support compromised by the role of imposing sanctions of detention and loss of liberty. Nowhere, to my knowledge, is this stark conflict of interests openly debated when attempting to make sense of and respond to extreme distress. Inevitably, care and compassion are entwined with control and coercion. As a society with a commitment to democracy we must develop more open reflective spaces to address these tensions. Currently our MHS often impose a paternalism resembling the forms and functions of control rather than care and compassion.

The foundations of the house of MHS

The epistemological foundations of the existing house are cemented in a search for categorical axioms. Psychiatry and psychology are guilty of advocating an atomistic view of human behaviour. Theories are privileged that propose distress can be understood through a reductionist process in the search for isolated constituent parts and our knowledge is based on a dualism separating mind and body. Psychiatry has looked in vain, despite very richly backed research, to identify genetic and biological causal explanations for mental health difficulties (Kendler, 2005; Joseph, 2003). Psychology tends to consider human behaviour in isolation from the wider social, political context in which it is embedded. Furthermore, psychology, like psychiatry, then searches for explanations for distress residing within the individual, for example, dysfunctional cognitive schema and fragile ego-strength. Our current philosophical and theoretical foundations for understanding distress are unstable and the cause of serious cracks in the structures from which our practices are developed. Equally of concern, an epistemology premised on positivism encourages a proliferation of misleading and misplaced practices, such as: the prioritising of randomised controlled trials as the 'gold standard' for the National Institute for Health and Clinical Excellence evidence (Midlands Psychology Group, 2011); the quadrupling of diagnostic categories over the past 60 years (Mayes & Horwitz, 2005); and the 10-fold increase in use of psychotropic medication over the past 20 years (Law, 2006). At the same time there has been a proliferation of psychotherapies and psychological techniques. The culture of care and compassion is increasingly obfuscated and manipulated by the allure of the latest brands and technical fixes.

We live our lives always within touching distance of madness; at times the distress surfaces, affecting us more publicly. We are never far from experiencing the depths of despair, yet equally, at times we can be close to a sense of meaning and purpose that enables us to create healthy spaces within which distress can be helpfully managed. The discerning line is much more delicately poised than we often wish to recognise. Madness co-exists alongside wellbeing, although we strive to tease them apart as if they were distinctly opposed entities. It is as though we have sectioned off a potential side of our humanity: madness. Staff work in MHS from a commitment to ease distress, however, our understanding of distress is obscured by processes of reifying, mystifying and professionalising the theories and practices of responding to madness. Through these processes we deny our own potential for madness and segregate it into those receiving diagnostic labels. We have simply made such experiences much more complicated than necessary, or most importantly, than helpful. Such segregation stops us from considering how our potential madness is always a reflection on the values and structures in society. Even with an honest and open appraisal of these values and structures, we cannot replace them overnight, although we can look to other theories for values to inform our practice. By considering values that go beyond our contemporary culture's fixation on the all-consuming individual, we can consider what influence this may have on the role of caring within MHS.

The structures and furnishings of the house

The existing house of MHS is constructed from two central pillars, psychotropic medication and talking treatments, both relatively modern developments. Interestingly, it was only 60 years ago that the use of medication for distress was not considered to be addressing pathological and organic causes located within the brain (Healy, 2006; Moncrieff, 2008). Rather, it was simply observed that some related medications appeared to have particular effects that may be considered prophylactic and ameliorative. Such accounts were based on what could be observed, which is a more honest account based on observable facts. Moncrieff (2008) has shown that during this period psychiatry transformed its role from the process of prescribing medications into identifying taxonomies of illnesses that purportedly could be correspondingly cured by medications. A century of richly invested research has failed to identify specific genetic causes of human distress. The diagnostic models of supposedly discrete conditions that psychiatry refers to as diagnoses and illness remain unreliable, have poor validity and are relatively meaningless (Kendler, 2005). Again, it is interesting to note that 20 years ago, as the relatively newer brands of medication described as 'atypicals' were promoted, they were considered to represent a breakthrough in addressing significantly distressing behaviour including auditory and visual hallucinations. Now we have evidence (Lewis & Lieberman, 2008) suggesting that the newer medications are no more effective than the older more-established medications, although they bring a range of different negative effects with them. A similar picture arises when the evidence for the effectiveness of antidepressants is considered. Outcomes for the use of antidepressant medication should be considered much more cautiously than the pharmaceutical companies would indicate (Healy, 2006; Kirsch, 2011). Moncrieff (2008) proposes a 'drug-centred' model of understanding the effects of medication as opposed to the present mainstream paradigm of illness, diagnoses and cure. This approach is more honest, meaningful and helpful for understanding the effects of psychotropic medications. One of the consequences of the over-reliance on the importance of medication in MHS is that staff become passive sentinels guarding and overseeing the delivery of medication cocktails. A second consequence is that it closes down other discourses such as the significance of abusive histories and current injustices. Staff are denuded of autonomy, they become diffident to a source of knowledge beyond their daily grasp. This helplessness extends across their work, limiting their sense of competence when qualities such as taking initiatives with practical support and enquiry through gentle, respectful curiosity are essential in providing support to people seeking help.

The second pillar of the existing house of MHS is psychotherapy, whilst not as influential as the structure of medication, it nonetheless contributes unnecessarily to restrictive practices in MHS. What is at the heart of all that is decent about talking approaches includes a real sense of support, comfort, clarifying and encouraging through conversations, many of the things David Smail (2001) has written about for many years. It is important to be clear here. I am arguing for more accessible, meaningful, engaging dialogue between staff and those seeking help. This includes much more supportive, personal and trusting conversations and, whenever possible, also includes practical, social and material assistance (Diamond, 2008). I am questioning the restrictive practices of select psychotherapies that purport to have a claim of expertise over human distress. There is a very established body of evidence, collected over many years (Bergin & Garfield, 1994; Epstein, 1995; Moloney, 2006) clarifying that when talking approaches are helpful, the overwhelming majority of good outcomes are due to common factors and not due to specific techniques for specific conditions. Clearly there are many implications from this evidence, but the point I would like to make here is that one consequence of the marketing and branding of psychotherapies is that many staff working in MHS do not feel confident to enter into supportive conversations with the people they are caring for and therefore shy away from doing so.

Working in the house

The dependency on the frameworks proposed by either medication or esoteric psychotherapies censors discussions required to consider additional meanings of distress. This process of dependency on the two pillars can be observed when an ephemeral, popular model or theory arises and for a short while is readily adopted. The temporary and local zeitgeist is usually short lived. Over the past 20 years this has occurred on several occasions, for example, the strengths model (Rapp, 1998). This advocated the inclusion of both the strengths and the personal significance and meaning associated for people seeking help. For a while, MHS embraced these values but without a more substantive philosophical underpinning that respects and embeds the values, their significance does not last. Within a short while the vast majority of discussions within multidisciplinary practice return to revolving around the questionable concept of symptoms of distress and details about histories of contact with MHS. Without reference to wider social factors, reviews of practice prioritise and problematise behaviour, any consideration of environmental factors is lost and clinical discussions often degenerate into catch-all pejorative phrases, such as attention-seeking and manipulative. This is because we have a lack of adequate frameworks to inform our practice.

Within Adult Mental Health Services in Nottingham, clinical psychology, amongst other things, has a history of working in psychiatric services. It has always encountered a challenge to uphold a psychological voice and implement psychological practice beyond merely providing individual psychotherapy. The question remains, where should psychologists position themselves in order to influence change, inside the existing structures or perhaps further afield? Positioned too far away renders any contribution isolated and unheard. If too close, psychologists run the risk of merely propping up the practice of psychiatry. Local clinical psychologists have tried to challenge the dominant discourse of psychiatry by adopting a critical constructive perspective in the various following ways: user involvement (Diamond, Parkin, Morris, Betinis & Bettersworth, 2003), values and practice (Houghton & Diamond, 2010), and establishing public debates (Keenan & Coles, 2012). They question the narrow dominant psychiatric discourse by producing regular summary information sheets entitled *Bite-Size* that provide socio-psychological accounts of the many clinical areas within MHS. *Bite-Size* is distributed widely across most staff groups in Nottingham Adult Mental Health Services.

The architecture of the ossified structures of the MHS monolith designed by psychiatry extends to cover any new and promising developments. Take the concept and practice of recovery (e.g., Repper & Perkins, 2003), which, despite its potential strengths and significant training initiatives based upon the concepts of recovery, has had only a questionable impact on practice. Many users of services now have the jaundiced view that recovery is simply another byword for rebranding the same old services. Rather than introducing new structures and blowing a freshness of ideas through our MHS house, recovery has become bogged down and left to mop up the puddles in the house from the shaky foundations and leaking roof.

Sometimes we lose sight of doing the more obvious decent things – why does this occur? Why, at times, is doing the decent thing not obvious to us all in mental health services? I think the limitations are more endemic, structural and embedded in the culture of MHS and power. All too often, we, as workers in MHS, defer, or re-refer requests for help due to insecurities and perhaps an excessive protection of practice. Take my profession, clinical psychology and psychotherapy, where on numerous occasions, psychotherapy services would not accept referrals for clients from MHS staff, justifying their actions on the grounds that the potential clients were insufficiently robust, of frail and fragile character, or were unable to access their cognitions. Interestingly, the psychotherapists considered it appropriate to pass such referrals to more generic psychology services for help and support. For me, it is the therapeutic response that is insufficiently robust when clients are denied the opportunity of a potential listening and supportive ear.

The behaviours I have experienced and described above are the consequences of a system that strips away all that is good about collaborative, supportive and caring responses to one another, leaving us in a state of occupational anomie.

Redesigning the house of MHS

What if, hypothetically, we were to redesign the house of MHS from a perspective of 'veiled ignorance' (Sandel, 2010) based on what we know about the efficacy and limitations of psychotropic medication and psychotherapy, but not knowing which of us in the future may require support from MHS? I suggest that we would design services that were much more inclusive, diverse and democratic, based on home truths that actively promote acting decently towards one another. In practice this would include a more judicious use of medication with clearer information available. The relationship and decision-making process between prescriber and recipient would be more open and interactive, with greater influence for the person receiving medication. Supportive conversations would replace esoteric psychotherapies. I have already stated that the latest brands of technique-driven talking treatments would be replaced by accessible supportive conversations that gave validity to the damage and traumas people suffer. Furthermore, all staff would be encouraged to support people using services to make sense of their experiences, make connections in society privately and publicly, and whenever possible, to achieve some element of control in their lives.

Critical and community psychology (Kagan, Burton, Duckett, Lawthorn & Siddiquee, 2011; Nelson & Prilleltensky, 2010; Orford, 2008) provides a significant framework that challenges the existing hierarchies and corresponding values in society. At its core, critical psychology identifies and challenges the dominant and powerful forces in society that act as sources of oppression, both quietening and marginalising those in society with fewer resources at their disposal. Equally it advocates redressing injustices arising from the poverties and inequalities that maintain the existing power structures and dominant hierarchies. There is a strong body of evidence highlighting the relationship between forms of oppression, social inequality and experiences of distress (Melzer, Fryers & Jenkins,

2004; Wilkinson & Pickett, 2009). Perhaps these are lofty aspirations for MHS but unless we acknowledge the damaging effects of oppression on distress, even though we may feel impotent to do anything about such forces, we are guilty of attending only to factors that support current theories and models of care. Core principles of critical community psychology are: diversity, innovation, liberation, commitment, critical reflection and humility. Rarely do clinical and applied psychology textbooks address the effects of professional power and interests, yet the social, political context in which we are embodied continually impresses and forms us. Critical and community psychology is equally concerned with trying to make a difference. It is as much about doing and reflecting as articulating theories. Ultimately it seeks to establish a democracy based on justice and equality across societies.

The epistemological foundations of our new design would be based on a phenomenological and heuristic enquiry framework of subjective meaning. Our explanations should be informed by a critical realism that embeds distress in historical, social and material settings, and not genetic, biological or intrapersonal determinism. Utilising a science that accepts that it is highly unlikely that we will ever have explanations that fully grasp human distress, it is, therefore, essential to embrace modesty and humility. We require a science that facilitates learning without seeking to establish itself as the conclusive authority. We also need to acknowledge that it is less meaningful, or reliable, to look to specific taxonomies such as diagnoses and their corollary, medication.

The structures and furnishings of the house are likely to include medication and talking treatments, but with much less emphasis on the esoteric, technical expert qualities of both. The potential benefits of medication would be incorporated but within a greatly reduced role, much closer to the framework advocated by Moncrieff (2008). Talking treatments would be less dependent on expert-therapists and more grounded in supportive conversations that respected historical, social and material contexts, very much along the lines advocated by Holmes (2010). The protective roof would require more preventative qualities that not only attended to care and compassion, but also addressed social inequalities and forms of oppression in society. Above all, future MHS must acknowledge the current tensions between providing care and exercising control. It is likely that both roles will be required in future societies, but should they be undertaken by the same service and profession? Society must also consider how to achieve greater transparency and scrutiny of acts of social control. Future MHS must create open, democratic spaces where all voices can be heard and justly responded to.

Rebuilding the house of MHS

This final section elaborates on the redesigning of the house of MHS by drawing further on ideas from critical community psychology and briefly provides an example of practice. The latter is a tentative exploration of ideas and practice to test out service development in MHS from a different set of values and priorities. As such it is a springboard for further action and always open to critical reflection. The emphasis of this section is on encouraging future ideas and practice backed by similar values.

Services must encourage staff to be gently curious through comforting, caring conversations. When staff were asked what initially motivated them to work with people experiencing distress, the vast majority said that they had wanted to make a difference, that they had considered they may be able to help and that they were simply interested in people. This is to their credit and has been, hitherto, spinal to the NHS. MHS are at serious risk of losing such admirable qualities.

I would like to describe an initiative that aimed to retrace and if possible regain some of the values and interests that initially inspired staff to work in MHS. It focuses on promoting and maintaining a socio-psychological presence on acute inpatient wards. The initiative hoped to get beyond simply delivering another staff training initiative that often tends to either preach to the converted or fall on deaf ears. Embracing the values and principles of critical community psychology, I was keen to explore what could be applied within inpatient services of MHS. Backed by a philosophy of learning that encourages us to maintain an open, reflective mind and a desire to work from home truths and to act decently, I wondered what could be done to encourage a more interactive, personally engaging atmosphere on wards. Whilst this example applies to the context of psychiatric admission wards, in general the philosophical values and underpinnings could apply to other MHS settings, such as the problematic nature of community treatment orders and the dilemmas facing community staff.

There have been many difficulties within inpatient MHS and Johnstone (2000) has identified significant structural abuses and abusers within psychiatry. The personal damages and distress encountered by inpatients in MHS is well documented (Rogers, Pilgrim & Lacey, 1993; Read & Reynolds, 1996). Psychiatric inpatient services have identified a number of problems in recent years (Sainsbury Centre for Mental Health, 2006), amongst others, accommodation issues, lack of involvement and extremely limited emotional support whilst living on wards.

Encouraged by the initiatives of Holmes (2010) to 'start small' but start somewhere, and buoyed by the evidence on non-specific factors in the outcomes of psychological therapy (Frank, 1991), I was keen to encourage more personal, meaningful engagement between staff and people using inpatient services. Holmes advocates the importance of building up support networks, a coming together of similar minds, sharing information that strips away technical and professional language in favour of plain speaking and acting collaboratively with modesty. Myself, a deputy ward manager and an occupational therapist introduced a ward staff development initiative, 'Working Therapeutically on Wards'. I have described the framework elsewhere (Diamond, 2008). Learning from critical and community psychology, we were keen to encourage a collaborative, participative learning environment, one that recognised that all staff brought with them strengths and qualities to share with one another. We, the facilitators, were keen to avoid being considered by staff as experts. Equally, we hoped to emphasise the importance of values and practice that were structured on theories that considered the environment as central to human behaviour and at least aspired to justice, and social equality. We considered ourselves to be kindred spirits, committed to making changes to the existing ward culture. We recognised the importance of supporting both one another and staff when faced with the tensions and dilemmas of institutional care.

It is not the aim of this chapter to elaborate on the contents of the staff development initiative, suffice to say, a significant number of staff from acute services undertook the two-day practice development. Our aim was to get beyond the fears, individually and institutionally, of trying something different. We all shared what it was like to try something a little different, being willing to make fools of ourselves, being open to failing and ultimately, as one participant summed up, 'willing to give it a go'. This initiative centred on the key considerations described below. Staff were encouraged to develop therapeutic working with people seeking their help by embracing the importance of being together, doing together and talking together. As facilitators we had learnt home truths from previous collaborations with people using MHS that the following were most valued.

- the importance of small talk and ordinary conversations
- being human and accepted
- engaging in personally meaningful activities
- combating discrimination
- encouragement with future social connections
- taking some control and having choices.

Although secondary to our principle aims, we included a pre-staff development and 18-month follow-up brief questionnaire that recorded significant increases in the levels of psychological practice provided by both individual staff and ward teams.

Whilst the initiative may look similar to most forms of staff training and development, the values and practice were structured on substantially different foundations and with more inclusive aims; as such, we hope the initiative contributes more meaningful, informative and sustainable changes. The initiative drew from critical community psychology (Kagan et al., 2011), namely, liberation, innovation and diversity, critical reflection and humility.

- liberation from the dogmatic dominant discourse of psychiatric biological determinism

- innovation and diversity to recognise our own limitations and to step beyond them into a less familiar setting to try something different

- critical reflection, humility and modesty: acknowledging a fear of looking silly in front of colleagues, embarrassment with potential failures, a willingness to acknowledge when working with uncertainty that we may be unsure what to do and recognising that our efforts may have limited, if any, success.

Critical reflection

This chapter has argued that if MHS are likened to a house, the foundations are weak, and the structures contain significant cracks. Consequently, the practices are often floundering. Clinical psychology must remain open to the critique that whilst it continues to work in this environment it props up the dominant oppressive psychiatric culture. In keeping with the analogy used in this chapter, the house, I take a leaf from Edward Hollis's wonderful book, *The Secret Lives of Buildings* (2009). Hollis provides accounts of the changing shape and functions of buildings over millennia, noting that the art of a building is not the architect's dream of all that is considered good, rather, the real beauty is the way buildings can transform their shape and function to serve people differently. Arguably, as far as we can see into the future, a house of MHS, in one form or another, will remain. If this is the case, future designs must incorporate the values of justice, equality and democracy. This chapter suggests developing the existing house to accommodate more democratic participation based on home truths that we are already aware of and a willingness to continue acting decently towards one another. In doing so, the reconstructed house of MHS would retain a mere passing resemblance to the one we currently know.

References

Bergin, A., & Garfield, S. (1994). *Handbook of Psychotherapy and Behavior Change.* New York: John Wiley.

Diamond, B. (2008). Opening up space for dissension: A questioning psychology. In A. Morgan, (Ed.), *Being Human: Reflections on mental distress in society* (pp. 174–189). Ross-on-Wye: PCCS Books.

Diamond, R. E., Parkin, G., Morris, K., Betinis, J., & Bettesworth, C. (2003). User involvement: Substance or spin? *Journal of Mental Health, 12,* 613–626.

Epstein, W. (1995). *The Illusion of Psychotherapy.* New York: Transaction Publishers.

Frank, J. (1991). *Persuasion and Healing: A comparative study of psychotherapy* (3rd ed.). Baltimore, MD: Johns Hopkins University Press.

Healy, D. (2006). *Let Them Eat Prozac: The unhealthy relationship between the pharmaceutical industry and depression.* London: New York University Press.

Hollis, E. (2009). *The Secret Lives of Buildings.* London: Portobello Books.

Holmes, G. (2010). *Psychology in the Real World: Community-based groupwork.* Ross-on-Wye: PCCS Books.

Houghton, P., & Diamond, B. (2010). Values-based practice: A critique. *Clinical Psychology Forum, 206,* 24–27.

Johnstone, L. (2000). *Users and Abusers of Psychiatry* (2nd ed.). London: Routledge.

Joseph, J. (2003). *The Gene Illusion: Genetic research in psychiatry and psychology under the microscope.* Ross-on-Wye: PCCS Books.

Judt, T. (2010). *Ill Fares the Land.* London: Allen Lane.

Kagan, C., Burton, M., Duckett, P., Lawthom, R., & Siddiquee, A. (2011). *Critical Community Psychology.* Chichester: BPS Blackwell.

Keenan, S., & Coles, S. (2012). The art of debate. *Clinical Psychology Forum, 233,* 19–22.

Kendler, K. (2005). Towards a philosophical structure for psychiatry. *American Journal of Psychiatry, 162,* 433–440.

Kirsch, I. (2011). *The Emperor's New Drugs: Exploding the antidepressant myth.* New York: Basic Books.

Law, J. (2006). *Big Pharma: How the world's biggest drug companies control illness.* London: Constable & Robinson.

Lewis, S., & Lieberman, J. (2008). CATIE and CUtLASS: Can we handle the truth? *British Journal of Psychiatry, 192,* 161–163.

Mayes, R., & Horwitz, A. V. (2005). *DSM-III* and the revolution in the classification of mental illness. *Journal of the History of the Behavioral Sciences, 41,* 249–267.

Melzer, D., Fryers, T., & Jenkins, R. (2004). *Social Inequalities and the Distribution of the Common Mental Disorders.* Hove: Psychology Press.

Midlands Psychology Group. (2011). Welcome to NICEworld. *Clinical Psychology Forum, 212,* 52–56.

Moloney, P. (2006). The trouble with psychotherapy. *Clinical Psychology Forum (Special Issue on Social Materialist Psychology), 162,* 29–33.

Moncrieff, J. (2008). *The Myth of the Chemical Cure: A critique of psychiatric drug treatment.* Basingstoke: Palgrave Macmillan.

Nelson, G., & Prilleltensky, I. (2010). *Community Psychology: In pursuit of liberation and well-being* (2nd ed.). New York: Palgrave Macmillan.

Orford, J. (2008). *Community Psychology: Challenges, controversies and emerging concensus.* Chichester: John Wiley.

Porter, R. (1991). *The Faber Book of Madness.* London: Faber and Faber.

Rapp, C. A. (1998). *The Strengths Model: Case management with people suffering from severe and persistent mental illness.* Oxford: Oxford University Press.

Read, J., & Reynolds, J. (1996). *Speaking Our Minds: An anthology.* London: Macmillan Press.

Repper, J., & Perkins, R. (2003). *Social Inclusion and Recovery: A model for mental health practice.* London: Baillière Tindall.

Rogers, A., Pilgrim, D., & Lacey, R. (1993). *Experiencing Psychiatry: Users' views of psychiatry.* London: Palgrave Macmillan.

Sainsbury Centre for Mental Health. (2006). *The Search for Acute Solutions: Improving the quality of care in acute psychiatric wards.* London: SCMH.

Sandel, M. (2010). *Justice: What's the right thing to do?* London: Penguin.

Smail, D. (2001). *The Nature of Unhappiness.* London: Robinson.

Wilkinson, R., & Pickett, K. (2009). *The Spirit Level: Why equality is better for everyone.* London: Penguin.

Chapter 21

A Beacon of Hope:
Alternative approaches to crisis –
learning from Leeds Survivor Led Crisis Service

Fiona Venner & Michelle Noad

Leeds Survivor Led Crisis Service (LSLCS) was founded in 1999 by a group of mental health service users, who had campaigned for an alternative to the medical model of psychiatric care for people in crisis. The service was initially run in partnership with Social Services and became a registered charity in 2001. The organisation was set up to be a place of sanctuary and as an alternative to hospital admission or statutory services for people in acute mental health crisis. As a survivor-led service, the organisation continues to be governed, managed and staffed by people who have experienced varying levels of mental distress themselves. We have developed our services based upon the knowledge we have gained through our own experiences of mental distress and use our expertise to help others within a non-diagnostic and non-medical philosophy (Venner, 2009; James, 2010). We also develop our practice in response to the needs articulated by our visitors and callers and their experiences of what is and is not effective in supporting people in acute mental health crisis.

The following chapter will describe the services provided by LSLCS and our practice as a survivor-led person-centred service. We will articulate how we differ from mainstream psychiatric services and our contrasting approaches to diagnosis, power and control, and working with risk. Direct quotes from our visitors and callers will illustrate how and why our services are successful, which will include a discussion on the contested idea of love as a therapeutic tool. We will demonstrate how we support people to resolve or better manage crisis and reduce the risks they present to themselves and other people. Finally we will argue that our approach is not only therapeutically effective, but cost effective.

LSLCS refers to the people who visit Dial House or are involved in group work as visitors and the people who call the Connect helpline as callers. These terms were chosen by visitors and callers themselves as preferable to service user, patient or client and will be used throughout this chapter.

What are the services provided by Leeds Survivor Led Crisis Service?

Connect

Connect is a telephone helpline open from 6 pm to 10.30 pm every night of the year. The service provides emotional support and information for people in distress. We receive around 5,000 calls per year. People can ring who are in crisis, anxious, depressed or lonely and they will be offered non-judgemental and empathic support or information about other services. Connect supports people in crisis, as well as providing a preventative service by supporting people before they reach the point of crisis. Connect also receives funding to provide emotional support to carers. The helpline is staffed by volunteers who have gone through a comprehensive and rigorous training programme and receive ongoing supervision, training and support.

Many of them have their own experiences of mental health problems. There is a paid supervisor on each shift.

Dial House

Dial House is a place of sanctuary open from 6 pm to 2 am every Friday, Saturday, Sunday and Monday. Visitors can access the service when they are in crisis. They can telephone to request a visit, or turn up at the door between 6 pm and 10.30 pm. Visitors can use the house as time out from a difficult situation or a home environment where they may feel unsafe or that may exacerbate their difficulties. Visitors can relax in a homely environment and can also receive one-to-one support from a crisis support worker.

Group work

The service hosts a number of weekly peer-led groups held at Dial House. Peer support allows people to share their experiences of coping with crisis in order to gain new perspectives. This idea for group work came from visitors and they have been supported to develop their skills to the point where they now plan and facilitate the groups themselves, with only minimal support from a group work support worker.

The 'My Time' groups aim to provide social contact and support to people whose crisis is due to chronic isolation and loneliness. 'My Time Wednesday' is an emotional support group where people can explore the effects of crisis and learn new coping strategies in a supportive environment. On Thursdays the social support group 'My Time Thursday' cook a meal and plan activities.

Background and what we believe

LSLCS supports people at acute risk of suicide and/or self-injury. During 2010, 64 per cent of visitors to Dial House were suicidal and self-injury was a presenting issue in 50 per cent of visits. This includes a small minority of people who self-injure in severe or life-threatening ways.

Most of our work is with people who have survived varying forms of trauma, most commonly sexual abuse. The most common issues presented at Dial House are those relating to people's experiences of current or past sexual violence (64 per cent in 2010).

We recognise that the people supported by us not only experience extreme distress because of trauma in early childhood but also because of trauma experienced in mental health services. The mainstream mental health system and the medical model of psychiatric practice have been widely critiqued as being oppressive and coercive (e.g., Bentall, 2003, 2009; Johnstone, 2000; Laurance, 2003). We are also aware of the stigma and discrimination experienced by those who struggle with their mental health. In response to this, our philosophy recognises that 'deprivation and oppression not only impact on people's ability to cope with distress, but can be the cause of distress' (LSLCS, 2007a).

Psychiatric diagnosis is a subject at the core of mental health critique (Tummey & Turner, 2008). However, our therapeutic approach is the person-centred approach (Rogers, 1951). This is non-diagnostic and treats the person as an individual and not as a label. Diagnosis and the person-centred approach are not compatible as conceptual frameworks. Carl Rogers, founder of the person-centred approach, objected to the use of diagnostic labels because they place the locus of evaluation outside of the person and in the hands of professionals (Rogers, 1951). Rogers states, 'there is a degree of loss of personhood as the individual acquires the belief that only the expert can accurately evaluate him and that therefore the measure of his personal worth lies in the hands of another' (Rogers, 1951, p. 224).

The person-centred approach is a phenomenological approach which recognises the validity of the subjective experience and reality of the individual. As Rachel Freeth puts it,

> Within the person-centred approach, phenomenology does not refer to a method of categorising mental experiences. It focuses on a person's subjective experience, as it is, without trying to impose a preconceived framework, define or explain it. The person-centred approach is concerned with how human beings experience the world and construct meaning. (2007, p. 976)

Most of our paid staff are qualified or qualifying person-centred counsellors or therapists. We describe the approach within our practice as follows:

- a belief in the organism's tendency to actualise
- we support the visitor/caller's direction
- the worker and visitor/caller co-create certain facilitative conditions.[1]

With regard to people's tendency to actualise (see Mearns & Thorne, 1999 for further discussion), we understand this to mean that people do the best they can, in the circumstances they are in, with the resources they have and are innately motivated towards growth. Carl Rogers (1951) used the metaphor of potatoes growing in an inhospitable environment to describe it:

> [Whilst the] actualizing tendency can, of course, be thwarted or warped ... it cannot be destroyed without destroying the organism ... They would never become plants, never mature, never fulfil their real potential. But under the most adverse circumstances, they were striving to become. Life would not give up, even if it could not flourish. (Rogers, 1980, p. 118)

When working with self-injury, our approach would be to think of the actualising tendency. We would respect that a caller or visitor is trying their absolute best with the resources that they have and in the circumstances that they find themselves. Even if somebody's self-injury is severe or even life threatening, we would view this as their attempt to survive and grow within the life that they have.

---

1 Keith Tudor supported the organisation to develop this format of describing the person-centred approach during a workshop in 2009.

Furthermore, we support the direction of our visitors and callers. This is often described as 'non-directivity'. This means that we respect the tendency of the individual towards growth and their creative attempt to survive even if we dislike the outcome. For example, when we support someone who is severely disfigured and disabled due to self-injury, we may find this shocking and distressing. However, we respect and understand that the self-inflicted injury was the person's attempt to survive unbearable, intolerable distress.

We refer above to the certain facilitative conditions of the person-centred approach. Carl Rogers defined these conditions as empathy, congruence (being genuine and authentic in the therapeutic relationship) and unconditional positive regard. We interpret this as an aspiration to treat all of our visitors and callers and each other with warmth, kindness, respect and compassion.

When we are working with someone, we support the whole person as the wonderful, complex, challenging being that they are and with whatever they present. In contrast to the medical model, we certainly would not view self-injury, hearing voices, flashbacks or hallucinations as a symptom of a person's disordered personality or illness. For example, if a woman describes inserting razor blades into her vagina, our response would not be to conceptualise this as part of an illness. Rather we would see this as an understandable and logical response in someone who has had a lifetime of sexual abuse and sexual violence and is creatively trying to find a way to stop it from happening again.

How we differ from mainstream psychiatric services

As a survivor-led, person-centred organisation in the voluntary sector, we are on the margins of the mental health system. We exist outside mainstream psychiatry. This position means that we attract people who have slipped through the net of mental health provision, been excluded from services, or with whom services have failed to engage. Some of our visitors have histories of violence, forensic histories and many have been labelled as having a personality disorder.

In contrast to mainstream mental health services, we aim to provide an anti-oppressive service. Our person-centred approach and our respect and attempts to live out values such as equality are at the core of such an anti-oppressive stance (see Dominelli, 1997 for further discussion).

Anxieties with regard to risks can derail such ideals; however, our service Mission Statement says that we aim 'to work sensitively and appropriately with people at risk' (LSLCS, 2007b). In December 2007, we won a Guardian Public Service Award for working with people with complex needs, which demonstrates our success in this area. The following sections demonstrate the ways that we are different to mainstream services which have contributed to this success.

Diagnosis/labelling

As an organisation set up to be an alternative to psychiatric services we are fiercely opposed to the use of psychiatric diagnoses. We pride ourselves on providing a non-medical approach to working with extreme mental distress. Our philosophy is about being alongside people in crisis, not treating them. We also believe passionately in the transformative and healing power of human connection. As our philosophy states,

> We believe that to deal with a crisis, a person must feel safe, listened to, and connected to other people. (LSLCS, 2007a)

The fact that we are a non-diagnostic alternative to the medical mainstream is something our visitors and callers value greatly. All the quotes that follow come from Leeds Survivor Led Crisis Service visitor and caller feedback, 2006–2010.

> *Dial House is mint! It's proper ace, it's decent, proper nice. Staff are really good, they listen and people are well nice to be around. It's cool to be around people who know what you have been through and who understand you – people who don't judge you.*

> *It is different to other services – it is easier to talk to staff. Staff are nice. They don't judge you or put a label on you – saying that's what's wrong with you.*

We are interested in the emerging concept of formulation as an alternative to diagnosis (Johnstone, 2008). In practice this would be developed collaboratively with the person and is an individual summary which holistically examines all areas of a person's life in order to try to identify the reasons behind their problems and to also determine any useful interventions. However, we are aware that at times formulation can be used as a mechanistic form of categorisation; we would see this as incompatible with the person-centred approach.

Power and control

The mental health system can disempower people further due to the lack of control that people often experience within services. For instance, psychiatry has been condemned for detaining people and treating them against their will (Johnstone, 2000). Furthermore, the numbers of people 'detained in hospital have soared by 50 per cent in a decade' (Laurance, 2003, p. xix).

Therefore, much of our appeal to our visitors and callers is that we are in the voluntary sector, as opposed to the public sector. This means that the organisation does not have any statutory powers, so people use our services entirely of their own volition. All our visitors and callers self-refer to Dial House, Connect and our group work. This is highly significant for mental health service users who may have been subject to coercion and compulsory detention under statutory services. The relationship between staff and our visitors and callers has a different, and arguably more positive, dynamic than the interaction of staff with patients who have been sectioned on a locked ward. As one of our visitors states:

> Most of all what I celebrate about your service is not being 'done to'. Others, statutory services, want power, they ask 'who are you?' establish the role and that's very disempowering. I've never had this at all from Connect or Dial House.

Risk

LSLCS's approach to managing risk can be summarised as trusting the innate capabilities of our visitors and callers and giving them as much control as possible in managing the risks they present to themselves and/or other people. We believe in engaging fully with people in relation to risk and allowing them to explore their absolute worst thoughts and feelings without over-reacting. We believe that this is a way of reducing risk. We believe that if you give someone the space to explore in depth, their thoughts, feelings and plans in relation to suicide, this will reduce the risk of it actually happening.

This also applies to risk to others. Over the years, we have supported people to explore difficult feelings, for example, that they want to set fire to their house, harm their brothers, abduct a baby, or steal cars. Our approach to this is to listen very carefully and sensitively question the person to help them work out why they are telling us this. Is it because they actually think they will do it and want us to try to stop them? Or is it because the thought terrifies them and they want to talk about it? Often the latter reduces the power of the thought and makes it less likely that it will happen. We would criticise standard risk assessment tools as reductive and unsubtle because they do not allow scope for such in-depth risk analysis.

LSLCS aims to provide an empowering service and we believe in giving people as much control as possible in managing risk. On several occasions we have supported people who routinely try to end their life at Dial House. This is understandable, as it is an environment where people feel safe and they do not want to end their life at home where their children or partner may find them. When people try to die at Dial House it is obviously both dangerous and distressing. The way we address this is to be very honest with the person and explain that while we do not want to exclude them from the service, what they are doing is unacceptable. We explain to the person that it is not fair to other visitors and staff, and that frequent attendance of ambulances will detract from the sanctuary element of the house. We would ask the person how they think they can continue to use the house in a way that is safe and support them to come up with their own plan for how we manage the risk they present.

Sometimes people may make choices such as having someone with them all the time or only being in the bathroom for a few minutes before we go in. This is interesting because in some ways it looks like special observations in hospital. We would not choose to follow someone around, or open the bathroom door. However, it is amazing how differently people feel about this when it is something they have chosen. So rather than being about containing worker anxiety, it is a way of empowering individuals to take responsibility for the risk they present.

In 12 years we have never had a single serious violent incident. Nor have we had any incidents whereby visitors have been violent to each other or to staff. Furthermore, we have never had a death or serious injury at Dial House. We work with extremely high levels of risk and we doubt that there are many mental health services with such an impressive record of lack of serious incidents. We firmly believe that this is entirely because of the way we treat our visitors and callers, the amount of trust we place in them and the amount of control they retain whilst at Dial House. Therefore, we agree with the approach practised by Maytree, a London-based sanctuary for people who are suicidal, who state: 'We believe that the seemingly high risk option of sticking with trust, often, in the end, carries lesser risks.'[2]

---

2 Maytree website: www.maytree.org.uk

Feedback from our visitors suggests that our approach is effective. Visitors report that that we have successfully supported them to reduce the risks they present to themselves:

I was on the verge of hanging myself, but by visiting the house, and having support, my life was turned around, and even though I still feel really depressed, I think I will be able to get through the night.

Connect helps me to work through my feelings and stop me from cutting and overdosing.

On many occasions, after leaving Dial House and having support has left me emotionally drained and I know I will not go home and do something like end my life. Also I may feel more rational; listening to other visitors also helps me gain perspective.

Why and in what ways are our services effective?

So, if we do not work with diagnoses, nor utilise all the tools, potions and paperwork statutory services have to offer, why and in what ways are our services successful? The survivor movement has pressed for a greater voice in services and assertion of their rights (see Laurance, 2003), therefore we feel that it is most appropriate for our visitors and callers to articulate what it is about our services that is most effective.

In order to ensure that we are providing a respectful, consistent, compassionate and empathic service, we undertake detailed evaluations of our services. Each year, we gather much informative feedback from our visitors and callers. This is collated from a variety of sources including visitor feedback books and questionnaires in Dial House, annual postal questionnaires and also by conducting reviews with regular visitors. We also have a focus group whereby current visitors and callers can contribute towards the development of the service. Furthermore, we have recently recruited two ex-Dial House visitors onto our Management Committee.

The feedback we receive is remarkably consistent and through this we have identified what we refer to as the five elements of effective support:

- listening
- treating people with warmth, kindness and respect

- people do not feel judged or assessed
- being in a different and calm environment
- peer support.

Again, the following quotes are from visitors and callers who have used our service between 2006 and 2010.

Listening

It is a sad indictment of both our society and our mental health system that our visitors and callers experience being attentively listened to as a revelation, although we receive such feedback all too often. The following quote demonstrates the transformative and healing power of feeling that somebody has listened and cares:

> It has made me feel wanted. I can talk to someone who listens. I leave feeling warm, rather than with a cold heart as if I've got nowhere.

Treating people with warmth, kindness and respect

> I'd like to thank all the staff for being supportive towards me, I find it a bit strange, 'cos I am not used to it.

In 2006, Leeds Survivor Led Crisis Service won its first award. This was the Guardian Public Service Award for customer service. The award submission required us to illustrate how we exceeded the expectations of the people who used our services. Our submission used the above quote to demonstrate how low service users' expectations are. The fact that we are kind, affectionate and respectful consistently exceeds the expectations of our visitors and callers:

> Just a short note to say thanks to K for helping me to wash my hair. It seems like such a simple thing to help with, but it is the fact that Dial House are there to help with everything including simple things which makes Dial House such a unique and fantastic place. Thanks again.

As the visitor herself states, it is a small task to support someone to wash their hair. Arguably it is the love underlying the act which has moved the visitor. The next visitor explicitly refers to the love they received at Dial House:

I would be in a real quandary without the kindness and empathy, and companionship which I experience when I come to Dial House. Thank you so much for all your love and support.

It is only having established our reputation and won five national awards that we are beginning to feel confident enough to publicly state that one of the ways our service is effective is that visitors and callers receive love from our staff and from each other. 'Love' is a contested word, which can carry both sexual and 'naff' connotations. Unconditional positive regard is one of the core conditions of the person-centred approach. Carl Rogers has stated that it could be fair to refer to unconditional positive regard as non-possessive love (see Tudor & Worrall, 2006, for discussion). Roger's use of the word could also be described as the form of love called *agape* – love for all of humankind. However, Rogers was also cautious about his use of this word.

Similar to Rogers, we have reservations about discussing love. Arguably, the only way that healing will occur is through the transformative impact of being truly in contact with another person. Yet, we are mindful of the challenges of explicitly referring to love. After all, many of our visitors have been sexually abused in the name of love by people who were supposed to be their caregivers and professed to love them. What we offer is something different; a non-possessive love that does not ask for anything in return.

It can be strange, and even painful, to receive love if you are not used to it. Being treated with compassion, care, kindness and affection can magnify what you did not have as a child and represent a painful contrast to the relationships you have experienced.

The very fact that we will even discuss love is undoubtedly one of the factors that differentiates us from a diagnostic approach to mental distress. This difference is reflected in our policies and our practice. One of the longest sections in our staff code of conduct concerns touch, as we often hug our visitors. We strive to be extremely thoughtful and mindful with regard to this physical representation of love, which would almost always be initiated by the visitor. Our code outlines that it is a personal choice if staff hug visitors. It states that staff must be aware of the visitor's history, gender issues and also self-aware regarding their own personal boundaries and history in relation to touch.

Occasionally, our approach causes difficulties. One of the authors had the experience of hugging a visitor, whom she believed was about to hug her. The visitor had in fact been going to shake her hand and was overwhelmed by the physical contact as it was the first time in 15 years that he had been hugged. This was a painful experience for the visitor, but one he was able to work through within the containing boundaries of Dial House and his relationship with the worker. It is now the case that whenever the visitor meets the worker, he jumps up and hugs her.

Many organisations, statutory and voluntary, simply apply a no-touching rule, and arguably this is safer as you will not encounter difficult scenarios such as the one described above. We would see our willingness to take risks in an area as contested as love and touch as our greatest strength. To withhold this would feel as though we were denying our visitors the potency of the human connectedness necessary for development and emotional healing.

People do not feel judged or assessed

> The crisis support workers at Dial House have been very supportive and non-judgemental towards my behaviours.

The person-centred approach asserts that all behaviour is understandable: 'Behaviour is basically the goal-directed attempts of the organism to satisfy its needs as experienced, in the field as perceived' (Rogers, 1951, p. 491). All behaviour, however challenging, is the person's attempts to meet their needs; or trying to do the best they can, in the circumstances they are in, with the resources they have. Holding this in mind enables us to respect the visitor's attempt to meet their needs, even if the manifestations of this are truly terrible.

Visitors and callers also tell us that the fact that we do not support them according to their diagnostic label is valued:

> When I've talked to people and tell them I have paranoid schizophrenia they have walked away, but you lot listen. Can tell people here what illness is – you don't give me a title [label].

> Staff are genuine and totally different to the rest of the system. Non-judgemental. Staff treat you better than in the rest of the system.

Being in a different and calm environment

> *Thank you for getting me away from the funny farm for a couple of hours, the peace and quiet was a nice change from the noisy, hectic, crazy ward.*

People can visit Dial House when they are inpatients, even if they are under section, providing they have permission to leave. The above quote powerfully illustrates that people in acute mental health crisis need a sanctuary or a place of asylum. The quote starkly highlights that this is often not how inpatient wards are experienced. The person refers to the noise and chaos of the ward and Dial House providing a welcome break from this. Laurance (2003) reports psychiatric wards as being dirty, overcrowded and unpleasant. However, Dial House provides an alternative environment:

> *The house has a special feel of welcome. I really like not having a TV in the main room. I like all the little extras like towels and fruit on the table.*

> *The house itself has a tremendous aura of peace. You feel better as soon as you close the door and shut out the world. There is food available should you need a meal, and staff to help you mix with other visitors and eventually to become calm.*

Peer support

Visitors gain as much support from each other as from staff at Dial House. It was a recognition of this that led us to develop our peer-led group work. Peer support can counter the stigma of having a mental health problem and reduce isolation and loneliness:

> *It gives me a break. By being around people in the same situation as you; you are not having to feel ashamed.*

> *Social time has helped my confidence. I couldn't trust strangers before coming here and now I have made some friends and met some lovely people.*

Cost effectiveness

In addition to the positive impact we have on the lives of our visitors and callers, we prevent people from the need to use statutory mental health services and the medical services provided by Accident and

Emergency. In 2009, our organisation was reviewed by our funders, NHS Leeds and Leeds City Council. One of the conclusions of their review was that there was considerable evidence that our services saved money of other parts of the health economy such as inpatient units, Accident and Emergency and the ambulance service. They also concluded that we supported other teams, such as the statutory Crisis Resolution Team, to function more effectively.

In recognition of both the cost effectiveness of our services and their therapeutic value for visitors and callers, we have received a significant increase in funding from NHS Leeds. Until recently, Dial House was not open on a Monday night. We have been given increased funding to expand the Dial House provision and to also undertake a project targeting people who present to accident and emergency departments in Leeds having self-injured. In the current financial climate, this is a great testimony to the efficacy of our non-medical approach to working with people in mental health crisis.

In addition to this, we have demonstrated our value further by having a Social Return on Investment (SROI) analysis undertaken about our organisation. SROI is a credible national tool which is used to demonstrate the impact of projects which are difficult to evaluate, such as regeneration schemes or community development teams. Through a process involving consultation with all stakeholders, an SROI consultant undertakes a cost-benefit analysis. By comparing the costs of an organisation to its benefits, you can demonstrate cost savings to the community and the long-term value of investment. An organisation ends up with an SROI ratio. Our ratio is £1 to £5.17. This means for every pound invested in Leeds Survivor Led Crisis Service, society gets £5.17 back. Or the £375,000 invested in our organisation over 2010–2011 becomes just under £2 million.

The challenges of mainstream funding

As outlined above, LSLCS receives almost all of its funding from the NHS and Leeds City Council. We are funded directly by the statutory sector to offer an alternative approach to that provided in statutory services. Despite being highly critical of diagnostic approaches to mental distress, most people are signposted to our services from secondary mental health care and we liaise extensively with the statutory Crisis Resolution Team and the Leeds Personality Disorder Clinical Network (LPDCN). Yet, we also remain firmly outside the statutory mental health system.

This interesting tension is highlighted by our relationship with LPDCN. Whether to partner LPDCN was a dilemma given we do not recognise the term 'personality disorder' or work within a diagnostic framework. The partnership succeeds because LPDCN respects the politics of the voluntary sector and understands that it is in the interest of their clients, who have traditionally been poorly served by mainstream psychiatry, that we are seen as outside the NHS. Both we and LPDCN refer to the partnership as at a distance. LPDCN funds our services, whilst respecting our autonomy.

It is essential that LSCLS is valued by staff working within mainstream services so they continue to signpost people to us. At the same time, we strive to maintain our identity as a radical, innovative alternative to statutory care. Achieving this balance is an ongoing challenge, requiring both passion and diplomacy.

Concluding comments

Over the last 12 years, we have been highly successful in providing a viable alternative to the medical model of care for people in acute mental health crisis. Our structure, team work, model, philosophy and practice enable us to work effectively with people who are in acute states of distress and at high risk. We believe our success is due to treating our visitors and callers with warmth, kindness and respect and having high expectations of them, whatever label they have been given. We believe this approach has a greater influence than any clinical technique.

This chapter is entitled 'A Beacon of Hope' because this is part of the title of an article written about us in *Mental Health Today* on the event of our tenth birthday (James, 2010). It is also a direct contrast to the hopelessness of being told that your personality is disordered or that you have a severe and enduring psychotic illness. At Leeds Survivor Led Crisis Service we attempt to hold hope for our visitors and callers even when they cannot hold it for themselves. We believe that people can and do recover from extreme distress. There are many inspiring examples within our team of people who have personal experience of mental health crisis. We have received feedback from our visitors that this in itself is a hopeful aspect of a survivor-led service.

> *I think Dial House staff are so dedicated to their work and the service users that they all deserve a medal or some form of recognition! At the minute I*

am not able to work due to my mental illness being at its worst ... However, in the future all being well, I hope to become a volunteer at Dial House. Survivor-led help is amazing because I know that people who talk to me here understand what I am going through. Thanks for being my glimmer of hope – every cloud has a silver lining and Dial House is mine. Smile.

This chapter has provided a brief overview of our services and philosophy and has described how we are now extremely well established as an alternative to mainstream services. We pride ourselves on being a person-centred survivor-led mental health crisis service. Although we differ in our approach to diagnosis, labelling, power, control and risk, we consistently receive positive feedback from our callers and visitors whilst maintaining professional relationships with statutory services.

Our work demonstrates that the restoration of positive mental health for those experiencing crisis relies on human connection, relationships and feeling that one is part of humanity. Our 'progressive' and 'radical' approach to mental distress has proven successful, cost effective and valuable. Therefore, we would recommend that our approach should inform the practice of all mental health professionals and should be at the centre of all future mental health services.

References

Bentall, R. P. (2003). *Madness Explained: Psychosis and human nature.* London: Penguin.

Bentall, R. P. (2009). *Doctoring the Mind: Why psychiatric treatments fail.* London: Penguin.

Dominelli, L. (1997). *Anti-racist Social Work* (2nd ed.). Basingstoke: Macmillan.

Freeth, R. (2007). *Humanising Psychiatry and Mental Health Care: The challenge of the person-centred approach.* Oxford: Radcliffe Publishing.

James, A. (2010). A beacon of hope. *Mental Health Today*, February, 18–19.

Johnstone, L. (2000). *Users and Abusers of Psychiatry* (2nd ed.). London: Routledge.

Johnstone, L. (2008). Psychiatric diagnosis. In R. Tummey & T. Turner (Eds.), *Critical Issues in Mental Health* (pp. 5–52). Basingstoke: Palgrave MacMillan.

Laurance, J. (2003). *Pure Madness: How fear drives the mental health system.* London: Routledge.

Leeds Survivor Led Crisis Service. (2007a). *Philosophy.* Leeds: LSLCS. Available to download from http://www.lslcs.org.uk/what-do-we-do/what-we-believe

Leeds Survivor Led Crisis Service. (2007b). *Mission Statement.* Leeds: LSLCS. Available to download from http://www.lslcs.org.uk/what-do-we-do/mission-statement

Mearns, D., & Thorne, B. (1999). *Person-Centred Counselling in Action* (2nd ed.). London: Sage.

Rogers, C. R. (1951). *Client-Centered Therapy.* London: Constable.

Rogers, C. R. (1980). *A Way of Being.* Boston: Houghton Mifflin.

Tudor, K., & Worrall, M. (2006). *Person-Centred Therapy: A clinical philosophy.* London: Routledge.

Tummey, R., & Turner, T. (Eds.). (2008). *Critical Issues in Mental Health.* Basingstoke: Palgrave MacMillan.

Venner, F. (2009). Risk management in a survivor-led crisis service. *Mental Health Practice, 13*(4), December, 18–22.

Contributors

Peter Beresford

Peter Beresford, OBE, is Professor of Social Policy and Director of the Centre for Citizen Participation at Brunel University. He is also a long-term user of mental health services and Chair of Shaping Our Lives, the national user-controlled organisation and network. He has a long-standing involvement in issues of participation, as writer, researcher, educator and campaigner and is co-editor of *Social Care, Service Users and User Involvement* (Jessica Kingsley Publishers, 2012).

Mary Boyle

Mary Boyle is Professor Emeritus of Clinical Psychology at the University of East London, where she was Director of the Clinical Psychology Masters and then Doctorate Programmes for over 20 years. She was also an NHS psychologist initially in adult services and more recently in women's health. Her main interests are in critical analyses of the medical model and the development of alternatives, and in feminist approaches to women's health. She has published widely in these areas.

Joan Busfield

Joan Busfield is a Professor in the Department of Sociology at the University of Essex. She has a long-standing interest in psychiatry and mental illness stemming from early training as a clinical psychologist at the Tavistock Clinic. Publications include: *Managing Madness* (Heinemann, 1996); an edited collection, *Rethinking the Sociology of Mental Health* (Blackwell, 2001); *Mental Illness* (Polity, 2011); and a paper 'Challenging claims that mental illness is increasing and mental well-being declining' (*Social Science and Medicine,* 2012). She has also researched the pharmaceutical industry. Papers include 'Pills, power, people: Sociological understandings of the pharmaceutical industry' (*Sociology*, 2006), and '"A pill for every ill": Explaining the expansion in medicine use' (*Social Science and Medicine*, 2010).

David Cohen

David Cohen is Professor of Psychopathology and Psychopharmacology at the School of Social Work of Florida International University, Miami, USA. He seeks to develop lines of critical thought as alternatives to biopsychiatric conceptions of distress and misbehaviour and to conventional views about the safety, efficacy, and purposes of psychiatric drug treatments. He held the 2012 Fulbright-Tocqueville Distinguished Chair to France. He is the author of *Mad Science* (with Stuart Kirk and Tomi Gomory) (Transaction Publishers, 2013), and the forthcoming *Ethical Psychopharmacology* (with Shannon Hughes).

Steven Coles

Steven Coles is a clinical psychologist in adult mental health services in Nottingham. He is questioning of how power is used and misused within mental health services and society. The stories recounted to him of fear, misery and madness have helped him to understand the social and material nature of these experiences; as well as how current cultural values and morality shape the responses of society and mental health services. Steven attempts to bring issues of power, the social material world and ethics to the forefront of his role, including publications, debates, conferences, as well as sharing and reflecting on ideas with staff, people within services and those outside the organisation.

Dirk Corstens

Dirk Corstens works as a psychiatrist and psychotherapist in Maastricht in the Netherlands at RIAGG Group, a community mental health centre. He was trained in psychodynamic, systems and cognitive psychotherapy and adapted the Voice Dialogue approach to voice hearing. He is chair of the Intervoice Board and has specialised in the treatment of voice hearers and conducts research on that subject.

John Cromby

John Cromby is in the Psychology Division, SSEHS, Loughborough University. Previously, he worked at the Universities of Bradford and Nottingham and in mental health, drug addiction and intellectual impairment settings. His research focuses on the ways that bodies and social processes come together to constitute experience, and involves engaging with topics such as the feelings associated with crime, death and paranoia; with methodological issues to do with measuring happiness and other emotions and feelings; and with basic psychological categories such as belief. Until 2012 he co-edited the journal *Subjectivity*, and he was co-editor of the books *Social Constructionist Psychology* (Open University Press, 1999) and *Theoretical Psychology: Global transformations and challenges* (Captus University Publications, 2011). With Dave Harper and Paula Reavey he wrote the textbook *Psychology, Mental Health and Distress* (Palgrave Macmillan, 2013).

Bob Diamond

Bob Diamond is a clinical psychologist and mental health advisor currently working in Higher Education. He is interested in enduring mental health difficulties and drawing on the ideas and practice from critical and community psychology. When previously working in adult mental health services, he sought to establish a psychological presence whilst questioning the oppressive dominance of psychiatry. He advocates more personally meaningful supportive services that acknowledge and, where possible, address historical, material and social injustices. He is a member of the Midlands Psychology Group.

Jacqui Dillon

Jacqui Dillon is a campaigner, writer, international speaker and trainer specialising in hearing voices, psychosis, trauma and recovery. Jacqui is Chair of the Hearing Voices Network, England, and Honorary Lecturer in Clinical Psychology at the University of East London. Jacqui's experiences of surviving childhood abuse and subsequently using psychiatric services inform her work and she is an outspoken advocate and campaigner for humane, trauma-informed approaches to madness and distress.

Anne Felton

Anne Felton is a lecturer in mental health nursing at the School of Nursing, Midwifery and Physiotherapy, University of Nottingham. Her practice and academic interests include risk, positive risk-taking, social inclusion and supervision within pre-registration education. Prior to joining the school she worked in rehabilitation adult mental health services.

Dave Harper

Dave Harper worked in NHS mental health services for a decade before moving to the University of East London where he is a Reader in Clinical Psychology. His research interests are in applying critical psychology and social constructionist ideas to the understanding both of distress (particularly paranoia and unusual experiences and beliefs) and the work of mental health professions. He is a co-author of *Deconstructing Psychopathology* (Sage, 1995) and *Psychology, Mental Health and Distress* (Palgrave MacMillan, 2013) and a co-editor of *Qualitative Research Methods in Mental Health and Psychotherapy* (Wiley, 2012). He also works clinically in Newham as part of the Systemic Consultation Service.

Guy Holmes

Guy Holmes works as a clinical psychologist in a CMHT in Shropshire. His book *Psychology in the Real World: Community-based groupwork* (PCCS Books) came out in 2010. He also co-edited *This is Madness* and *This is Madness Too* (PCCS Books, 1999, 2001) and has published in the areas of critical psychology, psychiatric medication, the medicalisation of human distress and toxic mental environments. More information can be found on www.psychologyintherealworld.co.uk

Sarah Keenan

Sarah Keenan is a clinical psychologist working in Nottingham City community mental health services with people who experience enduring mental health difficulties. Sarah's previous publications and clinical interests focus on how social context influences distress, and how and why these influences and expressions of distress are often medicalised or minimised within mental health services. Sarah has also taken an active role in helping to bring people together who have experiences of mental health services to share knowledge and support each other through informal meetings, formal debates on key issues and the successful *Psychosis in Context* conference series.

Leicester Living with Psychiatric Medication Group

The Living with Psychiatric Medication (LWPM) Group meet in Leicester and are a collection of individuals interested in psychiatric medication who meet fortnightly to talk, share experiences and engage in action projects. They were inspired to come together and form LWPM in 2006 and have been evolving ever since, joining a growing network of similarly orientated community groups. Alongside their social action projects they have presented at several national conferences and previously published in *OpenMind* magazine.

Eleanor Longden

Eleanor Longden is a postgraduate researcher at the University of Leeds and a current board member of Intervoice: The International Network for Training, Education and Research into Hearing Voices. She has lectured and published worldwide on recovery-orientated approaches to psychosis, dissociation and complex trauma and is a faculty member of the International Centre for Recovery Action in Practice Education and Research (ICRA), an honorary member of the French Hearing Voices Network, and a trustee of the UK Soteria Network.

John Mason

John Mason was born in London. He graduated MB, ChB, BSc, at the University of Manchester and then returned to London where he held a series of hospital appointments and obtained membership of the Royal College of Psychiatrists in 2006. He has since completed MSc studies on the 'Philosophy of Mental Disorder' at King's College London and the Institute of Psychiatry. Most recently he has entered further studies in psychodynamic psychotherapy at the Tavistock Clinic.

Rufus May

Rufus May works as a clinical psychologist in Bradford. He is interested in holistic approaches to mental health problems and believes everybody can flourish with the right support network. His interest is rooted in his own experiences of psychosis and recovery in his late teens, and finding a medical approach unhelpful. Stories of hope, friendship and social activities helped him rebuild his life. His interests include community development, healing from trauma, bodywork, mindfulness, communication skills and inner dialogue work. More information is available at www.rufusmay.com. He is an organiser of Evolving Minds, a public meeting that looks at different approaches to wellbeing. His work was featured in the Channel 4 documentary 'The Doctor Who Hears Voices'.

Midlands Psychology Group

The Midlands Psychology Group (MPG) is a group of psychologists: clinical, counselling and academic. The group members call themselves social materialist psychologists. This is not necessarily a formally worked-out philosophical stance. Most psychology is individual and idealist. It takes the individual as a given unit of analysis, and treats the social as a somewhat optional and often uniform context. And, in what is still at root a Cartesian move, it treats the material world as straightforwardly present, but simultaneously subordinate to the immaterial cognitions by which we reflect upon it. It is by contrast to this that the psychology proposed by the Midlands Psychology Group is social materialist. For more information about the MPG please see http://www.midpsy.org/

Joanna Moncrieff

Dr Joanna Moncrieff is a Senior Lecturer in the Department of Mental Health Sciences at University College London and she also works for North East London Foundation as a consultant psychiatrist. Her main interest is in the nature of psychiatric drug treatment, and she is the author of two books on the subject, *The Myth of the Chemical Cure* published by Palgrave Macmillan (2008) and *A Straight Talking Introduction to Psychiatric Drugs* published by PCCS Books (2009), as well as numerous papers and book chapters. She is the co-chairperson of the Critical Psychiatry Network.

Alastair Morgan

Alastair Morgan is a Senior Lecturer in Mental Health and Social Care in the Faculty of Health and Wellbeing at Sheffield Hallam University. He is the editor of *Being Human: Reflections on Mental Distress in Society* (PCCS Books, 2008), and the author of *Adorno's Concept of Life* (Continuum, 2007). He worked for a number of years in mental health in the voluntary sector and the NHS, particularly with marginalised and excluded groups. He has a full academic training in philosophy with a special interest in critical theory and particularly the first generation of the Frankfurt School.

Michelle Noad

Michelle Noad (BSc) graduated from Leeds Metropolitan University in 2011 with First Class Honours in Counselling and Therapeutic Studies. Whilst studying, Michelle became aware of the widespread oppression and stigma related to mental heath and became interested in alternative and non-medical approaches to working alongside mental distress. These interests led her to Leeds Survivor Led Crisis Service where she currently works as the Administrator and as a Crisis Support Worker. She also co-facilitates a Hearing Voices group. Michelle dedicates this chapter to her late grandfather Harry and also to her late nephew Reece-Harry.

Nottingham Mind Medication Group

The Mind Medication Group is a self-help group for people in Nottinghamshire who use, or have used psychiatric drugs and feel caught up in a 'psychiatric medication bubble'. It aims to help people discover new ways of coping and feeling less dependent on medication in order to live more fulfilling lives. The group also aims to challenge the power imbalance between service users and the psychiatric system by increasing access to information about medication through inviting speakers to attend the group, and through raising awareness about the effects of psychiatric medication within the wider community.

David Pilgrim

David Pilgrim trained and worked in the NHS as a clinical psychologist before completing a PhD in Psychology (about psychotherapy in the NHS) and then a Masters in Sociology. Since then he has worked around the boundary between these two disciplines, taking a particular interest in mental health in its social context. Currently he is Professor of Health and Social Policy, Department of Sociology, Social Policy and Criminology, University of Liverpool.

Becky Shaw

Becky Shaw grew up in rural Nottinghamshire then trained as a teacher. A series of traumatic events, including abuse and a war zone, led to her accessing the psychiatric system. Becky founded and still runs a peer-support group, delivers training and conducts research; all of which play an important part in her recovery. Her belief is that having knowledge gives individuals choice and control in their support, care and lives, which led to her first published book, *Wonderfully Strange,* which continues to sell well, receiving great reviews from professionals, carers and readers who have also suffered emotional turmoil.

Theo Stickley

Theo Stickley is a mental health nurse and Associate Professor of Mental Health at the University of Nottingham. He has been involved in developing methods of meaningful collaboration with service users in nurse education for the last 12 years. He has been a motorcyclist for nearly all his adult life and claims that being a 'biker' is an integral part of his identity. Theo is a member of the Nottingham Society of Artists and is committed to regular life-drawing. He is also a gardener and is mostly proud of the quality of the compost he produces.

Philip Thomas

Philip Thomas worked as a consultant psychiatrist in the NHS for over 20 years, before leaving clinical practice in 2004 to focus on writing and academic work. He has published many scholarly papers mostly in peer-reviewed journals. He works in alliance with survivors of psychiatry, service users and community groups, nationally and internationally. He is a founder member, and from 1999 to 2011 was co-chair of, the Critical Psychiatry Network. His first book, *Dialectics of Schizophrenia* (Free Association Books)was published in 1997, and he co-authored *Postpsychiatry* (Oxford University Press) with Pat Bracken in 2005. He is currently working on two books, one about critical psychiatry and one about madness, meaning and culture.

Floris Tomasini

Floris is a philosopher with an interest in continental philosophy, environmental philosophy, bioethics, philosophy of psychiatry, disability and death. He is currently working as a research fellow on a Welcome Trust grant at the University of Leicester (Harnessing the Power of the Criminal Corpse).

Fiona Venner

Fiona Venner has been the manager of Leeds Survivor Led Crisis Service since 2005. Fiona has worked in mental health since the early 1990s, always in the voluntary sector and in acute settings. This has included working with homeless people with mental health problems in London and managing the Suicide and Self Harm Team at 42nd Street, a Manchester-based charity supporting young people. Fiona worked at Leeds Mind prior to her current job and has worked as a volunteer therapist within various Leeds counselling services. Fiona runs marathons and lives in Leeds with her partner and Persian cats.

Jan Wallcraft

Jan Wallcraft is a freelance researcher whose work is informed by experience as a mental health service user and activist. She has worked in service user involvement for a range of NGOs in England. She has a PhD from South Bank University London examining narratives of first experiences with psychiatric hospitalisation. Currently she is a Fellow of Birmingham and Hertfordshire Universities. Jan is also a consultant on service users' perspectives with the World Psychiatric Association. She is lead editor of the *Handbook of Service User Involvement in Mental Health Research* (Wiley, 2009).

Index

The Critical Examinations Series
Edited by Craig Newnes

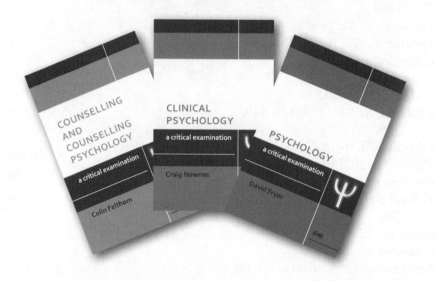

'Critique' is the crux of good academic work, and functions as the hinge point between scholarship, professional activity and practice. Each theory is only as strong as its capacity to withstand sustained critical examination of the assumptions it makes about the world, and so each of these books has been constructed in such a way as to anticipate what would be made of their arguments by the most searching reader.

Ian Parker, Professor of Psychology, Discourse Unit, Manchester Metropolitan University

Counselling and Counselling Psychology:
A critical examination
Colin Feltham (April 2013)

Clinical Psychology: A critical examination
Craig Newnes (June 2013)

Psychology: A critical examination
David Fryer (Spring 2014)

Psychotherapy: A critical examination
Keith Tudor (Spring 2015)